APMLE

APMLE

PART 1
Comprehensive Review

A convenient, effective and high-yield review course for Part 1.

An essential study guide for the American Podiatric
Medical Licensing Examination (APMLE) Part1

Podiatry Boards Prep

Print information available on the last page.

Rev. date: 10/07/2015

To order additional copies of this book, contact:
Xlibris
1-888-795-4274
www.Xlibris.com
Orders@Xlibris.com
712665

CONTENTS

Anatomy 1

Neuroscience...15

Osteology/Ossification 38

Bones: General Features...41

Bones: Particular Features 71

Medial Side of the Thigh..147

Gluteal Region 158

Back of the Thigh 179

Popliteal Fossa 190

Leg 203

Anterior Compartment of the Leg... 207

Dorsum of the Foot...217

Lateral Compartment of the Leg.. 227

Posterior Compartment of the Leg.. 234

Sole of the Foot 249

Segmental Cutaneous Innervation of the Lower Limb..270

Lymphatics of the Lower Limb...272

Joints of the Lower Limb 274

Histology 316

Biochemistry.. 324

Cell Biology 346

Cell and Muscle Physiology 366

Endocrinology 374

GI Physiology..389

Renal Physiology 394

Respiratory Physiology... 397

Immunology 401

General Pathology..415

Pathology..423

Dermatology 428

Endocrinology 433

Gestroenterology 439

Hematology..448

Nephrology..461

Neurology..468

Pulmonology...474

Miscellaneous 481

Pharmacology..484

ANATOMY

HEAD AND NECK

* *Pharyngeal arches*: mesoderm + neural crest
- **1st arch:** formed muscles of mastication, tensor tympani, tensor palatine, incus, malleus, maxilla, mandible, and mandibular nerve (CN-5-III)
- **2nd arch:** formed muscles of facial expression, stapedius, stapes,
- styloid process, lesser horn and upper body of hyoid and facial nerve (CN-7)
- **3rd arch:** formed stylopharengeus muscle, greater horn and lower
- body of hyoid and glossopharyngeal nerve (CN-9)
- **4th arch:** formed cricothyroid muscles, right subclavian artery, laryngeal cartilage, and superior laryngeal nerve (a branch of vagus nerve [CN-10])
- **5th arch:** obliterated normally
- **6th arch:** all laryngeal muscles *except* cricothyroid muscle, laryngeal cartilage, and recurrent laryngeal nerve (a branch of vagus nerve [CN-10])
- It is very easy to remember the **nerve supply of different derivatives of all arches. The cranial nerve derived from a particular arch is responsible for supplying them**!

* *Pharyngeal pouches*: endoderm
   1. Epithelial lining of auditory tube and middle ear cavity
   2. Epithelial lining of crypts of palatine tonsil
   3. **Thymus, inferior parathyroid gland** (*absent in DiGeorge*)
   4. Ultimobranchial body, superior parathyroid gland

- Neural crest cells migrate into the ultimobranchial body to form parafollicular cells of thyroid gland (secrete calcitonin).

* ***Pharyngeal grooves***: ectoderm
- Epithelial lining of external auditory meatus All other grooves are obliterated

* ***Paranasal Sinuses***
- Sphenoidal – in superior meatus
- Maxillary, frontal, anterior, and middle ethmoidal – in middle meatus
- Posterior ethmoidal – in superior meatus
- Hiatus semilunaris (in middle meatus) – frontal, maxillary, and anterior ethmoidal sinus
- Bulla ethmoidalis (in middle meatus) – middle ethmoidal sinus

* ***Ansa Cervicalis (C1, 2, 3)***
- Supply three strap muscles – sternohyoid, omohyoid (both bellies), sternothyroid
- Remaining two strap muscles – thyrohyoid, giniohyoid (supplied by C1 fiber)

- Posterior belly of digastric and stylohyoid – supplied by CN-7 (facial N)
- Anterior belly of digastric and mylohyoid – supplied by CN-5-III (mandibular N)

- ***Tongue***: anterior 2/3 – general sensation – CN-5-III (mandibular N) taste sensation – CN-7 (facial N)
       posterior 1/3 – general and taste sensation – CN-9
- *All the muscles of tongue* innervated by CN-12 *except* palatoglossus.
- Palatoglossus is innervated by CN-10.
- **Test for CN-12 lesion:** on protrusion of tongue, tongue deviates ***toward*** the site of lesion
- Protrusion of tongue – genioglossus muscle

- ***All muscles of mastication*** are innervated by mandibular N.

- ***All muscles of pharynx*** supplied by CN-10 ***except*** tensor palatine

- Tensor palatine (mandibular N) elevates the soft palate to avoid regurgitation of food/liquid in nasopharynx during swallowing.

* *Muscles of Larynx*
- Lateral cricoarytenoid – adduct vocal cord
- Posterior cricoarytenoid – abduct vocal cord
- Thyroarytenoid – sphincter of vestibule, narrowing the laryngeal inlet
- Cricothyroid – lengthen and stretch the vocal cord
- *Paired laryngeal cartilage* – arytenoid, corniculate, and cuneiforms
- *Single laryngeal cartilage* – cricoid, thyroid, and epiglottis
- **All muscles of larynx** are supplied by recurrent laryngeal nerve
- *except* cricothyroid (superior laryngeal nerve).

* *Important Points about Cranial Nerve Lesions*
- **CN-1 (olfactory N):** loss of smell
- **CN-2 (optic N):** different signs and symptoms according to the site of the lesion (see neuroscience notes)
- **CN-3 (occulomotor N):** loss of accommodation, ptosis, outward deviation (LR)
- **CN-4 (trochlear N):** weakness of downward and inward eye movement (SO)
- **CN-6 (abducent N):** inability to look laterally (weak LR, inward deviation)
- **CN-5 (trigeminal N):** the jaw deviates to the weak side when the mouth is opened, loss of corneal reflex, loss of sensation on face
- **CN-7 (facial N):** ipsilateral paralysis of *all* facial muscles (Bell's palsy)
- **CN-8 (vestibulocochlear N):** unilateral sensorineural deafness, vestibular symptoms (balance and postural problem)
- **CN-9 (glossopharyngeal N):** loss of sensation on posterior 1/3 of tongue, loss of gag reflex (gag reflex – sensory [CN-9]; motor [CN-10])
- **CN-10 (vagus N):** uvula deviates *opposite* side of lesion
- **CN-11 (accessory N):** loss of shoulder shrugging (trapezius) and weakness of sternocleidomastoid
- **CN-12 (hypoglossal N):** tongue deviates *toward* the site of lesion on protrusion
- All cranial nerve lesion produce defect on the same side *except*

- CN-10 (vagus N)
- Pupillary Reflex: sensory (CN-2); motor (CN-3)
- Corneal Reflex: sensory (CN-5, ophthalmic division); motor (CN-3)

THORAX

- Breast: lateral ½ - axillary lymphnode medial ½ - parasternal lymphnode
- 1–7: true ribs
- 8–10: false ribs – attached to the costal cartilage of the rib
- 11–12: false ribs – no anterior attachment (floating ribs)

- Intercostal Muscles Blood Supply

Anterior Intercostal Arteries 12 pairs – 11 intercostal and 1 subcostal	*Posterior Intercostal Arteries* 12 pairs – 11 intercostal and 1 subcostal
- Pairs 1–6: internal thoracic - Pairs 7–9: musculophrenic - No anterior intercostal artery in 11 and 12 space. It is supplied by branches of posterior intercostal arteries	- Pairs 1–2: superior intercostal artery (branch of subclavian) - Pairs 3–12: branch of thoracic aorta
- Drain into internal thoracic and musculophrenic veins	- Drain into azygos system of veins

- Collateral between internal thoracic artery and aorta produce rib notching in coarctation of the aorta
- Bottom of the pleura is two ribs lower than the bottom of the lung

	Bottom of Lung	Bottom of Pleura
Midclavicular line	6th rib	8th rib
Midaxillary line	8th rib	10th rib
Paravertebral line	10th rib	12th rib

- Any penetrating injury below fourth intercostal space on the right side can injure the liver
- Roots of phrenic nerve – C3, 4, 5
- Bronchopulmonary segments – ten on the right, eight on the left

Borders of Heart
- **Right** – right atrium (3rd to 6th ribs)
- **Left** – left ventricle (2nd to 5th rib)
- **Superior** – right and left auricles + conus arteriosus of right ventricle
- **Apex** – tip of the left ventricle
- **Ant wall** – right ventricle
- **Post wall** – left atrium
- **Diaphragmatic wall** – left ventricle

- **Pericardial space** – space between epicardium and parietal pericardium

Right and Left Atrium
- *Auricle*: pectinate muscles (rough part)
- *Crista terminalis*: ventricle ridge that separates smooth and rough parts
- *Sinus venerum*: smooth walled (formed by SVC and IVC)

Right and Left Ventricle
- Trabaculae carneae (same as pectinate muscle)
- Papillary muscles
- Chordea tendinae
- Infundibulum (right ventricle)
- Aortic vestibule (left ventricle)

Right Coronary Artery
- SA node, AV node
- Right atrium, right ventricle
- Part of left atrium and ventricle
- *Posterior part of the interventricular septum* (In left dominant, it is supplied by left circumflex artery)

- **■ *Left Coronary Artery***
- Left anterior descending: most part of interventricular septum, apex of the left ventricle
- Circumflex: left atrium, left ventricle, lateral wall

- **■ *Venous Drainage of the Heart***
- Great cardiac vein: travel with anterior interventricular artery
- Middle cardiac vein: travel with posterior interventricular artery (both open in coronary sinus)
- Venae cordis minimae (Thebesian vein) and anterior cardiac vein
- *directly open* in the chambers of heart
- Coronary sinus travel in posterior coronary sulcus and open in right atrium

- ***Thoracic Duct*:** starts in the abdomen from cisterna chyli (L2, 3 level)
- Drain: **lef**t upper limb (UL)
    left thorax, left head and neck (H&N), pelvis, abdomen and lower limb (LL)
- Empty in left brachiocephalic vein
- Found in posterior and superior mediastinum

- **■ *Right Lymphatic Duct***
- Drain: right thorax and right H&N, right UL
- Empty in right brachiocephalic vein

- **■ *Azygos System of Veins***
- Right side – azygos
- Left side – hemiazygos and accessory hemiazygos (both drain to azygos vein)
- The posterior thoracic and abdominal walls are drained by the azygos system of veins
- Azygos – arise from the posterior aspect of IVC (inferior vena cava)
- Hemiazygos – arise from the left renal vein
- Azygos veins empty into superior vena cava
- **Openings in the Diaphragm:** caval (T8 plus right phrenic nerves) esophageal (T10 plus vegus nerve) aortic (T12 plus azygos vein and thoracic duct)

UPPER LIMB

- *Musculocutaneous N (C5 to C7)*: all the muscles of the anterior compartment of arm (biceps, brachialis, coracobrachi)

- *Long thoracic N (C5 to C7)*: serratus anterior

- *Axillary N (C5, C6)*: deltoid and teres major muscle (deltoid – origin: clavicle and acromion)

* **Median N (C5 to T1):** supracondylar region of humerus
- All muscles of anterior compartment of forearm except one and a half muscles (flexor carpi ulnaris and ulnar half of the flexor digitorum profundas)
- Three thenar muscles and 1ˢᵗ and 2ⁿᵈ lumbricals
- **If injured:** *ulnar deviation* of hand *on flexion*

* **Ulnar N (C7 to T1):** medial epicondyle of humerus
- Flexor carpi ulnaris
- Ulnar half of flexor digitorum profundas
- 3ʳᵈ and 4ᵗʰ lumbricals
- All introssei muscles

* **Radial N (C5 to T1):** shaft of the humerus
- The posterior muscles of arm and forearm (there are no muscles in the posterior of the hand)

- *Upper trunk (C5, C6)*: axillary N, musculocutaneous N
  Erb's palsy – muscles of **shoulder and anterior arm** (waiter's tip)
  Arm – medially rotated and adducted
  Forearm – extended and pronated

- *Lower trunk (C8, T1)*
  Klumpke's palsy – loss of the muscles of forearm and **hand**

- *Lumbricals (4)*: flex metacarpophalangeal joint and extend interphalangeal joint
- *Introssei (7)*: **four** dorsal (abduct fingers) and three palmar (adduct fingers)

Thenar muscles	Hypothenar muscles
Abd. Pollicis bravis	Abd. digiti minimi
Flex. Pollicis bravis	Flex. digiti minimi
Opponens pollicis	Opponens digiti minimi

* **Abductors of Thumb**
- Abd pollicis bravis – median N
- Abd pollicis longus – radial N (posterior interosseous nerve), so patient can abduct his hand in median N injury

* **Flexors of Thumb**
- Flex pollicis bravis – median N
- Flex pollicis longus – median N (anterior interosseous nerve)

* **Adductors of Thumb**
- Adductor pollicis – ulnar N

- Therefore, muscles of thumb get nerve supply from all three nerves (radial, median, and ulnar)

* *Test for Injury of Different Nerves*
- *Axillary N:* loss of abduction of the arm to the horizontal level
- *Radial N:* loss of extensors, wrist drop
- *Median N:* loss of opponens; patient can't oppose thumb (can't count with fingers)
- *Ulnar N:* loss of abd and add of fingers (interossei); ask patient to
- hold paper in between two fingers
- *Long thoracic N:* winging of the scapula

ABDOMEN

- *Layers of the Abdominal Wall* (From Outside to Inside)
  1. Skin
  2. Superficial fascia
  3. Deep fascia
  4. External (ext) oblique
  5. Internal (int) oblique
  6. Transversus abdominis

    7.   Transversalis fascia

    8.   Parietal peritoneum

*   **Superficial fascia:** There are two types of superficial fascia. One is *Camper's* fascia, which is mainly composed of fat, and another is *Scarpa's* fascia, which is membranous. Scarpa's fascia is continuous with fascialata of the thigh, Dartos fascia of the scrotum, and Colle's fascia of the perineum.

▪   **Muscles of abdominal wall:** All three muscles of the abdomen consist of its covering fascia, muscles, and its aponeurosis.

▪   The free border of the external oblique aponeurosis forms the

▪   *inguinal ligament.*

▪   *Superficial inguinal ring* is an opening in the ext oblique aponeurosis.

▪   Int oblique and transversus aponeurosis muscles fibers join to form

▪   *conjoint tendon.*

▪   *Deep inguinal ring* begin as an outpouching of the transversalis fascia.

▪   Arcualte line: between umbilicus and pubis

▪   Above arcuate line: rectus sheath is covered by all three muscles' aponeuroses, both anteriorly and posteriorly

▪   Below arcuate line: covered only anteriorly by three muscles' aponeuroses; posteriorly, it is covered by transversalis fascia only

*   ***Boundaries of Inguinal Canal***

▪   *Roof*: int oblique and transversus abdominis

▪   *Ant wall*: aponeuroses of ext oblique and int oblique

▪   *Floor*: inguinal ligament

▪   *Post wall*: transversalis fascia (weaker part) and conjoint tendon (reinforce medial part)

*   ***Boundaries of Femoral Canal***

▪   Anterior – inguinal ligament

▪   Posterior – pubis

▪   Medial – lacunar ligament

▪   Lateral – femoral vein

▪   **Direct inguinal hernia** – abdominal contents herniate through a weak point in the fascia of the abdominal wall and into the inguinal canal

- **Indirect inguinal hernia** – abdominal contents protrude through the deep inguinal ring (failure of closure of processus vaginalis)
- **Femoral hernia** – inferior and lateral to the pubic tubercle
- **Processus vaginalis** – developmental outpouching of the peritoneum: it precedes the testis in their descent down within

- the gubernaculum, and closes—the remaining portion around the testis becomes **tunica vaginalis**
- Psoas major – chief flexor of hip

- Foregut: up to first part of duodenum
- Midgut: up to proximal two-thirds of the transverse colon
- Spleen is *not* a derivative of foregut, but it is **supplied by foregut artery** (branch of celiac artery)

- **Greater omentum:** gastrophrenic, gastrocolic, and gastrosplenic ligaments
- **Lesser omentum:** hepatoduodenal and hepatogastric ligaments
- **Greater and lesser peritoneal sacs** are separated by the *hepatogastric ligament on the right* (*surgical access to lesser sac*) and by the *gastrosplenic ligament on the left*
- **Epiploic foramen:** an opening into omental bursa (lesser sac); a finger in the epiploic foramen touches the hepatoduodenal ligament anteriorly and IVC posteriorly
- Free edge of lesser omentum (**hepatoduodenal ligament**) contain
- three structures: hepatic portal vein, common bile duct, and hepatic artery
- The **spleenorenal ligament** contains the splenic artery and vein.
- The **gastrosplenic ligament** contains short gastric vessels and left gastroepiploic vessels.
- The **hepatogastric ligament** contains the right and left gastric
- arteries **near** the stomach.
- *Retroperitoneal organs*: duodenum, ascending colon, descending colon, kidneys, and adrenal glands
- **Branches of celiac trunk: lef**t gastric artery (lesser curvature),
- common hepatic artery, and splenic artery
- **Hepatic artery:** proper hepatic artery, cystic artery, gastroduodenal artery, right gastric artery (lesser curvature)
- **Splenic artery: lef**t gastroepiploic artery, dorsal pancreatic artery,

- short gastric artery

* ***Blood Supply of Stomach***
- *Left gastric*: proximal lesser curvature
- *Right gastric*: distal lesser curvature
- *Left gastroepiploic*: proximal greater curvature
- *Right gastroepiploic*: distal lesser curvature
- *Short gastric*: short greater curvature above splenic artery

* ***Portosystemic Anastomoses*** (Branch of Portal Vein + Branch of Systemic Vein)
  1. *Lower esophagus*: esophageal branch of left gastric (portal) and azygos vein (systemic)
  2. *Upper anal canal*: superior rectal vein (portal) and middle / inferior rectal veins (systemic)
  3. *Umbilicus*: vein of ligamentum teres (portal) and superior / inferior epigastric vein (systemic)
  4. *Bare area of liver*: hepatic/portal vein (portal) and inferior phrenic vein (systemic)
  5. *Patent ductus venosus (rare)*: left branch of portal vein (portal) and IVC (systemic)
  6. *Retroperitoneal*: colonic veins (portal) and body wall veins (systemic)

* ***Kidney***
- Pronephros – cervical intermediate mesoderm (fourth week of gestation)
- Mesonephros – thoracic and lumbar intermediate mesoderm (fifth week)
- Metanephros – lumbar and sacral intermediate mesoderm (fifthweek)
- **Tubule regress and duct persists**
- Pronephros – nonfunctional
- **Mesonephric duct forms (Wolffian duct)** – epididymidis, ductus (vas) deferens, ejaculatory duct, seminal vesicle
- Metanephros – *ureteric bud* (also known as *metanephric duct*, diverticulum of metanephric duct) and metanephrogenic blastema
- **Ureteric bud forms** – ureters, renal pelvis, collecting ducts, major and minor calyces

- **Metanephrogenic blastema (lumbar and sacral mesoderm) forms** – renal tubules (PCT, DCT, loop of Henle, Bowman's capsule) and definitive glomerulus

- Upper and largest part of urogenital sinus becomes **urinary bladder**

- **Male urethra:** prostatic, membranous, and proximal penile derived from urogenital sinus; distal penile derived from glans of penis
- **Female urethra:** upper two thirds derived from mesonephric duct; lower one third derived from urogenital sinus

- **Prostate gland** in male is also derived from urogenital sinus

* *Relationship of Ureters*
- Lies on anterior surface of psoas major
- Crossing ext iliac as they pass over the pelvic brim
- *Posterior to the uterine artery in female*

* *Blood Supply of Kidney*
- Interlobar arteries
- Arcuate artery
- Interlobular artery (branch of arcuate artery)
- Afferent arterioles leads to capillary tuft of glomeruli

* *Blood supply of urinary bladder*: internal iliac artery

* *Content of Superior Perineal Pouch*
- Bartholin's gland (*in female*)
- Cura of penis or clitoris
- Bulb of penis or bulb of vestibule
- Ischiocavernous muscle
- Bulbospongious muscle

* *Content of Deep Perineal Pouch*
- Bulbourethral gland (*in male*)
- Sphincter urethrae muscle
- Deep transverse perineal muscle

- **Descent of the testis**: The testis develops in the extraperitoneal layer (between layer 7 and 8) and descends from abdomen into scrotum. When it starts descending from the abdomen into the scrotum, its covers of fascia comes in its way. Three fascias (internal spermatic fascia, cremasteric fascia, and external spermatic fascia) cover it from *inside to outside* respectively. These three fascias derived from transversalis, internal oblique, and external oblique fascias respectively. Skin and Scarpa's fascia make scrotum. When the testis starts decent, it brings part of the peritoneum with it (processus vaginalis) which is obliterated after birth.

* **Testis**: seminiferous tubule + stroma (contain interstitial cells [*Leyding cells*])
- *Seminiferous tubule*: site of spermatogenesis
- *Sertoli cells*: irregular columnar cells extend from the basal lamina to the lumen
    - Provide blood-testes barrier
    - Tight junction between Sertoli cells divide seminiferous tubule in two compartment: basal compartment (spermatogonia) and adluminal compartment (spermatocytes and spermatids)
- Spermatogonia are near basal lamina and between two sertoli cells (all germ cells are between two sertoli cells)
- Sperm undergoes maturation in epididymis
- Seminal vesicles secrete fluids that contain fructose and serve as an energy source for the sperm.

* **Ovary**: cortex: ovarian follicles medulla: nerves and blood vessels
- **Ovarian follicles:** composed of oocytes surrounded by follicular (granulosa) cells
    - *Primordial follicle*: primary oocytes surrounded by single layer of flattened follicular cells
    - *Primary follicle*: primary oocytes + one or more layers of cuboidal like follicular cells
    - *Secondary follicle*: follicular cavity (antrum), cumulus oophorus, corona radiata, thica interna (secrete androgens that convert into estradiol by granulosa cells), thica externa, zona pellucida around the oocyte (zona pellucida is PAS positive)
    - *Graafian follicle*: mature follicle extends through cortex

- *Ovulation*: increase in antral fluid causes rupture of follicle and ovum along with corona radiata passes out of the ovary
- Follicular cavity changes occur leads to formation of *corpus lutem*
- Thica interna – *thica lutin interna* (in corpus lutem) – secrete estrogen
- Thica externa – *granulosa lutin cells* (in corpus lutem) – secrete progesterone
- Corpus lutem persists until three months by hCG secreted by embryo. After the 40th day, the placenta produces progesterone necessary to maintain pregnancy

- **Spermatogenesis:** primordial germ cells *arrive in the indifferent gonad at week 4* and **remain dormant until puberty**
  - *At puberty*, primordial germ cells differentiate into type-A spermatogonia, which serve as stem cells throughout adult life
  - **Oogenesis:** primordial germ cells *arrive in the indifferent gonad at week 4* and **differentiate into oogonia**
  - Oogonia enter miosis-I to form primary oocytes. *All primary oocytes formed by 5th month of fetal life,* **remain arrested in prophase (diplotene) of miosis-I until puberty**
  - *At puberty*, complete miosis-I and become secondary oocyte and polar body
  - Secondary oocyte *arrested in metaphase of miosis-II and is ovulated*
  - *At fertilization*, secondary oocyte complete miosis-II to form mature oocyte and polar body

  - **Miosis-I:** synapsis (pairing), crossing over, disjunction (**without** centromere splitting)
  - **Miosis-II:** *no* synapsis, *no* crossing over, disjunction **with** centromere splitting

NEUROSCIENCE

Basic Concepts

* Our cerebral cortex has ultimate control over the body!
* Our body sends sensation to our cortex so sensory fibers are always afferent (goes toward the brain)
* Our cortex sends information to different parts of the body to do their function so motor fibers are always efferent (goes away from brain)
* No matter which fibers (afferent or efferent), both cross the midline so our brain controls the opposite side of our body! The right side of the brain controls the left side of body! So any lesion to our brain produces contralateral (opposite side) defects. The exception to this rule is the cerebellum. Cerebellar fibers cross midline twice, so cerebellar lesions produce ipsilateral (same side) defects.
* For cranial nerves (CN), most of the CN nuclei are located in the brain stem so these nuclei work as LMN for those CN and their control (cerebral cortex) work as UMN for them.
* UMN lesion – spastic paralysis, usually contralateral
* LMN lesion – flaccid paralysis, usually ipsilateral
* Cerebral cortex control opposite side of our body, involvement of CN in cerebral cortex lesion is contralateral and ipsilateral in brainstem lesion.
* Important parts of our brain – cerebral cortex, brain stem (midbrain, pons, and medulla) and cerebellum. Other small parts are basal ganglia, thalamus, hypothalamus, and internal capsule. Spinal cord is also a part of CNS!

- Forebrain – telencephalon (cerebral cortex, basal ganglia, lateral ventricles, and olfactory bulb) and diencephalon (prethalamus,

thalamus, hypothalamus, subthalamus, epithalamus, pretectum, and the posterior pituitary gland)

- Midbrain – mesencephalon (midbrain, cerebral aqueduct)

- Hindbrain – metencephalon (pons and cerebellum) and myelencephalon (medulla); the 4th ventricle forms from both metencephalon and myelencephalon

- Anterior pituitary gland – is an outgrowth of oral ectoderm (Rathke's pouch). Remnant of Rathke's pouch forms craniopharyngioma that compress optic chiasm and produce bitemporal heteronymous hemianopsia

- Neural crest form – adrenal medulla, primary sensory neurons and postganglionic autonomic neurons (cell bodies in ganglia [peripheral nervous system {PNS}])
- Neural tube form – skeletal motor neurons and preganglionic autonomic neurons (cell bodies in SC [central nervous system {CNS}])

- Schwann cells make myelin for PNS
- Oligodendrocytes make myelin for CNS
- Optic N (CN-2) is an outgrowth of brain so its myelin is formed by oligodendrocytes. CN-2 is affected in multiple sclerosis

- Sympathetic outflow – T1 to L2 (*descending hypothalamic fibers drive all Pre- ganglionic sympathetic nerve fibers*)

- Parasympathetic outflow – *CN-3, 7, 9, 10* and S-2, 3, 4

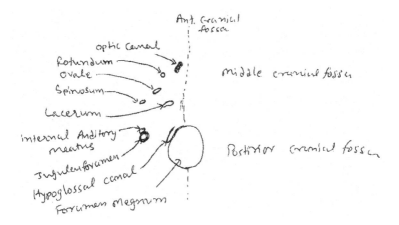

- Optic canal – CN-2 (optic N) and ophthalmic artery
- Rotundum – maxillary N (CN-5 second division), V2
- Ovale – mandibular N (V3), ophthalmic division V1 pass through superior orbital fissure
- Spinosum – middle meningeal artery (epidural hematoma)
- Lacerum – nothing
- Internal auditory meatus – CN-7, 8
- Jugular foramen – CN-9, 10, 11, sigmoid sinus
- Hypoglossal canal – CN-12
- Foramen magnum – CN-11, vertebral artery, spinal cord – brain stem junction

- *Spinal cord (SC)*

- *Cell bodies* of sensory *fibers* – dorsal root ganglion (so not in SC)
- *Cell bodies* of motor *fibers* – ventral horn of gray matter of SC

- *Dorsal root of spinal cord* – sensory fibers
- *Ventral root of spinal cord* – motor fibers

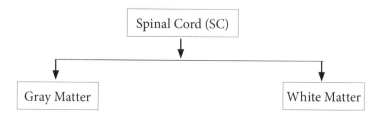

- Cell bodies, their dendrites and tracts the proximal part of axons

- Ascending and descending

Dorsal Horn (Sensory)	Ventral Horn (Motor)	Intermediate Horn (Cerebellar tract)
All incoming sensory fibers enter in dorsal horn (dorsolateral part of the SC)	α and γ motorneurons	Present between T1 to L2 only
	α innervate extrafusal fibers of skeletal muscles	Clarke's nucleus send unconscious proprioception to the cerebellum
	γ innervate intrafusal fibers of muscle spindles	
	Both neurons leave the SC by way of ventral root	

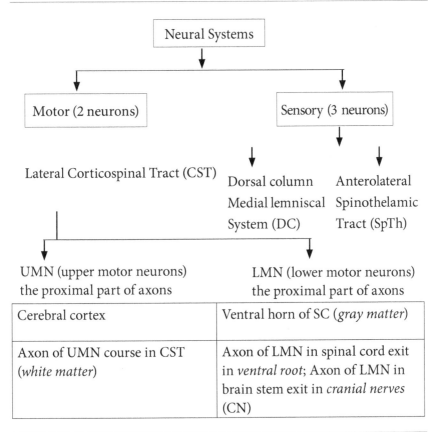

The following table continues from the diagram:

UMN (upper motor neurons) the proximal part of axons	LMN (lower motor neurons) the proximal part of axons
Cerebral cortex	Ventral horn of SC (*gray matter*)
Axon of UMN course in CST (*white matter*)	Axon of LMN in spinal cord exit in *ventral root*; Axon of LMN in brain stem exit in *cranial nerves* (CN)

Occupy venteromedial position during their course	Play roles in reflexes (α and γ) α – contraction of muscles γ – carry stretch sensation to SC
Cross at lower medulla (Pyramidal Decussation)	UMN and LMN lesions are opposite to each other. See below signs of UMN

- UMN has *net inhibitory effect* on reflex; therefore in UMN lesion, there is hyperreflexia, spastic paralysis, and Babinski sign present (extension of toes)

- *Dorsal column – medial lemniscal system (DC)*: three neurons

- Discriminative touch, joint position sense, vibratory and pressure sensation from the trunk and limbs

- Fasciculus gracillis (LL): found at all level of SC (LL = lower limb)
- Fasciculus cuneatus (UL): found only at upper thoracic and cervical level of SC

- Cell bodies of 1st neuron – DRG (DRG = dorsal root ganglion)
- Cell bodies of 2nd neuron – lower medulla
- Cell bodies of 3rd neuron – thalamus (VPL = ventral posterolateral nucleus of thalamus)
- Fibers of *2nd neuron cross at lower part of medulla*
- From VPL, it goes to somatosensory cortex in to the postcentral gyrus

- *Lesion of the dorsal column*: loss of two point discrimination, joint position sense, vibratory and pressure sensation; astereognosis – loss of ability to identify the characteristic of an objects; diagnosis (Dx): Romberg's sign (patients sway when they close their eyes) and vibratory sensation by 128 Hz tuning fork (If patient has cerebellar damage, patient will sway even with their eyes open)

- Fibers of 2nd neurons *must* cross midline in *both* (DC and SpTh) sensory systems

- *Anterolateral spinothelamic tract system*: three neurons

- Pain, temperature (temp), and crude touch sensation from the extremities and trunk

- Cell bodies of 1st neuron – DRG
- Cell bodies of 2nd neuron – dorsal horn gray matter
- Cell bodies of 3rd neuron – thalamus (VPL)
- Fibers of *2nd neuron cross at spinal cord*

- Because the pain and temp information crosses almost as soon as it enters the SC, any unilateral lesion of the SpTh in the SC or brain stem will result in a contralateral loss of pain and temp

- SpTh fibers run closely to the SC and can affect 1st in SC cavitations (Syringomyelia). Cavitations usually occur at cervical level so bilateral loss of pain and temp in UL occurs first.

- Descending hypothalamic fibers run with SpTh *without* crossing at brain stem therefore any lesion of SC above T2 produces Hornor's syndrome (ipsilateral)

- *Amyotrophic lateral sclerosis (ALS, Lou Gehrig's disease)* is a pure motor system disease and affects *both* UMN and LMN and typically begins at cervical level of spinal cord. It occurs due to mutation in superoxide dismutase gene. Increased levels of glutamate is seen in a patient with ALS. Rulizole is currently the only FDA-approved drug for ALS (see figure below).

- *Brain stem*: home of nine cranial nerves
- Midbrain – 3rd and 4th (4th is the only CN that exit from dorsal brain stem)
- Pons – 5th, 6th, 7th, 8th
- Medulla – 9th, 10th, 12th
- *Motor nuclei of CN situated *medially* and sensory nuclei situated lateral to motor nuclei
- ③ Pure motor CN – 3, 4, 6, 11, 12
- Pure sensory CN – 1, 2, 8
- Mixed CN (both motor and sensory function) – 5, 7, 9, 10

- *Lesion in brain stem*: loss occurs on contralateral side of any three long tracks (one motor and two sensory), Hornor's syndrome (always ipsilateral) and ipsilateral CN lesion

- *Medial longitudinal fasciculus (MLF)* fiber bundle is a center for *horizontal gaze* connect vestibular nuclei and nuclei of CN-3, 4, 6
- Lesion of MLF leads to disrupt vestibule-occular reflex
- *MLF is *located in pons and midbrain* in *midline

- Solitary nucleus (7, 9, 10) – taste and visceral sensation
- Nucleus ambiguus (9, 10) – motorneurons (muscles of soft palate, larynx, pharynx, and upper esophagus)
- Dorsal motor nucleus of CN-10 – visceral motorneurons (major parasympathetic nucleus of the brain stem; viscera of thorax, foregut, and midgut)
- Midbrain: superior colliculus (*vertical gaze*) and inferior colliculus
- (auditory information – lateral lemniscus)

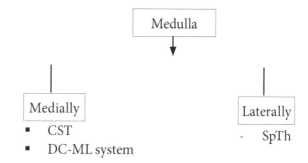

- *Blood Supply of Brain Stem:*

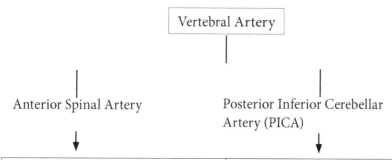

Ventrolateral 2/3 of cervical spinal cord	Cerebellum
Ventrolateral part of medulla (CST and DC-ML system)	Dorsolateral part of medulla (SpTh)
Occlusion of vertebral or anterior spinal artery produce Medial medullary syndrome	Occlusion of PICA produce Lateral medullary syndrome (Wallenberg's syndrome)
Both above tract symptoms Hypoglossal N (CN-12)	Inferior cerebellar peduncle (ICP) lesion (Ipsilateral limb ataxia) Above tract symptoms (pain and temp loss) Descending hypothalamic fibers lesion (Hornor's syndrome) Spinal nucleus of CN-5 lesion Vestibular nuclei lesion Ambiguus nucleus (CN-9, 10) lesion

- Two vertebral arteries joined to form basilary artery
- Labyrinthine artery – a branch of basilar artery, supplies inner ear

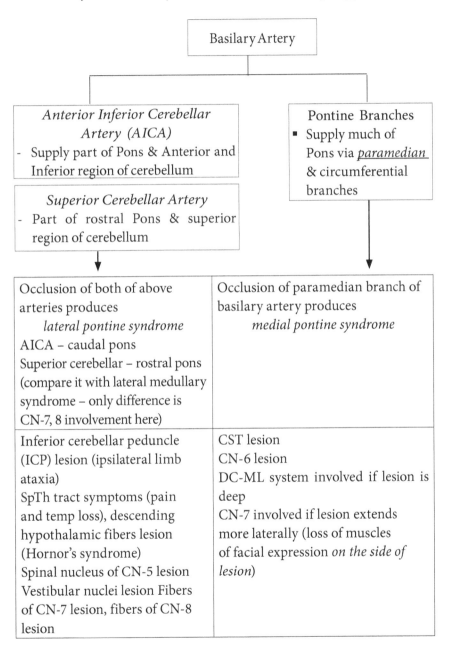

Basilary Artery	

| *Anterior Inferior Cerebellar Artery (AICA)*
- Supply part of Pons & Anterior and Inferior region of cerebellum | Pontine Branches
- Supply much of Pons via *paramedian* & circumferential branches |
| *Superior Cerebellar Artery*
- Part of rostral Pons & superior region of cerebellum | |

Occlusion of both of above arteries produces
    lateral pontine syndrome
AICA – caudal pons
Superior cerebellar – rostral pons (compare it with lateral medullary syndrome – only difference is CN-7, 8 involvement here)
	Occlusion of paramedian branch of basilary artery produces
	    medial pontine syndrome

Inferior cerebellar peduncle (ICP) lesion (ipsilateral limb ataxia) SpTh tract symptoms (pain and temp loss), descending hypothalamic fibers lesion (Hornor's syndrome) Spinal nucleus of CN-5 lesion Vestibular nuclei lesion Fibers of CN-7 lesion, fibers of CN-8 lesion	CST lesion CN-6 lesion DC-ML system involved if lesion is deep CN-7 involved if lesion extends more laterally (loss of muscles of facial expression *on the side of lesion*)

- At rostral end of midbrain, the basilary artery divides into a pair of posterior cerebral arteries

- *How will you identify all different syndromes on exam? – By looking at involvement of different cranial nerves.* Involvement of CN-12 (medial medullary syndrome); CN-9, 10 (lateral medullary syndrome); CN-7, 8 (lateral pontine syndrome); CN-6 (medial pontine syndrome); and CN-3 (medial midbrain syndrome)

> **Posterior Cerebral Artery**
> - branches supply midbrain

↓

> Occlusion of branches of posterior cerebral artery produce medial midbrain syndrome (Weber's syndrome)

↓

> - CST lesion
> - Corticobulbar tract lesion (Contralateral spastic paralysis of lower ½ of face
> - Fibers of CN-3 – ipsilateral oculomotor nerve palsy (dilated pupils, ptosis, lateral strabismus

- Pontocerebellar angle syndrome: caused by acoustic neuroma (Schwannoma) of CN-8 – *absence of long tracts signs* indicates that the lesion must be outside of brain
- Parinaud syndrome: pineal gland tumor compressing superior colliculus. The most common sign is paralysis of upward (vertical) gaze (sunset sign) combined with bilateral pupillary abnormality

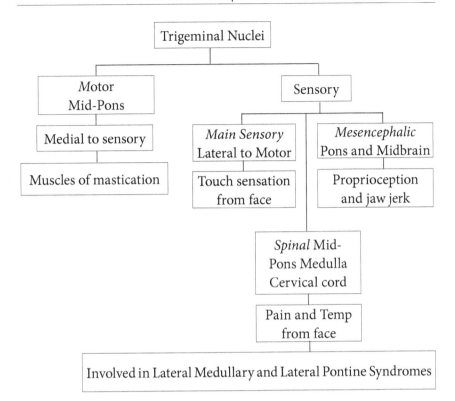

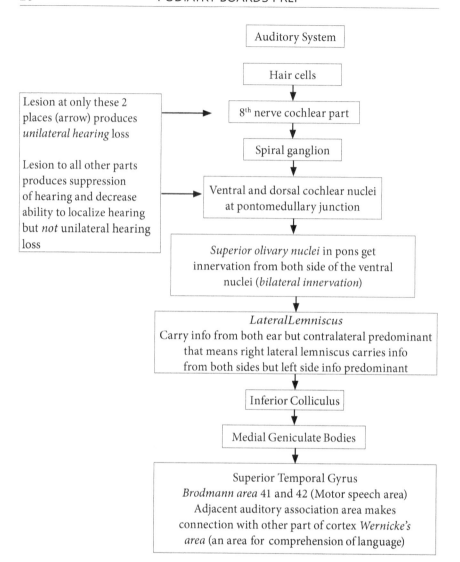

- High frequency sounds – base of cochlea
- Low frequency sounds – apex of cochlea

- **Vestibular System**
- *Urticle and saccule*: linear acceleration – positional changes in the head relative to gravity
- *Ampullary crest*: angular acceleration – results from circular
- movement of head
- Head turns right leads to *both* eyes move left

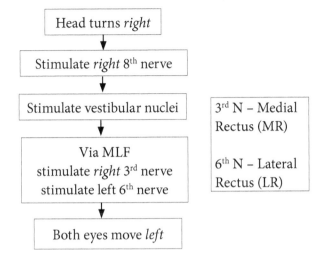

- *Nystagmus*: unilateral vestibular nerve *or* nuclei lesion produce nystagmus

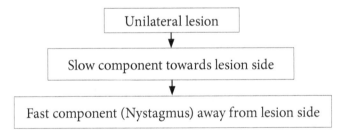

9. *Caloric Test*

- Pouring *cool water* (mimic nerve lesion) into ear – nystagmus *opposite side*
- Pouring *warm water* (mimic nerve stimulation) into ear – nystagmus *same side*

10. *Horizontal Gaze*

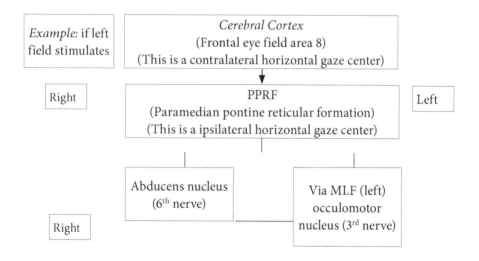

So if the left frontal eye field is stimulated, activation of the pontine gaze center occurs on right and saccadic horizontal eye movements of *both* eyes occur to the right.

- Left frontal eye field lesion – both eyes can't look to the right (but slow drift occurs to the left)
- Left MLF lesion – left eye can't look to the right, and therefore, right eye exhibits nystagmus
- Right abducens nucleus *or* right PPRF lesion – both eyes can't look
- to the right (but slowly drifts to the left)
- Right 6th nerve lesion – right eye can't look to the right

11. *Visual System*

- *Pathway*: retina → optic nerve (nasal and temporal fibers) → optic chiasm → optic tract → LGB (lateral geniculate body) → optic radiation (lateral fibers and medial fibers) → cerebral cortex (occipital lobe – cuneus and lingual)

- Nasal field projects on temporal fibers and temporal field projects on nasal fibers.
- Nasal fibers cross at optic chiasm, but temporal fibers don't cross.

- Upper field projects on lower retina and lower field projects on upper retina.
- Image from *lower* retina → *l*ateral fiber → make Mayer's *l*oop (temporal lobe)
- Image from upper retina → medial fiber (pass through parietal lobe)
- Calcarine sulcus (occipital lobe) – cuneus (*up* – *u*pper retina – medial fiber) and lingual (below cuneus – lower retina – lateral fiber)

- All lesions *past the chiasm* produce contralateral (homonymous) defects.
- *Only optic chiasm lesions* produce *heteronymous.*
- Destruction of macula produces central scotoma.
- Hemianopsia = loss of half visual field
- Anopsia = loss of total visual field

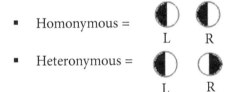

- Homonymous =

      L   R
- Heteronymous =

      L   R

Examples	Lesion of Visual System Pathway	Defect
Right	optic N (nasal + temporal fibers)	right eye anopsia
Right	temporal fiber	right nasal hemianopsia
	optic chiasm	bitemporal heteronymous hemianopsia
Right	optic tract	left homonymous hemianopsia
Right	optic radiation (medial + lateral)	left homonymous hemianopsia
Left	lateral fibers of optic radiation	right homonymous superior quadrantanopsia
Left	medial fibers of optic radiation	right homonymous inferior quadrantanopsia
Left	cerebral cortex (visual)	right homonymous hemianopsia with macular sparing

- Lesion of optic N produces blindness (anopsia) but lesion of visual cortex (occlusion of posterior cerebral artery) leads to contralateral homonymous hemianopsia with macular (central) vision spared (macula has collateral blood supply from middle cerebral artery).
- Macular atrophy (elderly people) leads to loss of central vision.

* *Important point about facial N (CN-7) lesion*: *Upper face muscles* (which wrinkle forehead and shut eyes) get *bilateral cortical innervation* whereas lower face has unilateral cortical innervations. Therefore, a *cortical lesion* leads to *only* drooping of angle of mouth on contralateral side whereas a *facial nerve lesion* leads to ipsilateral paralysis of *all* facial muscles (Bell's palsy).

- Most people (80%) are right-handed, so the left hemisphere is more highly developed. Speech and language functions are also predominantly organized in the left hemisphere; therefore, left middle artery occlusion produce aphasia (Broca's, Wernicke's, or both).

7. *Middle Cerebral Artery (MCA)*
- Bulk of *lateral surface* of hemisphere
- Genu and posterior limb of internal capsule
- Basal ganglia
- *Occlusion of MCA*: contralateral spastic paralysis and anesthesia of *lower face and UL*, aphasia (in left MCA occlusion), left side neglect (in right MCA occlusion), contralateral superior quadrantanopsia (occlusion of branches that supply Mayer's loop of visual radiation)

- *Anterior Cerebral Artery (ACA)*
- *Medial surface* of frontal and parietal lobes that include motor and sensory areas for the *pelvis and lower limb*
- Anterior four-fifths of corpus callosum
- Anterior limb of internal capsule
- *Occlusion of ACA*: contralateral spastic paralysis and anesthesia of LL, urinary incontinence, transcortical apraxia (The patient cannot move the left arm in response to verbal command. This is because left hemisphere [language dominant] has been disconnected from the motor cortex of right hemisphere, both of which are connected through corpus callosum.)

- *Posterior Cerebral Artery (PCA)*
  - Occipital lobe and posterior two thirds of temporal lobe on *medial surface* of hemisphere
  - Thalamus, splenium of corpus callosum
  - Subthalamic nucleus
  - *Occlusion of PCA*: homonymous hemianopsia of the contralateral visual field with macular sparing, left PCA occlusion produce alexia *without* agraphia (Can't read but can write. This is because involvement of the splenium of the corpus callosum prevents visual information from intact right occipital cortex to language comprehension cortex in the left hemisphere; therefore, patient can see word in the left visual field but can't understand what words mean.)

- *Frontal Lobe*
  - Primary motor cortex (area 4)
  - Premotor cortex (area 6)
  - Frontal eye field (area 8)
  - Motor speech areas of Broca (areas 44, 45; inferior frontal lobe)
  - Precentral gyrus – primary motor cortex contain motor homunculus
  - *Frontal lobe syndrome*: lesion in the frontal area – can't concentrate,
  - apathy (severe emotional indifference), abullia (slowing of intellectual faculties, slow speech, decrease participation in social interaction), emergence of infantile suckling or grasp reflex in adult, personality change, expressive aphasia, inability to make voluntary eye movements toward contralateral side (frontal eye field – contralateral horizontal gaze center)

- *Parietal Lobe*
  - Primary somatosensory cortex (postcentral gyrus; areas 3, 1, and 2)
  - Posterior parietal association cortex (area 5 and 7)
  - Wernicke's area (area 39 and 40; area 22 is in temporal lobe)
  - Area 22 – spoken word; area 39 – written word
  - *Parietal lobe lesion*: receptive aphasia, transcortical apraxia, asomatognosia (left side neglect; lesion in area 7, 39, and 40), conductive aphasia (arcuate fasciculus – large fiber bundle that connects areas 22, 39, and 40 to Broca's area)

- *Gerstmann's syndrome*: lesion to angular gyrus (area 39) – alexia with agraphia (can't read and can't write) but patient can understand spoken words

- *Temporal Lobe*
- Auditory cortex (area 41 and 42)
- Wernicke's area 22
- *Temporal lobe lesion*: unilateral lesion to auditory cortex leads to only little loss of auditory sensitivity but have some difficulty in localizing sound, problem with memory, receptive aphasia (area 22)

- *Occipital Lobe*
- Primary visual cortex (area 17)
- Visual association cortex
- Bilateral visual cortex lesion produces cortical blindness. This means the patient can't see but pupillary reflexes are intact (center for pupillary reflex is in pretectal area in the midbrain; pupillary reflex – sensory [CN-2] and motor [CN-3]).
- Visual association cortex → *forms and color* → parvocellular-blob
- system → "cone stream" project on blob zone of primary visual cortex → *temporal lobe (area 20 and 21)*
- Unilateral lesion to areas 20 and 21: achromatopsia (complete loss of color vision in contralateral hemifield; the patient sees everything in shades of gray), prosopagnosia (inability to recognize face), visual agnosia (inability to recognize visual pattern including object)
- Visual association cortex → *motion and depth* → magnocellular
- system → "Rod stream" project on the stripe zone of primary visual cortex → *Parietal lobe (area 18 and 19)*
- Unilateral lesion to areas 18 and 19: deficit in perceiving visual motion (visual field, color vision, and reading are unaffected)

- *Olfactory system*: central projection of olfactory structures reach parts of the temporal lobe and amygdala (pyeariform cortex is a primary olfactory cortex)
- Fracture of the cribriform plate (occur in head injury) can tear the olfactory nerve fibers. As olfactory nerve is an outgrowth of the CNS, it is covered by meninges, and tearing of olfactory nerve

fiber may tear meninges, causing CSF leaking through cribriform plate into nasal cavity

- *Limbic system*: hippocampal formation on the medial aspect of temporal lobe (include hippocampus, dentate gyrus, subiculum and adjacent entorhinal cortex), amygdala (located rostral to hippocampus) and septal nuclei

12. *Cerebellum*
- Major input – ICP and MCP (inferior and middle cerebellar peduncle)
- Major output – SCP (superior cerebellar peduncle)
- Granule cells are the only excitatory cells within the cerebellar cortex
- Purkinje cells are the only outflow from the cerebellar cortex. It sends fibers to deep cerebellar nuclei
- Climbing fibers from inferior olivary nucleus of contralateral medulla provide direct excitatory input to the Purkinje cells
- Mossy fibers provide an indirect excitatory input to the Purkinje cells

13. *Spinocerebellar pathway*: send unconscious proprioception

14. Fibers of the spinocerebellar tract *cross two times in central nervous system*; therefore, cerebellar injuries produce loss of function on ipsilateral (same side). As these fibers are involved in unconscious proprioception, patient tends to fall on same side of cerebellar lesion (cerebellar injuries always produce ipsilateral loss of function).

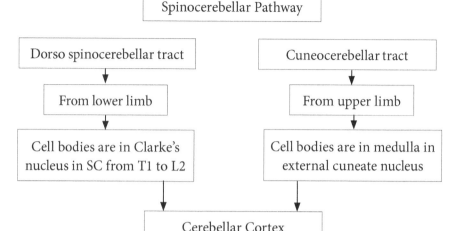

- *Deep Cerebellar Nuclei and Cerebellar Area*
- Flocculo nodular lobe → *fastigeal nucleus* → vestibular nucleus → elicit positional changes of eyes and trunk in response to movement of head
- Intermediate hemisphere → *interpositus nucleus* → red nucleus
- and reticular formation → influence LMN via rubrospinal and reticulospinal tracts to adjust posture and affect movements
- Lateral hemisphere → *dentate nucleus* → thalamus (VL), then cortex
- → influence LMN via CST, which affect voluntary movements, especially, sequence and precision

15. The cerebellum is involved in planning and fine tuning of skeletal muscles' contraction; therefore, cerebellar lesions produce intention tremor (tremor occurs during voluntary movements).
16. Basal ganglia initiate and provide gross control over skeletal muscle movements; therefore, basal ganglia lesions produce dyskinesia (movement disorder) and slow initiation of movement; tremors at rest.
17. *Basal ganglia*: striatum (caudate nucleus and putamen), globus palidus, substantia nigra (substantia nigra is in the midbrain)

- Disinhibition: One population of inhibitory neurons inhibits second population of inhibitory neurons.
- *Direct pathway*: Net effect is excitation of cortex and promotion of movement.

- *Indirect pathway*: Net effect is inhibition (decrease cortex excitation).

- ACh – stimulates indirect pathway (ACh found within striatum)
- Dopamine – stimulates direct pathway and inhibits indirect pathway

18. Indirect pathway lesion: chorea, athetosis, hemiballismus
19. Direct pathway lesion: Parkinsonism
20. Hemiballismus: wild flinging movement (violent projectile movements) of half of the body – typically observed in upper limb – usually seen in hypertensive patient
21. Tourette's syndrome: also a basal ganglia disease involves facial and vocal ticks that progress to jerking movements of the limb – frequently associated with explosive, vulgar speech – *treatment*: pimozide

- *Thalamus*: process and relay sensory information selectively to various parts of the cerebral cortex

- Involvement of thalamus in CV stroke identified by contralateral painful anesthesia means burning *or* aching on one half of the body. It is often accompanied by mood swings.

- *Hypothalamus*: One of the most important functions of the hypothalamus is to link the nervous system to the endocrine system via the pituitary gland. It synthesizes and secretes neurohormones (hypothalamic-releasing hormones), and these, in turn, stimulate or inhibit the secretion of pituitary hormones.

- *Hypothalamic Nuclei*
    - Medial preoptic nucleus (urinary bladder contraction, decreased heart rate, and decreased blood pressure)
    - Paraventricular and supraoptic nuclei (synthesize ADH and oxytocin)
    - Anterior hypothalamic nucleus (thermoregulation, sweating, thyrotropin inhibition)
    - Lateral nucleus (thirst and hunger)
    - Suprachiasmatic nucleus (visual input from retina; plays role in the circadian rhythm [twenty-four-hour light-dark cycle])
    - Arcuate nucleus (produce LH and FSH releasing hormones)

- ■ Venteromedial nucleus (satiety center and regulate food intake, neuroendocrine control; lesion to this produces obesity)
- ■ Dorsomedial hypothalamic nucleus (GI stimulation)
- ■ Mammillary bodies – memory
- ■ Posterior nucleus – increase blood pressure, pupillary dilation, and shivering (lesion to this produces hypothermia)
- ■ Preoptic area – responsive to androgens and estrogen; influences the production of sex hormone by anterior pituitary; lesion to preoptic area before puberty arrests sexual development; after puberty causes amenorrhea *or* impotence
- ■ Ventrolateral preoptic nucleus – They are primarily active during non-REM sleep and inhibit other neurons that are involved in wakefulness.

- ▪ *Epithalamus*: pineal body—synthesizes melatonin, serotonin, cholecystokinin; environmental light regulates the activity of the pineal gland

22. *Internal capsule*: anterior limb, genu, and posterior limb; course takenbyallfibersthatareleaving *or* entering cortex; thalamocortical (limbic system) in anterior limb; corticobulbar (cranial nerve sign) in genu; CST and all somatosensory thalamocortical projections in posterior limb

- ▪ Six layers of cerebral cortex:
  1. Molecular layer
  2. External granular layer
  3. External pyramidal layer
  4. Internal granular layer
  5. Internal pyramidal layer
  6. Multiform layer

- ▪ Internal pyramidal layer gives rise to axons that form CST and corticobulbar tract
- ▪ Pyramidal layer well-developed in frontal lobe
- ▪ Granular layer well developed in parietal, occipital, and temporal lobes. It is a site for termination of major sensory neurons

- *Reticular formation* is a poorly-differentiated area of the brain stem, centered roughly in the pons. The ascending reticular activating system connects to areas in the thalamus, hypothalamus, and cortex, while the descending reticular activating system connects to the cerebellum and sensory nerves.
- It controls respiration, cardiovascular responses, behavior arousal, and *sleep*—lesion to this produces coma and death.
- Three nuclei (raphe, locus cerulus and periaqueductal gray)
- Raphe nuclei: synthesize serotonin (5-HT). Serotonin seems to be the culprit in many of our modern psychopharmaceutical problems such as anorexia, depression, and sleep disorders; SSRI works here.
- Locus cerulus: located within the dorsal wall of the rostral pons in the lateral floor of the fourth ventricle, synthesize norepinephrine, involved with physiological responses to stress and panic and in arousal, decreases NE level in REM sleep
  Both of above nuclei are degenerate in Alzheimer's disease.

- Periaqueductal gray: opioid receptors

23. Wernicke–Korsakoff syndrome: Combined manifestation of two disorders, Korsakoff's psychosis and Wernicke's encephalopathy. Wernicke's encephalopathy is characterized by confusion, nystagmus, ophthalmoplegia, ataxia, coma, and death. Korasakoff's psychosis is characterized by anterograde and retrograde amnesia, hallucination, and confabulation. Wernicke's encephalopathy results from severe acute deficiency of thiamine (Vitamin B1), whilst Korsakoff's psychosis is a chronic neurologic sequel after Wernicke's encephalopathy. In the United States, it is usually found in malnourished chronic alcoholics who undergo prolonged intravenous (IV) therapy without Vitamin B1 supplementation. Lesion is believe to be found in mamillary body and the medial dorsal thalamus.

24. Klüver-Bucy syndrome: Occurs when both the right and left medial temporal lobes of the brain malfunction. Amygdala (main site for the pathogenesis of this syndrome)—placidity (docility) (lowered aggressive behavior), hyperorality (put everything in mouth), dietary changes, hypersexuality, hypermetamorphosis (an irresistible impulse to notice and react to everything within sight), memory loss

OSTEOLOGY/OSSIFICATION

The sacrum (*five fused sacral vertebrate*) appears 4th month; after birth, fourteen secondary centers appear; *thirty-five total centers of ossification*

Pelvic Bone (*ilium, pubis, ischium*)

* Primary centers: 2–5th
* fetal month; ossifies from three primary centers; age ten, formation of tri-radiate cartilage
* Secondary centers at puberty: iliac crest, acetabulum, pubic body, ischial tuberosity
* Fusion of all parts: 15–25 years old

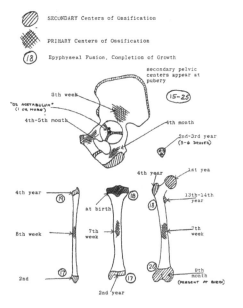

Femur (*knee joint; earliest we see secondary center, birth*)
* Primary center: shaft (7th week)
* Secondary center: distal end (9 months), head (1st year), greater trochanter (4th year), lesser trochanter (13–14 year)
* Completion: 18–20 years old

Patella: center appears, 2–3 years old; growth completes at puberty

Tibia

* Primary center: shaft (7 week)

- Secondary center: proximal end (birth), distal end (1–1½ years), sometimes tibial tuberosity/medial malleolus
- Osgood-Schlatter disease: too much action on growth plate at tibial tuberosity
- Completion: proximal end (16–18 years old), distal end (15–17 years)

Fibula

- Primary center: shaft (8th week)
- Secondary center: distal epiphysis (1st year), proximal epiphysis (3rd year)
- Completion: distal end (15–17 years), proximal end (17–19 years)

Calcaneus (*Only tarsal bone with primary and secondary centers*)

- Primary center: *3rd mo.*
- Secondary center: tuberosity (6–8 years); a.k.a. calcaneal apophysis
- Sever's disease: heel pain, overuse injury at calcaneal apophysis
- Fusion: 14–16 years

Talus- 6th mo.

- Accessory bone: *os trigonum* Navicular (*last tarsal bone to begin ossification*): 3–5 years
- Accessory bone: *tibiale externum* Cuboid: *birth-6 months* Medial cuneiform: *1–2 years* (sometimes two primary centers; dorsal/plantar) Lateral cuneiform: 1st year Intermediate cuneiform: 3rd year Metatarsals

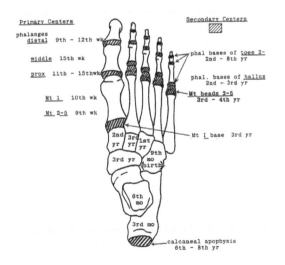

- Primary centers: shaft (I = 10 week, II-V = 9 week)
- Secondary centers: base of metatarsal I (3rd year) and heads II-V (3–4th year) Phalanges
- Primary centers: distal head (9–12 week), middle head (15 week), proximal head (11–15 week)
- Secondary centers: hallux base (2–3rd year), II-V base (2–8th year) Sesamoids in MPJ: 10–12 years

Sesamoid/Accessory Bones

- Fibular and tibial sesamoid of 1st MPJ, imbedded in *flexor hallucis brevis tendons*, plantar aspect of 1st MPJ, ossifies 9–11 years
- Os peroneum (peroneal sesamoid): associated with *peroneus longus tendon*, inferolateral angle of cuboid
- Os tibiale externum (tibialis posterior sesamoid): associated with *tibialis posterior tendon*, near navicular tuberosity
- Os trigonum (talus accessorius): *posterior to lateral tubercle of posterior process* of talus
- Os intermetatarsalis I: between bases of met I-II
- Os vasalianum: tuberosity of 5th metatarsal
- Os intercuneiform: between medial and intermediate cuneiform

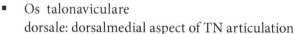

- Os calcaneus s e c o n d a r i u s: between calcaneus and cuboid
- Os sustentaculi: associated with sustentaculum tali of calcaneus
- Os talonaviculare dorsale: dorsalmedial aspect of TN articulation
- Os cuboid secondarius: where cuboid, navicular, calcaneus meet

Pars peronea metatarsalis I: inferomedially between base of 1st met and medial cuneiform

BONES: GENERAL FEATURES

The bones of the lower limb should be at hand during the study of the anatomy of the lower limb. The student has to know the general features of the bones before dissection of the soft tissues.

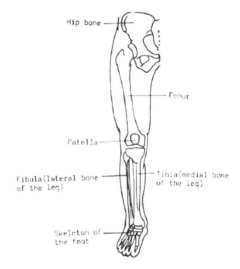

Fig. 1: Skeleton of the lower limb.

The skeleton of the lower limb is formed by the following bones (fig. 1):

A - Pelvic girdle: which is formed by the *hip bone.*

B - Skeleton of the thigh: which is formed by the *femur.*

C - Skeleton of the leg: which is formed by two bones: The *tibia* medially and the *fibula* laterally.

D - Skeleton of the foot: which is formed of three regions. Arranged in a proximodistal direction, they are:

1- *Tarsus:* is formed of 7 tarsal bones.

2- *Metatarsus:* is formed of 5 metatarsal bones.

3- *Phalanges:* 14 in number.

HIP BONE

The hip bone (Os innominatum) forms the *pelvic girdle* which connects the skeleton of the lower limb with the axial skeleton. The two hip bones articulate together at the symphysis pubis. But, posteriorly, the two hip bones are separated by and articulate with the sacrum at the sacoiliac joints.

The hip bone is an irregular bone which is formed of three parts: ilium, pubis and ischium (fig. 2). The three parts are separated by cartilage at young age and fuse together at puberty.

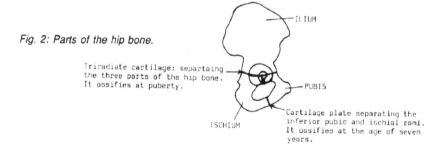

Fig. 2: Parts of the hip bone.

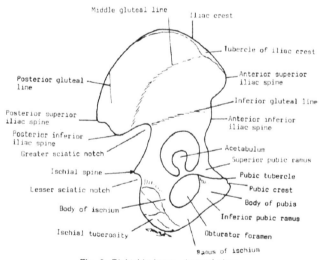

Fig. 3: Right hip bone - Lateral view.

Ilium

This is the upper part of the hip bone. It includes the upper part of the acetabulum and the bone above it (figs. 3, 4).

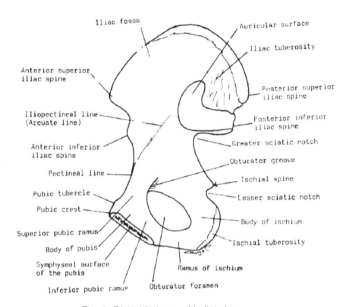

Fig. 4: Right hip bone - Medial view.

It has four borders:

A- **Iliac crest:** is the upper border of the ilium. Its anterior end forms a projection called the *anterior superior iliac spine* while its posterior end forms the *posterior superior iliac spine.* The iliac crest is sinuous; its anterior part being concave inwards while its posterior part is concave outwards (fig. 5).

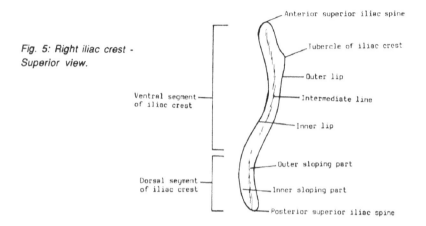

Fig. 5: Right iliac crest -
Superior view.

For descriptive purposes, the iliac crest is differentiated into ventral and dorsal segments:

Ventral segment: includes the anterior two-thirds of the iliac crest. It is concave inwards and has an outer lip, an intermediate line and an inner lip. Two inches behind the anterior superior iliac spine, the outer lip presents a prominence called the *tubercle of iliac crest.* The tubercle lies nearly along the midaxillary line.

Dorsal segment: includes the posterior third of the iliac crest. It is concave outwards and is formed of outer and inner sloping parts separated by a ridge.

B - **Anterior border:** is a short border which begins at the *anterior superior iliac spine.* It ends just above the acetabulum where it forms another projection called the *anterior inferior iliac spine* (fig. 3).

C- **Posterior border:** is an irregular border which begins at the *posetrior superior iliac spine.* If followed for a short distance, it forms another junction called the *posterior inferior iliac spine.* Then it forms, the upper part of a large notch called the *greater sciatic notch* (fig. 3). Its lower end is continuous with the posterior border of the ischium.

D- **Medial border:** is called the *arcuate or iliopectineal line* of the hip bone. This border forms the greater part of the pelvic brim on each side. Its junction with the pubis forms a projection called the *iliopectineal or iliopubic eminence* (fig. 4).

The ilium has three surfaces:

A - Gluteal surface: is the wide outer surface of the ilium (fig. 3). This surface is bounded by the iliac crest above, the acetabulum below, the anterior border anteriorly and the posterior border posteriorly. This surface is divided into four areas by thee *gluteal lines:*

1- *Posterior gluteal line:* extends vertically from the posterior inferior iliac spine to the iliac crest. Its lower part is ill-defined.

2- *Middle gluteal line:* extends in an arched form from the upper border of the greater sciatic notch upwards and forwards towards the anterior superior iliac spine.

3- *Inferior gluteal line:* extends forwards in an arched form from the apex of the greater sciatic notch towards the upper part of the anterior inferior iliac spine.

B - Iliac fossa: is a smooth and gently concave surface which is directed forwards and medially (figs. 4, 6). It is bounded by the iliac crest superiorly, anterior border anteriorly and medial border (arcuate line) posteriorly.

C - Sacropelvic surface: is an irregular surface which lies behind and below the iliac fossa with the medial border intervening. This surface is bounded by the dorsal segment of the iliac crest superiorly and posteriorly and by the posterior border posteriorly and inferiorly. Anteriorly and superiorly, it is bounded by the medial border (arcuate or iliopectineal line) which separates it from the iliac fossa.

The sacropelvic surface is differentiated into three parts (fig. 6):

1- *Iliac tuberosity:* is the rough raised area below the dorsal segment of the iliac crest.

2- *Auricular surface:* is so called because it resembles the auricle of the external ear. This surface articulates with the auricular surface of the sacrum to form the sacroiliac joint (plane synovial joint).

3- *Pelvic surface:* is the lower part of the sacropelvic surface; and is so called because it forms a part of the lateral wall of the true pelvis.

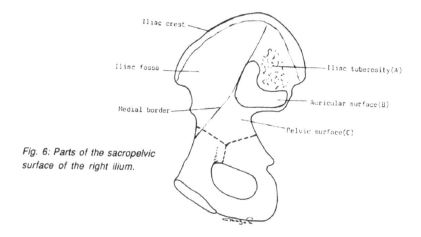

Fig. 6: Parts of the sacropelvic
surface of the right ilium.

Pubis

This is the anterior and inferior part of the hip bone. It includes the anterior part of the acetabulum and extends to the symphysis pubi.

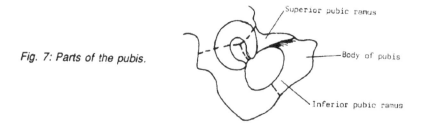

Fig. 7: Parts of the pubis.

The pubis is formed of three main parts: body and two rami (fig. 7):

A - Body of the pubis: is flattened and has three surfaces:

1- *Anterior surface:* directed anteroinferiorly towards the thigh.

2- *Posterior surface:* directed posterosuperiorly towards the pelvis.

3- *Symphyseal surface:* directed medially where it shares in the symphysis pubis.

The upper border of the body is called the *pubic crest.* The crest forms a part of the pelvic brim; and ends laterally in a small but well-defined bony projection called the *pubic tubercle.*

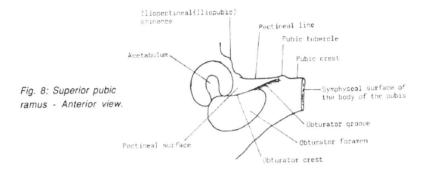

Fig. 8: Superior pubic ramus - Anterior view.

B - Superior pubic ramus: is the part of the pubis extending from the body to the acetabulum. This ramus is triangular in cross section, having three surface which are separated by three borders (fig. 8): The surfaces are:

1- *Pectineal surface:* a triangular surface which is directed anterosuperiorly. It extends from the pubic tubercle to the iliopectineal eminence.

2- *Pelvic surface:* which is directed posterosuperiorly, forming a part of the wall of the true pelvis.

3- *Obturator surface:* which is directed posteroinferiorly towards the obturator foramen. This surface is grooved obliquely to form the *obturator groove.*

The borders of the superior pubic ramus are:

1- *Pectineal line (Pectin pubis):* a sharp ridge extending from the pubic tubercle to the iliopectineal eminence. This line separates the pectineal and pelvic surfaces. It forms a part of the pelvic brim.

2- *Obturator crest:* a rounded ridge separating the pectineal and obturator surfaces.

3- *Inferior border:* separates the obturator and pelvic surfaces. This border forms a part of the margin of the obturator foramen.

C - Inferior pubic ramus: is shorter than the superior ramus, and extends downwards and laterally from the body to join the ischial ramus where they form together the *conjoined ramus.* The conjoined rami of both sides form the *pubic arch*. The inferior pubic ramus has two surfaces separated by two borders. The surfaces are:

1- **Anterior (Outer) surface:** which is directed anterioinferiorly towards the thigh.

2- **Posterior (Inner) surface:** which is directed posterosuperiorly towards the pelvis.

The borders are:

1- **Medial (Anterior) border:** which forms a part of the pubic arch.

2- **Lateral (Posterior) border:** which forms a part of the margin of the obturator foramen.

Ischium

This is the posterior and inferior part of the hip bone. It includes the lower part of the acetabulum and is formed of a body and one ramus (fig. 9).

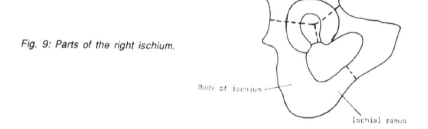

Fig. 9: Parts of the right ischium.

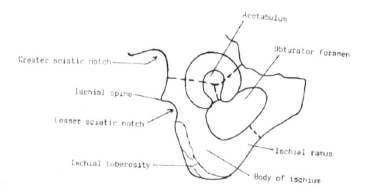

Fig. 10: General features of the right ischium.

A - Body of ischium: is the mass of bone forming the lower part of the acetabulum and the bone below it. It is continuous inferiorly with the ischial ramus. It has three surfaces separated by three borders. The surfaces of the body are:

1- **Dorsal surface:** which is directed backwards and upwards. Superiorly, it is continuous with the gluteal surface of the ilium. Its lower part forms a rough impression called the *ischial tuberosity* (described later).

2- **Outer (Femoral) surface:** which is directed antereolaterally towards the thigh.

3- **Inner (Pelvic) surface:** which is directed posteromedially towards the pelvis.

The borders of the body are:

1- **Posterior border:** is an irregular border which is continuous superiorly with the posterior border of the ilium where it forms the lower part of the *greater sciatic notch* (fig. 10). Then, it forms a sharp well-defined triangular projection called the *ischial spine*. Below the spine, it forms a small notch called the *lesser sciatic notch*.

2- **Lateral border:** which forms the lateral border of the ischial tuberosity.

3- **Anterior border:** which forms a part of the margin of the obturator foramen.

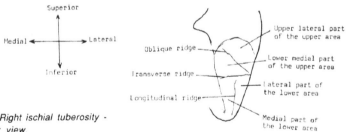

Fig. 11: Right ischial tuberosity - Posterior view.

Ischial tuberosity: is a marked elongated impression on the dorsal surface of the body of the ischium which is wider above and taparing below (fig. 11). It is divided by a *transverse ridge* into two areas:

1- **Upper quadrangular area:** which is divided by an *oblique ridge* into two parts:

    a- Upper lateral part.
    b- Lower medial part.

3- **Lower triangular area:** which is divided by a *longitudinal ridge* into two parts:
    a- Lateral part.
    b- Medial part.

B - **Ischial ramus:** extends from the lower part of the body to join the inferior pubic ramus, forming together the conjoined ramus. The ischial ramus has two surfaces separated by two borders. The surfaces are:

1- **Anterior (Outer) surface:** which is directed outwards towards the thigh.

2- **Posterior (Inner) surface:** which is directed inwards towards the pelvis and perineum.

The borders are:

1- **Superior border:** which forms a part of the margin of the obturator foramen.

2- **Inferior border:** which forms a part of the pubic arch.

Acetabulum

This is a cup-shaped depression on the lateral side of the hip bone, including parts of the three components of the hip bone. It articulates with the head of the femur to form the hip joint.

Fig. 12: Parts of the right acetabulum.

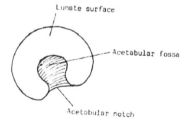

The margin of the acetabulum shows an inferior deficiency called the *acetabular notch* (fig. 12). The floor of the acetabulum shows a nonarticular area called the *acetabular fossa*. The acetabular fossa is incompletely surrounded by a C-shaped articular strip called the *lunate surface.*

The contribution of the three parts of the hip bone to the acetabulum is not equal. The pubis only forms the anterior fifth of the lunate surface. The ilium forms the superior two-fifths of the lunate surface. The ischium forms the posterior two-fifth of the lunate surface in addition to the acetabular fossa (fig. 2).

Obturator Foramen

This is an oval roughly triangular foramen which is bounded by the different parts of the pubis and ischium (figs. 3, 4).

Sexual differences in the hip bone: The hip bone shows sexual differences more than any other bone in the body. Details of the differences between the male and female hip bones are described with the true pelvis (See Abdomen).

How to identify to which side a given hip bone belongs
1- Ilium is directed superiorly.

2- Pubis is directed anteriorly.

3- Acetabulum is directed laterally.

FEMUR

The femur is a long bone which is formed of an upper end, a shaft and a lower end (figs. 13, 14).

Upper End

This end is formed of four parts: head, neck, greater trochanter and lesser trochanter.
1- **Head:** is directed upwards and medially with a slight forward inclination. It forms more than half (about two-thirds) of a sphere. Just below and behind its centre, the head presents a small depression called the *fovea* of the head of the femur.

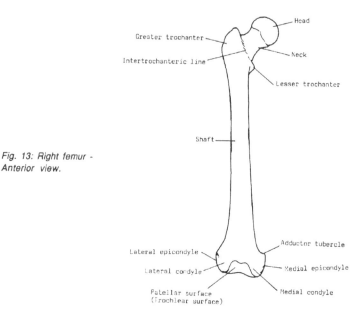

*Fig. 13: Right femur -
Anterior view.*

2- **Neck:** is about two inches long and forms an angle with the shaft. This angle is called the *angle of femoral inclination* and is about 127 degrees (fig. 15). This angle is greater in males than females due to the greater transverse diameter of the pelvis and consequent greater inclination of the shaft of the femur in females.

At the junction of the neck with the shaft anteriorly, the neck presents a line called the *intertrochanteric line* (fig. 13). At the junction with the shaft posteriorly, the neck presents a prominent ridge called the *intertrochanteric crest* (figs. 14, 16). The middle part of the crest presents a prominence called the *quadrate tubercle.*

3- **Greater trochanter:** is a large bony prominence which lies on the upper end of the shaft at its junction with the neck. It is quadrangular, having anterior, lateral and medial surfaces. It has an upper border which forms a projection at its posterior end called the *posterosuperior angle.* Posteriorly, the greater trochanter is bounded by the upper part of the intertrochanteric crest. The lateral surface presents an *oblique ridge* which extends downwards and forwards from the posterosuperior angle. The medial surface presents a depression called the *trochanteric fossa* (fig. 16).

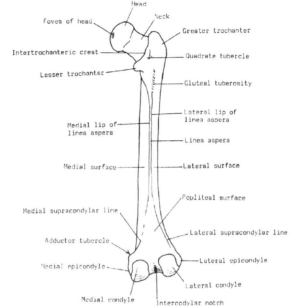

Fig. 14: Right femur - Posterior view.

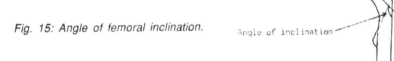

Fig. 15: Angle of femoral inclination.

4- **Lesser trochanter:** smaller than the greater trochanter, it is a conical bony projection which lies posteromedially at the junction of the neck with the shaft. It is continuous with the lower end of the intertrochanteric crest.

Shaft

The shaft is curved with a slight anterior convexity. It is cylindrical for the greater part of its extent; but its upper third is slightly expanded while its lower third is greatly expanded.

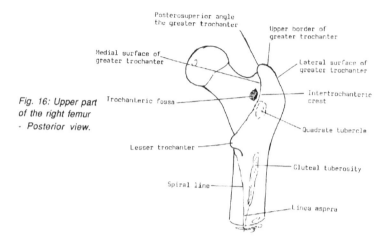

Fig. 16: Upper part of the right femur - Posterior view.

The middle third of the shaft has three surfaces and three borders. The surfaces are:

1- **Anterior surface:** gently convex and directed anteriorly.

2- **Lateral surface:** directed posterolaterally.

3- **Medial surface:** directed posteromedially.

The borders are:

1- **Lateral border:** an ill-defined border directed laterally.

2- **Medial border:** an ill-defined border directed medially.

3- **Posterior border:** which is called the *linea aspera*. It is a prominent and thick ridge which has medial and lateral lips.

The upper third of the shaft presents a fourth surface which called the *posterior surface.* This surface is bounded medially by a rough line called the *spiral line.* This line connects the lower end of the intertrochanteric line with the medial lip of the linea aspera. Laterally, the posterior surface is bounded by a rough prominent ridge called the *gluteal tuberosity* which is continuous inferiorly with the lateral lip of linea aspera.

The lower third of the shaft also presents a fourth posterior surface which is called the *popliteal surface of the femur* (fig. 14). This surface is triangular with its apex directed upwards at the lower end of the linea aspera. It is bounded laterally by a prominent line called the *lateral supracondylar line* which is continuous with the lateral lip of the linea aspera. Meially, it is bounded by a prominent line called the *medial supracondylar line* which is continuous with the medial lip of the linea aspera. However, the upper part of the medial supracondylar line is smooth and ill-defined. The lower part of this line ends in a projection above the posterior part of the medial condyle which is called the *adductor tubercle*.

Lower End

This end is formed of two large masses called the medial and lateral *condyles* of the femur. Anteriorly, the two condyles are continuous together; but posteriorly they are separated by a large gap called the *intercondylar notch (or fossa)*.

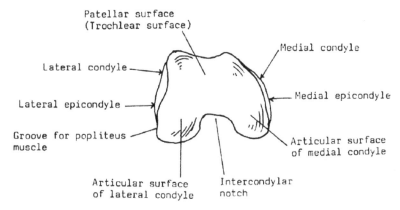

Fig. 17: Articular surfaces of the lower end of the right femur.

The two condyles are partially covered by a ^ - shaped articular surface which articulates with the patella and condyles of the tibia to form the knee joint (fig. 17). The anterior part of the articular surface is called the *patellar or trochlear surface* which lies in front of both condyles and articulates with the patella. The remainder of the articular surface forms two strips which extend into the inferior and posterior surfaces of the two condyles.

The *lateral condyle* is larger than the medial condyle and is more in line with the shaft. The most prominent part on its lateral surface is called the *lateral epicondyle* (fig. 18). Just below and behind the lateral epicondyle, the lateral surface presents a *groove for popliteus muscle (popliteal groove)*.

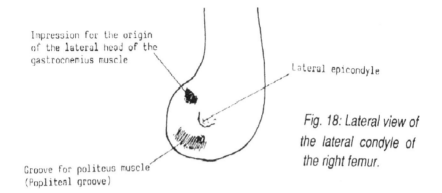

Fig. 18: Lateral view of the lateral condyle of the right femur.

The *medial condyle* is smaller than the lateral condyle, but is more deflected medially. The most prominent part on its medial surface is called the *medial epicondyle.*

The *intercondylar notch* has a lateral wall which is formed by the medial surface of the lateral condyle. The notch has a medial wall which is formed by the lateral surface of the medial condyle. The notch is separated from the popliteal surface by a line called the *intercondylar line.*

Angle of femoral torsion: Like the humerus, the longest axes of the upper and lower ends of the femur are not in line with each other. The neck of the femur is directed upwards and medially with a slight forward inclination. Accordingly, the long axis of the neck forms an angle with the transverse axis of the lower end. This angle is called the *angle of femoral torsion* which is 14 to 16 degrees, but wide variations do occur.

Fig. 19: Angle of femoral torsion.

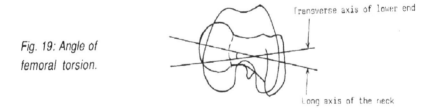

How to identify to which side a given femur belongs

1- The head is directed upwards and medially.

2- The shaft is convex anteriorly.

Patella

This is the largest sesamoid bone in the body, developing in the insertion of the quadriceps femoris. It is a flattened triangular bone with its *apex* directed downwards and its *base* directed upwards (figs. 20, 21). It has *three borders:* upper border (base of the patella), lateral border and medial border. It has *two surfaces:* anterior and posterior. The anterior surface is rough. The posterior surface is divided into an *upper articular area* and a *lower nonarticular area.*

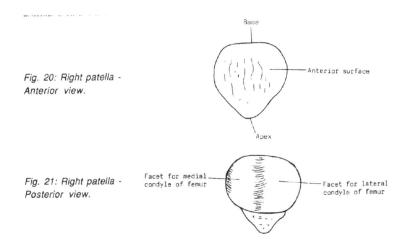

Fig. 20: Right patella - Anterior view.

Fig. 21: Right patella - Posterior view.

The articular surface of the patella articulates with the patellar (trochlear) surface of the femur to form a part of the knee joint. It is divided into lateral and medial parts by a blunt vertical ridge. The *lateral part* is larger and articulates with the lateral condyle of the femur while the *medial part* is smaller and articulates with the medial condyle of the femur. The medial part presents a small longitudinal medial strip which articulates with the medial condyle of the femur only in full flexion of the knee joint. The ridge between the lateral and medial parts articulates with the middle depressed part of the trochlear (patellar) surface of the femur.

TIBIA

This is the medial and stronger bone of the leg. It is a long bone which has an upper end, a shaft and a lower end (figs. 22, 23).

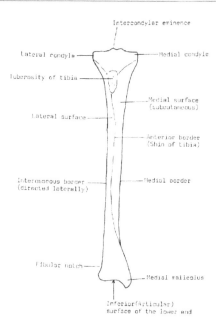

Fig. 22: Right tibia -
Anterior view.

Upper End

This end is much larger than the lower end and is formed of medial and lateral *condyles.* The two condyles carry upper articular surfaces which articulate with the corresponding femoral condyles in the knee joint (fig. 24). The articular surfaces of both condyles are separated by a nonarticular strip called the *intercondylar area.* The middle part of this area is raised to form the intercondylar eminence. The *intercondylar eminence* presents two upward projections called the medial and lateral *intercondylar tubercles.* The part of the area in front of the eminence is called the *anterior intercondylar area* while the part behind the eminence is called the *posterior intercondylar area.*

The *medial condyle* is larger than the lateral condyle. Its superior articular surface is large and oval; and articulates with the medial condyle of the femur. Its posterior surface shows a shallow transverse groove (for insertion of semimembranosus).

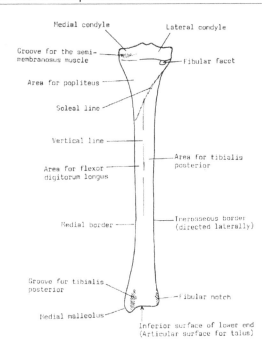

Medial condyle

Lateral condyle

Groove for the semi-membranosus muscle

Fibular facet

Area for popliteus

Soleal line

Vertical line

Area for tibialis posterior

Fig. 23: Right tibia - Posterior view.

Area for flexor digitorum longus

Interosseous border (directed laterally)

Medial border

Groove for tibialis posterior

Fibular notch

Medial malleolus

Inferior surface of lower end (Articular surface for talus)

The *lateral condyle* is smaller than the medial condyle. Its superior articular surface is small and circular; and articulates with the lateral condyle of the femur. The posterolateral part of its inferior surface carries a circular articular facet called the *fibular facet* which articulates with the head of the fibula to form the superior (proximal) tibiofibular joint (palne synovial joint).

The front of the upper end of the tibia presents a well-define projection called the *tibial tuberosity.* The upper part of the tuberosity is smooth while its lower part is rough and subcutaneous.

The greater parts of both condyles are subcutaneous and can be felt on both sides of the knee.

Shaft

The shaft gradually decreases in thickness as followed from the upper to lower end. It is triangular in cross section, having three borders and three surfaces (fig. 29). The borders are:

1- **Anterior border:** is prominent, forming the *shin of the tibia.* This border is slightly sinuous; and begins at the tuberosity and ends at the medial malleolus. This border is easily felt as it is subcutaneous throughout its whole extent.

2- **Medial border:** is also subcutaneous throughout its whole extent. It begins below the groove for semimembranosus muscle and descends vertically to the posterior margin of the medial malleolus.

3- **Interosseous border:** is a sharp border which is directed laterally (towards the fibula). It extends from the fibular facet down to the anterior margin of the fibular notch on the lower end. This border is connected to the interosseous border of the fibula by the interosseous membrane of the leg.

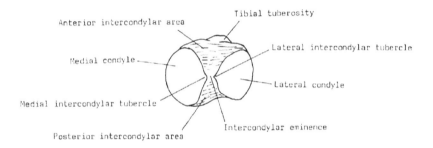

Fig. 24: Upper end of right tibia - Superior view.

The surfaces of the shaft are:

1- **Medial surface:** between the anterior and medial borders. This surface is easily felt as it is almost completely subcutaneous.

2- **Lateral surface:** between the anterior and interosseous borders. The lower part of this surface deviates to the front of the lower part of the shaft following the deviation of the anterior and interosseous borders.

3- **Posterior surface:** between the interosseous and medial borders. The upper part of this surface is crossed by an oblique ridge called the *soleal line.* The area above the soleal line is nearly triangular. The area below the soleal line is divided into medial and lateral parts by a *vertical line.* The posterior surface presents a *nutrient foremen* close to the upper part of the vertical line.

Lower End

This end is smaller than the upper end and has five surfaces: anterior, posterior, medial, lateral and inferior surfaces.

The *anterior surface* is continuous with the lateral surface of the shaft. The *posterior surface* is continuous with the posterior surface of the shaft. The *medial surface* is continuous with the medial surface of the shaft and forms a downward projection called the *medial malleolus* which is also subcutaneous. The *lateral surface* is depressed to form the *fibular notch*.

This notch is firmly attached to the lower part of the shaft of the fibula by a strong interosseous tibiofibular ligament, forming the inferior (distal) tibiofibular joint (fibrous joint or syndesmosis). The *inferior surface* is an articular surface which articulates with the body of the talus in the ankle joint. This surface is continuous with the articular surface of the medial malleolus which also shares in the ankle joint.

The posterior surface of the medial malleolus shows a well-defined longitudinal groove (for the tendon of tibialis posterior). The lower end or tip of the medial malleolus presents a shallow depression.

How to identify to which side a given tibia belongs
1- The upper end is larger than the lower end.

2- The tibial tuberosity is directed anteriorly.

3- The medial malleolus is directed medially.

FIBULA

This is the lateral bone of the leg. It is a slender and weak bone as compared with the tibia. Therefore, it has no role in weight bearing and only serves for muscle attachments. It is formed of an upper end, a shaft and a lower end (figs. 25, 26, 27, 28). The upper end is called the *head* of the fibula while the lower end is called the *lateral malleolus*.

Upper End (Head of Fibula)

This end is expanded and carries a circular facet which articulates the fibular facet of the lateral condyle of the tibia to form the superior tibiofibular joint (plane synovial joint). It forms an upward projection called the *styloid process* or *apex of the head.* The constriction which marks the junction of the head with the shaft is called the *neck* of fibula.

Shaft

The shaft is also described as having three borders and three surfaces (fig. 29). The borders are:

1- **Anterior border:** is best identified if followed from the lower to the upper end. It begins from the apex of a triangular subcutaneous area on the lateral aspect of the lower part of the shaft above the lateral malleolus. This border can be easily followed up to the head of the fibula.

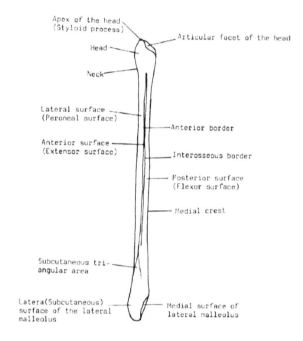

Fig. 25: Right fibula - Anterior view.

Apex of the head (Styloid process)

Articular facet of the head

Head

Neck

Lateral surface (Peroneal surface)

Anterior border

Anterior surface (Extensor surface)

Interosseous border

Posterior surface (Flexor surface)

Medial crest

Subcutaneous triangular area

Latera(Subcutaneous) surface of the lateral malleolus

Medial surface of lateral malleolus

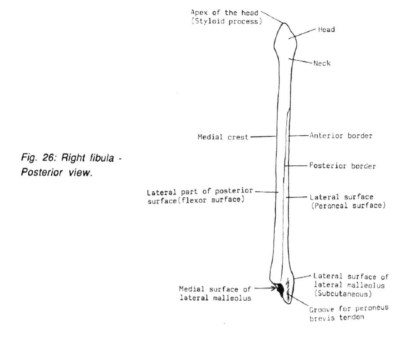

Fig. 26: *Right fibula - Posterior view.*

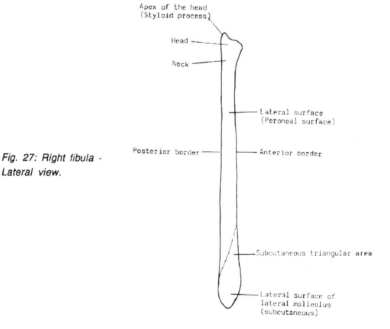

Fig. 27: *Right fibula - Lateral view.*

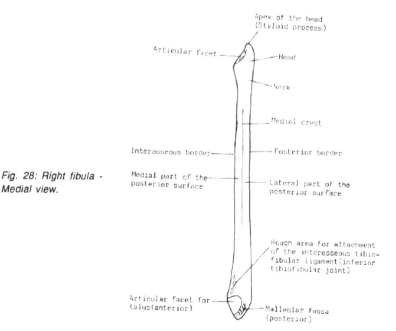

Fig. 28: Right fibula -
Medial view.

2- **Interosseous border:** lies close to the medial side of the anterior border, so that the two borders are almost fused in the upper part of the shaft where the intervening anterior surface is greately narrowed. This border is directed medially (towards the tibia) and is connected to the interosseous border of the tibia by the interosseous membrane of the leg.

3- **Posterior border:** is also best identified if followed from the lower to the upper end. It extends from the back of the lateral malleolus up to the head, but is ill-defined in the upper part of the shaft.

The surfaces are:

1- **Anterior surface:** is a narrow surface between the anterior and interosseous borders. Its upper part is very narrow where the two borders come close together. This surface is called the *extensor surface* as it gives origin to extensor muscles.

2- **Lateral surface:** is a wide surface between the anterior and posterior borders. The lower part of this surface deviates backwards to reach the back of the lateral malleolus. Tis surface is called the *peroneal surface* as it gives origin to the peronei longus and brevis.

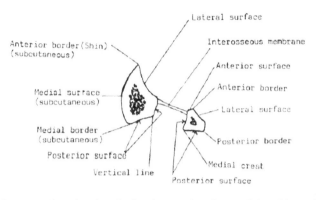

Fig. 29: Cross section showing the borders and surfaces of the tibia and fibula.

3- **Posterior surface:** is a wide surface between the posterior and interosseous borders. The upper two-thirds of this surface are divided into lateral and medial parts by a prominent ridge called the *medial crest* which is more marked than the borders of the bone and may be mistaken for any of the borders. The posterior surface is called the *flexor surface* as it gives origin to flexor muscles. The lower part of the posterior surface deviates to the medial aspect of the lower end where it forms a rough impression that gives attachment to the interosseous tibiofibular ligament, forming the inferior tibiofibular joint (fibrous joint or syndesmosis).

The posterior surface presents a *nutrient foramen* close to the upper part of the medial crest.

Lower End (Lateral Malleolus)

This end is flattened from side to side. Its lateral surface is subcutaneous and continuous with a triangular subcutaneous area on the lateral aspect of the lower part of the shaft (fig. 27).

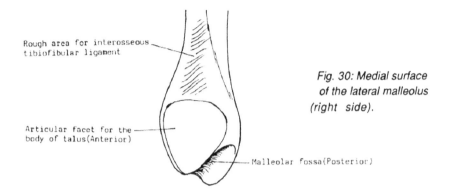

Rough area for interosseous tibiofibular ligament

Fig. 30: Medial surface of the lateral malleolus (right side).

Articular facet for the body of talus(Anterior)

Malleolar fossa(Posterior)

The medial surface of the lateral malleolus is differentiated into an anterior articular part and a posterior nonarticular part (fig. 30). The anterior articular part articulates with the lateral surface of the body of the talus in the ankle joint. The posterior nonarticular part is depressed to form the *malleolar fossa*.

The back of the lateral malleolus shows a longitudinal groove (for the tendon of peroneus brevis). The lower end (tip) of the lateral malleolus shows a small notch and reaches to a lower level than the medial malleolus.

How to identify to which side a given fibula belongs

1- The head is directed upwards.

2- The articular surface of the lateral malleolus is directed medially.

3- The malleolar fossa lies posterior to the articular surface of the lateral malleolus.

SKELETON OF THE FOOT

The skeleton of the foot is formed of three regions: tarsus, metatarsus and phalanges arranged in a proximodistal direction (figs. 31, 32).

Tarsus

This region is formed of seven tarsal bones which are irregularly arranged into a proximal row and a distal row with one bone intervening between the two rows medially.

The *proximal row* is formed of two bones: talus and calcaneus, the talus lying above the calcaneus.

The *distal row* is formed of four bones which are arranged mediolaterally as follows: medial cuneiform, intermediate cuneiform, lateral cuneiform and cuboid.

The seventh tarsal bone is the *navicular bone*. This bone is interposed between the proximal and distal rows, lying on the medial side and intervening between the talus and three cuneiform bones.

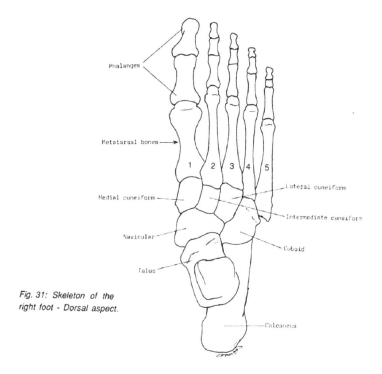

Fig. 31: Skeleton of the
right foot - Dorsal aspect.

Talus: is formed of a head, neck and body. The *head* is directed forwards and slightly downwards and medially. The *neck* is the constriction just behind the head. Its plantar (inferior) surface is deeply grooved, forming the *sulcus tali*. This sulcus forms the roof of a tunnel between the talus and calcaneus known as the *sinus tarsi*. The *body* is the expanded part behind the neck.

Calcaneus: is the bone of the heel, lying below the talus (fig. 33). Its upper surface presents a groove called the *suclus calcancei* which together with the sulcus tali form the *sinus tarsi* as previously decsribed.

The anterosuperior part of the bone forms a medial shelf-like projection called the *sustentaculum tali* as it carries, supports and articulates with the head of the talus.

The plantar (inferior) surface is rough; and posteriorly it presents a rough elevation called the *calcanean tuberosity.* The tuberosity is divided into a large *medial tubercle* and a smaller *lateral tubercle.*

The medial surface is smooth and concave.

The lateral surface is rough and presents an ill-defined projection called the *peroneal tubercle.*

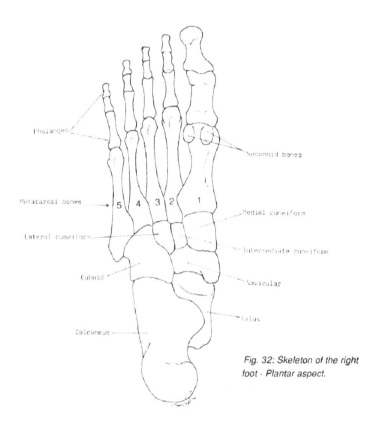

Fig. 32: Skeleton of the right foot - Plantar aspect.

Navicular: is interposed between the head of the talus and the three cuneiform bones. It has a rough convex dorsal surface and a rough concave plantar surface. It forms a medial projection which is called the *tuberosity* of navicular bone.

Cuneiform bones: are three wedge-shaped bones which are arranged as *medial, intermediate* and *lateral* cuneiform bones. They are interposed between the navicular and the bases of the first, second and third metatarsal bones.

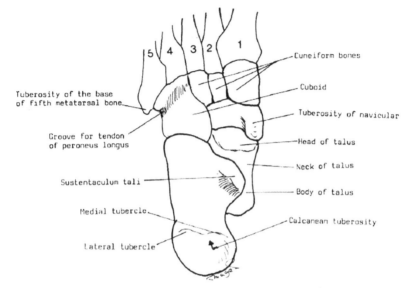

Fig. 33: Some general features of the tarsus - Plantar view.

Cuboid bone: is the lateral bone of the distal row. It is interposed between the calcaneus and the bases of the fourth and fifth metatarsal bones. It has a rough dorsal surface. Its plantar surface presents a well-defined oblique *groove* (for the tendon of peroneus longus). Its lateral surface is rough and presents the beginning of the groove for peroneus longus. Just behind the groove, the lateral surface forms a projection called the *tuberosity* of cuboid bone which usually carries a *facet* for a sesamoid bone or cartilage in the tendon of peroneus longus.

Metatarsus

This region is formed of five *metatarsal bones* arranged first to fifth from the medial to the lateral side. This means that the first metatarsal bone is in line with the big toe while the fifth is in line with the little toe.

Each metatarsal bone is a long bone which is formed of three parts: proximal end or base, shaft and distal end or head.

The base of the fifth metatarsal bone forms a posterolateral projection which is called the *tuberosity of the base of fifth metatarsal bone.*

Phalanges

These are the bones of the toes (digits). They are 14 in numbers: two for the big toe and three for each of the lateral four toes.

The big toe contains two phalanges: proximal phalanx and distal (terminal) phalanx. Each of the lateral four toes contains three phalanges: proximal phalanx, middle phalanx and distal (terminal) phalanx.

Each phalanx is a long bone which is formed of a proximal end or base, shaft and a distal end or head.

BONES: PARTICULAR FEATURES

HIP BONE

Particular features of the bones are only to be studied after complete dissection of the lower limb. The bones should be at hand during study of their particular features.

Ilium

Iliac crest
- The outer lip gives attachment to the deep fascia of the thigh (fascia lata). Its anterior part, including the tubercle of iliac crest, gives origin to the tensor fasciae latae (fig. 34). Its anterior half gives insertion to the lower digitations of the obliquus externus abdominis (fig. 36). Behind the external oblique, it gives a slip of origin of latissimus dorsi. The interval between the external oblique and latissimus dorsi forms the base of the lumbar triangle.
- The anterior two-thirds of the intermediate line give partial origin to the obliquus internus abdominis.
- The anterior two-thirds of the inner lip give partial origin to the transversus abdominis. Its posterior part gives partial origin to the quadratus lumborum and attachment to the anterior and intermediate layers of the thoracolumbar fascia (fig. 35).
- The outer sloping part of the dorsal segment gives origin to the highest fibers of gluteus maximus while the inner sloping part gives partial origin to the erector spinae (sacrospinalis).

Anterior border
- The inguinal ligament is attached to the upper part of the anterior superior iliac spine while the lower part of the spine gives origin to the sartorius.

- The straight head of rectus femoris takes origin from the upper part of the anterior inferior iliac spine while the lower part of the spine gives attachment to the iliofemoral ligament. This is a very strong ligament which prevents hyperextension of the hip joint.

Posterior border

- The posterior superior iliac spine can be felt in the floor of a skin dimple in the back just above the buttock (fig. 235). It lies opposite the middle of the sacroiliac joint, at the level of the second sacral spine.
- The sacrotuberous ligament is partially attached to the posterior border.
- The greater sciatic notch is described later.

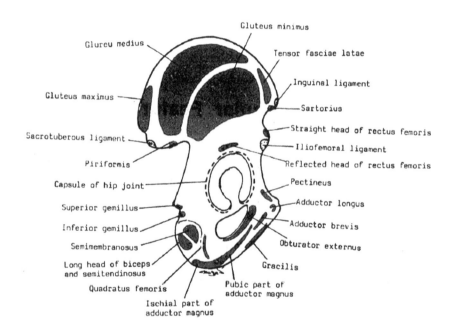

Fig. 34: Right hip bone - Lateral view.

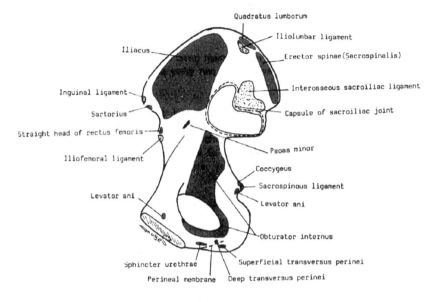

Fig. 35: Right hip bone - Medial view.

Medial border

- Forms the greater part of the pelvic brim.
- The iliopectineal (iliopubic) eminence gives insertion to the tendon of psoas minor.

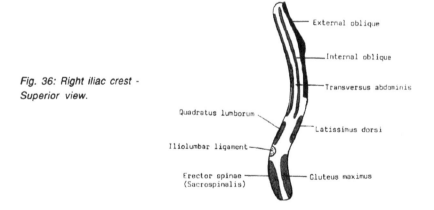

Fig. 36: Right iliac crest - Superior view.

Gluteal surface

- The tensor fasciae latae takes origin from a strip close to the anterior part of the outer lip of iliac crest.

- The gluteus maximus takes partial origin from the upper part of the area behind the posterior gluteal line. The lower part of this area gives attachment to the sacrotuberous ligament and a slip origin to the piriformis.
- The gluteus medius takes origin from the area between the iliac crest and posterior and middle gluteal lines.
- The gluteus minimus takes origin from the area between the middle and inferior gluteal lines.
- The reflected head of rectus femoris takes origin from an impression below the inferior gluteal line and just above the acetabulum.

Iliac fossa
- Forms the posterolateral wall of the false (greater) pelvis.
- Its upper two-thirds give origin to the iliacus muscle.
- The iliac branch of iliolumbar artery runs on the floor of the fossa deep to the iliacus muscle, giving a nutrient artery to the bone.

Sacropelvic surface
- The iliac tuberosity gives attachment to the interosseous sacroiliac ligament which is one of the strongest ligaments in the body.
- The auricular surface articulates with the auricular surface of the sacrum to form the sacroiliac joint (plane synovial joint). Its anterior and inferior margins give attachment to the ventral sacroiliac ligament.
- The pelvic surface forms a part of the lateral wall of the true (lesser) pelvis. It gives partial origin to the obturator internus. It presents a groove between the auricular surface and the greater sciatic notch which is called the *preauricular sulcus*. This sulcus gives attachment to the ventral sacroiliac ligament and is more marked in female bones as a result of the slight mobility of the sacroiliac joint during late pregnancy and labour.

Pubis

Body
- The pubic crest gives origin to the rectus femoris and pyramidalis and attachment to the conjoint tendon and fascia transversalis.
- The pubic tubercle gives attachment to the inguinal ligament and insertion to the tendon of cremaster.

- The adductor longus takes origin by a stout rouded tendon from the front of the body of the pubis just below the pubic tubercle. The front of the body gives partial origin to the gracilis, adductor brevis and obturator externus arranged mediolaterally below the origin of adductor longus, their origin extending to the inferior pubic ramus.
- The posterior surface of the body is related to the urinary bladder from which it is separated by the retropubic fat in the retropubic space. It gives origin to the puborectalis part of the levator ani and the anterior part of obturator internus. Its lower margin gives attachment to the pubovesial and puboprostatic ligaments in male; and to the pubovesical and pubourethral ligaments in female.

Superior pubic ramus
- The pectineal line gives attachment to the lacunar ligament medially and pectineal ligament laterally. It also gives attachment to the conjoint tendon and fascia transversalis.
- The upper part of the pectineal surface gives origin to the pectineus.
- The posterior (pelvic) surface is lined by the parietal pelvic peritoneum.
- The obturator groove is converted by the obturator membrane into a tunnel called the *obturator canal.* This canal transmits the obturator vessels and nerve from the pelvis to the thigh.

Inferior pubic ramus
- The gracilis, adductor brevis and obturator externus arranged mediolaterally take origin from the anterior surface of the inferior pubic ramus, their origin extending up to the lower part of the body.
- The inner surface gives origin to the obturator internus close to the margin of the obturator foramen. Its medial part is related to the crus and dorsal nerve of the penis in male and to the crus and dorsal nerve of clitoris in female; and gives attachment to the perineal membrane.
- The medial border gives attachment to the fascia lata and to the membranous layer of superficial fascia of the perineum. This border is more everted in male as the crura of the penis are much larger than those of the clitoris.

-   The lateral border forms a part of the margin of the obturator foramen and gives attachment to the obturator membrane.

Ischium

Body

-   The outer (femoral) surface gives partial origin to the obturator externus close to the obturator foramen.
-   The inner (pelvic) surface gives partial origin to the obturator internus close to the obturator foramen. The obturator internus and its covering obturator fascia separate the body of the ischium from the ischiorectal fossa.
-   The greater sciatic notch is converted into the *greater sciatic foramen* by the sacrotuberous and sacrospinous ligaments.
-   The tip of the ischial spine gives attachment to the sacrospinous ligament and origin to the coccygeus muscle close to the front of the ligament. The pelvic surface of the spine gives origin to the most posterior part of the levator ani. The tip of the spine is crossed dorsally by the internal pudendal vessels while its base is crossed by the nerve to the obturator internus.
-   The lesser sciatic notch is converted into the *lesser sciatic foramen* by the sacrotuberous and sacrospinous ligaments. The upper margin of the notch gives origin to the superior gemillus while its lower margin gives origin to the inferior gemillus.
-   The anterior border of the body forms a part of the margin of the obturator foramen and gives attachment to the obturator membrane.
-   The dorsal surface of the body presents a transverse shallow groove above the ischial tuberosity which is related to the tendon of obturator internus and two gemilli, a bursa intervening between the tendon and the bone.

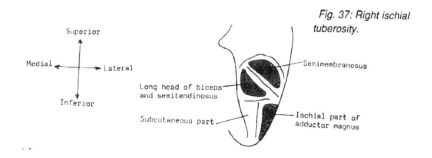

Fig. 37: Right ischial tuberosity.

Ischial tuberosity

- The upper lateral part of the upper area gives origin to the semimembranosus.
- The lower medial part of the upper area gives a common origin to the long head of biceps and semitendinosus.
- The lateral part of the lower area gives origin to the ischial part of adductor magnus.
- The medial part of the lower area is described to be subcutaneous. It does not give origin to muscles and is separated from the skin by fibrofatty tissue. This part, with its fellow of the opposite side, support the body in the sitting position.
- The lateral border of the tuberosity gives origin to the quadratus femoris.
- The medial border of the tuberosity gives attachment to the sacrotuberous ligament.

Ischial ramus

- The anterior (outer) surface gives partial origin to the obturator externus close to the obturator foramen. It gives origin to the pubic part of adductor magnus and the lower part of the gracilis muscle.
- Its posterior (inner) surface gives partial origin to the obturator internus close to the obturator foramen. The perineal part of this surface gives attachment to the perineal membrane and is related to the stuctures in the superficial and deep perineal spaces.
- Its upper border forms a part of the margin of the obturator foramen and gives attachment to the obturator membrane.
- Its lower border gives attachment to the fascia lata and membranous layer of superficial fascia of the perineum.

Acetabulum

- The lunate surface articulates with the head of the femur in the hip joint.
- The acetabular fossa is filled with fat which is covered by synovial membrane.
- The margins of the acetabular notch give attachment to the transverse ligament of the acetabulum which converts the notch into the *acetabular foramen.* The foramen transmits nerves and vessels to the hip joint (See chapter 16).
- The margins of the acetabulum and transverse ligament give attachment to the labrum acetabulare and capsule of the hip joint outside the labrum acetabulare. This means that the labrum is completely intracapsular.

Obturator Foramen

- This foramen is closed by the obturator membrane except at the obturator groove where it leaves a gap for the obturator canal. The obturator canal transmits the obturator vessels and nerve to the thigh.
- Its margins give origin to the obturator externus outside the obturator membrane and obturator internus inside the obturator membrane.
- The obturator foramen is larger and oval in male bones, but is smaller and triangular in female bones.

Ossification of the Hip Bone

The hip bone ossifies in cartilage from three primary and six or more secondary centres (fig. 38).

Primary centres: are three in number, one for each part of the hip bone:
1- A primary centre for the ilium which appears in the second month of intrauterine life.

2- A imary centre for the ischium which appears in the fourth month of intrauterine life.

3- A primary centre for the pubis which appears in the fifth month of intrauterine life.

As ossification spreads out, the three parts become separated by a Y-shaped cartilage called the *triradiate cartilage* in the region of the acetabulum. This cartilage ossifies and disappears at puberty (13-15 years) The inferior pubic ramus is separated from the ischial ramus by a cartilage plate which ossifies and disappears at the age of 7 years.

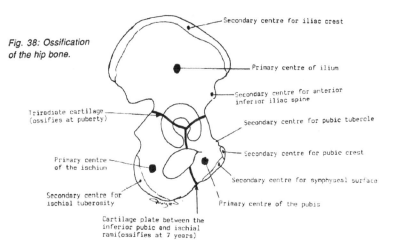

Fig. 38: Ossification of the hip bone.

The secondary centres appear at the age of 18 years and join the rest of the hip bone at the age of 25 years.

FEMUR

Upper End

A - *Head:*
- Articulates with the acetabulum to form the hip joint. The head is completely intracapsular.
- The fovea of the head gives attachment to the ligament of the head of the femur which carries blood supply to the head and has no role in the stability of hip joint.

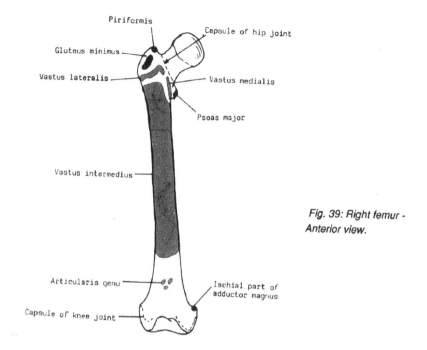

Fig. 39: Right femur - Anterior view.

B - Neck

- The capsule of hip joint is attached to the intertrochanteric line anteriorly; so the neck is completely intracapsular as seen from the front (figs. 39, 41). But, posteriorly the capsule is attached to the neck of the femur one cm medial to the intertrochanteric crest; so the neck is partly intracapsular and partly extracapsular as seen from the back (figs. 40, 42).

- In addition to the capsule, the intertrochanteric line gives attachment to the iliofemoral ligament. This is a very strong V- or Y-shaped ligament which prevents hyperextension of the hip joint. The upper part of the intertrochanteric line gives origin to the upper fibers of the vastus lateralis while its lower part gives origin to the upper fibers of the vastus medialis (fig. 43).

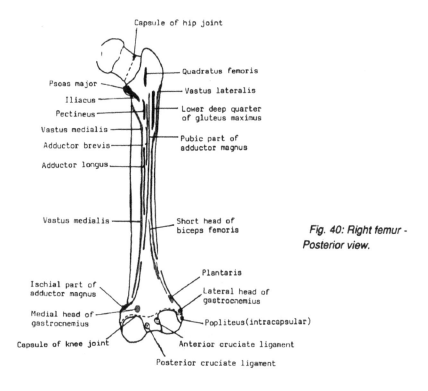

Fig. 40: Right femur - Posterior view.

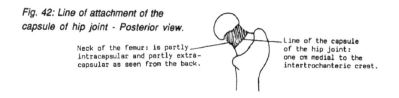

Fig. 41: Line of attachment of the capsule of hip joint - Anterior view.

Neck of the femur: is completely intracapsular as seen from the front.

Fig. 42: Line of attachment of the capsule of hip joint - Posterior view.

Neck of the femur: is partly intracapsular and partly extra-capsular as seen from the back.

Line of the capsule of the hip joint: one cm medial to the intertrochanteric crest.

- The quadrate tubercle and lower part of intertrochanteric crest give insertion to the quadratus femoris (fig. 44).

C - *Greater trochanter*

- Its upper border lies one hand's breadth below the tubercle of the iliac crest, opposite the centre of the head of the femur. This border gives insertion to the piriformis muscle.
- Its anterior surface gives insertion to the gluteus minimus (fig. 43).
- The gluteus medius is inserted into the posterosuperior angle and the oblique ridge on the lateral surface of the greater trochanter (figs. 44, 45).
- The trochanteric fossa gives insertion to the obturator externus. The obturator internus is inserted into the medial surface of the greater trochanter above the trochanteric fossa.

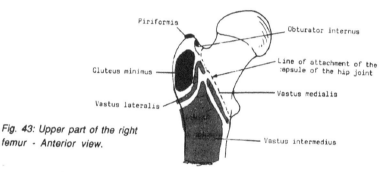

Fig. 43: Upper part of the right femur - Anterior view.

D - *Lesser trochanter*

- gives insertion to the iliopsoas. The psoas major is inserted into the lesser trochanter. The iliacus is inserted mainly into the psoas tendon, but the insertion of the iliacus extends for a short distance to the bone below the lesser trochanter.

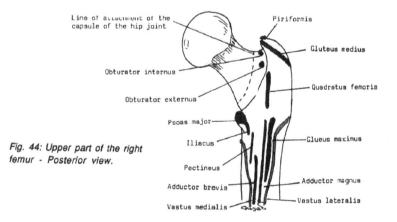

Fig. 44: Upper part of the right femur - Posterior view.

Shaft

is thickly covered by muscles. The vastus intermedius takes a wide origin from the upper three-fourths of the anterior and lateral surfaces of the shaft. The medial surface does not give origin to muscles but is thickly covered by the vastus medialis. The distal part of the anterior surface gives origin to bundles of the articularis genu and is related to the suprapatellar bursa which intervenes between the quadriceps tendon and the bone.

The vastus lateralis has a linear origin from the upper part of the intertrochanteric line, root of the greater trochanter, lateral margin of the gluteal tuberosity and lateral lip of linear aspera.

The vastus medialis has a linear origin from the lower part of the intertrochanteric line, spiral line, medial lip of linea aspera and upper part of the medial supracondylar line.

The gluteal tuberosity gives insertion to the lower deep quarter of gluteus maximus (figs. 44, 45).

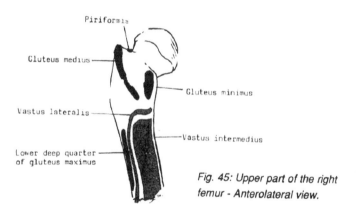

Fig. 45: Upper part of the right femur - Anterolateral view.

The pectineus is inserted into the back of the shaft, along the upper part of a line between the lesser trochanter and linea aspera. The adductor brevis is inserted into the lower part of this line, lateral to the pectineus; its insertion extending to the upper part of the linea aspera (fig. 44).

The adductor longus is inserted into the linea aspera, medial to the adductor brevis; but its insertion extends lower down than the brevis.

The adductor magnus has a linear insertion into the medial margin of the gluteal tuberosity, linea aspera, medial supracondylar line and adductor tubercle. The adductor tubercle receives the tendon of insertion of the ischial part of adductor magnus. The linear insertion of the adductor magnus is interrupted by tendinous arches which bridge over the perforating branches of the profunda femoris artery as they cross the linea aspera. Opposite, the upper part of the medial supracondylar line, the insertion is also interrupted by a large tendinous arch which bounds the adductor opening transmitting the femoral vessels from the adductor canal to the popliteal fossa.

The posteromedial surface presents a nutrient foramen close to the linea aspera. This foramen transmits the nutrient artery to the femur which is usually a branch of the second perforating artery.

The short head of bicep femoris takes origin from the lower part of the linea aspera and upper part of the lateral supracondylar line.

The linea aspera and supracondylar lines give attachment to the medial, posterior and lateral intermuscular septa of deep fascia of the thigh.

The popliteal surface of the femur forms the upper part of the floor of the politeal fossa where it is closely related to the popliteal artery, with some fat between the artery and the bone. The medial head of gastrocnemius takes origin from the popliteal surface just above the medial condyle while the plantaris takes origin from the popliteal surface just above the lateral condyle (fig. 40).

Lower End

The lateral epicondyle gives attachment to the fibular collateral (lateral) ligament of the knee joint. The lateral head of gastrocnemius takes origin from an impression on the lateral surface of the lateral condyle just above and behind the lateral epicondyle; this origin lies outside the knee joint (extracapsular) (fig. 46). The popliteus takes origin by a rounded tendon from the anterior part of the popliteal groove on the lateral surface of the lateral condyle below the lateral epicondyle. This origin is inside the knee joint (intracapsular but extrasynovial) (fig. 46).

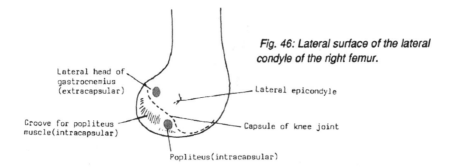

Lateral head of gastrocnemius (extracapsular)

Groove for popliteus muscle(intracapsular)

Lateral epicondyle

Capsule of knee joint

Popliteus(intracapsular)

Fig. 46: Lateral surface of the lateral condyle of the right femur.

The medial epicondyle gives attachment to the tibial collateral (medial) ligament of the knee joint.

The greater parts of both condyles are subcutaneous laterally and medially.

The capsule of knee joint is attached medially to the medial margin of the articular surface of the medial condyle. But, laterally the capsule is attached to the lateral surface of the lateral condyle above the groove for popliteus muscle which is intracapsular and below the origin of the lateral head of gastrocnemius which is extracapsular (fig. 46). The capsule is attached posteriorly to the upper margins of both condyles and intercondylar line. Anteriorly, the capsule of knee joint is defficient where it is replaced by quadriceps tendon, patellar retinacula, patella and ligamentum patellae (fig. 47).

The intercondylar notch is intracapsular but extrasynovial. Its lateral wall is formed by the medial surface of the lateral condyle; its posterior part giving attachment to the anterior cruciate ligament (fig. 48). Its medial wall if formed by the lateral surface of the medial condyle; its anterior part giving attachment to the posterior cruciate ligament.

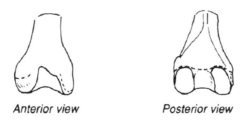

Anterior view   Posterior view

Fig. 47: Line of attachment of the capsule of knee joint.

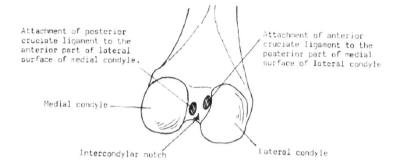

Fig. 48: Attachments of the cruciate ligaments to the intercondylar notch of the right femur-Posterior view.

Ossification Of The Femur

The femur ossifies in cartilage from one primary and four secondary centres (fig. 49):

Primary centre: appears in the middle of the shaft in the seventh week of intrauterine life.

Secondary centres
1- A centre for the lower end which appears in the ninth month of intrauterine life.

   This centre is of mediocolegeal importance as it is a sign of foetal maturity.
2- A centre for the head which appears in the first year after birth.
3- A centre for the greater trochanter which appears in the fourth year.
4- A centre for the lesser trochanter which appears in the thirteenth year.

The greater and lesser trochanters fuse with the shaft just after puberty. The head fuses with the neck at 14-16 years in females and 17-19 years in males.

The lower end fuses with the shaft at 16-18 years in females and 18-20 years in males. Accordingly, the lower end of the femur is the growing end of the bone. The epiphyseal line of the lower end lies transversely at the level of the adductor tubercle.

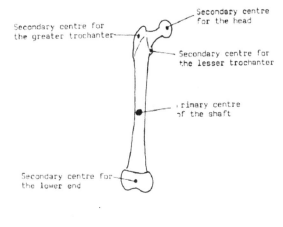

Secondary centre for the head

Secondary centre for the greater trochanter

Secondary centre for the lesser trochanter

Primary centre of the shaft

Secondary centre for the lower end

Fig. 49: Ossification of the femur.

Patella

Anterior surface: is subcutaneous, but is covered by a thin expasnsion from the quadriceps tendon to the ligamentum patellae. This surface is partly separated from the skin by the subcutaneous prepatellar bursa.

Posterior surface

- The upper articular area articulates with the patellar (trochlear) surface of the femur in the knee joint. This area is divided by a vertical ridge into a larger lateral part and a smaller medial part. The larger lateral part articulates with the lateral condyle of the femur. The smaller medial part articulates with the medial condyle of the femur. The small articular strip close to the medial border articulates with the medial condyle during full flexion of the knee joint.
- The lower nonarticular area together with the apex of the patella give attachment to the ligamentum patellae.

Upper border (Base): gives attachment to the part of quadriceps tendon which receives the insertions of the rectus femoris and varsus intermedius.

Medial border: gives attachment to the medial patellar retinaculum which is the part of the quadriceps tendon that receives the insertion of the vastus medialis.

Lateral border: gives attachment to the latelar patellar retinaculum which is the part of the quadriceps tendon that receives the insertion of the vastus lateralis.

Ossification: The patella appears as a cartilage model through the quadriceps tendon in the third month of intrauterine life. It ossifies from several centres which appear at the age of 3-6 years and soon fuse with each other. Ossification is completed at puberty.

TIBIA

Upper End

- The upper surfaces of both condyles are partly separated from the corresponding femoral condyles by the menisci.
- The anterior intercondylar area gives attachment to the following structures arranged anteroposteriorly: anterior horn of medial meniscus, anterior cruciate ligament and anterior horn of lateral meniscus (fig. 52).
- The posterior intercondylar area gives attachment to the following structures arranged anteroposteriorly: posterior horn of lateral meniscus, posterior horn of medial meniscus and posterior cruciate ligament (fig. 52).

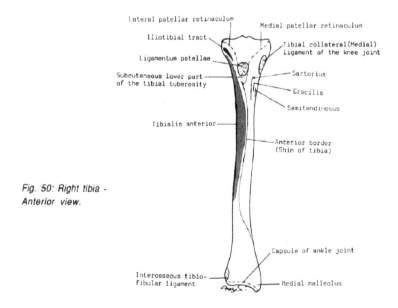

Fig. 50: Right tibia - Anterior view.

- Posteriorly, the capsule of knee joint is attached to the posterior border of the intercondylar area and posterior borders of both condyles. Medially, the capsule is attached to the medial border of the medial condyle and laterally to the lateral border of the lateral condyle.
- The margins of the triangular area above the tibial tuberosity give attachment to the medial and lateral patellar retinacula which replace the capsule of knee joint anteriorly (fig. 50). This triangular area is separated from the ligamentum patellae by fat and deep infrapatellar bursa.
- The smooth upper part of the tibial tuberosity gives attachment to the ligamentum patellae. The rough lower part of the tuberosity is subcutaneous, separated from the skin by the subcutaneous infrapatellar bursa.
- The iliotibial tract is attached to the oblique ridge on the front of the lateral condyle (fig. 50).
- The semimembranosus is inserted into the groove on the back of the medial condyle (fig. 51).

Shaft

Anterior border: is called the shin of the tibia because it is completely subcutaneous. This border gives attachment to the deep fascia of the leg. The lower part of this border gives attachment to the medial end of the superior extensor retinaculum.

Medial border: is also subcutaneous and gives attachment to the deep fascia of the leg. Its middle third gives partial origin to the soleus muscle.

Interosseous border: gives attachment to the interosseous membrane of the leg.

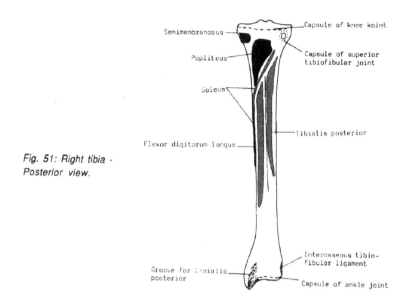

Fig. 51: Right tibia - Posterior view.

Medial surface: is almost completely subcutaneous. Its upper part gives insertion to the sartorius, gracilis and semitendinosus arranged anteroposteriorly (fig. 50). Behind the three muscles, it gives attachment to the tibial collateral (medial) ligament of the knee joint. The lower part of this surface is crossed obliquely by the great saphenous vein and saphenous nerve.

Lateral surface: Its upper two-thirds give origin to the tibialis anterior. The lower part of this surface deviates anteriorly and is related to the following structures deep to the superior extensor retinaculum arranged mediolaterally: tibialis anterior, extensor hallucis longus, anterior tibial vessels, deep peroneal (anterior tibial) nerve, extensor digitorum longus and peroneus tertius.

Posterior surface: The triangular area above the soleal line gives insertion to the popliteus (fig. 51). The soleal line gives partial origin to the soleus muscle. It also gives attachment to the fascia covering the popliteus muscle. The area below the soleal line and medial to the vertical line gives origin to the flexor digitorum longus. The area below the soleal line and lateral to the vertical line gives partial origin to the tibialis posterior.

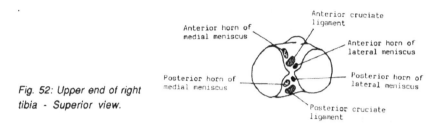

Fig. 52: Upper end of right
tibia - Superior view.

The lower part of the posterior surface is related to the following structures deep to the flexor retinaculum arranged mediolaterally: tibialis posterior, flexor digitorum longus, posterior tibial vessels, tibial (posterior tibial) nerve and flexer hallucis longus.

The vertical line gives attachment to the second septum of deep fascia of the leg. The nutrient foramen close to the vertical line transmits the nutrient artery of the tibia which is a branch of the posterior tibial artery.

Lower End

- Its **anterior surface** is a downward continuation of the lateral surface of the shaft and is related to the same structures as previously described.
- Its **posterior surface** is a downward continuation of the posterior surface of the shaft and is related to the same structures as previously described.
- The medial surface of the **medial malleolus** is subcutaneous while its lateral surface articulates with the talus in the ankle joint. The groove on the back of the medial malleolus is related to the tendon of tibialis posterior (fig. 51). The front of the medial mallelous is related to the great saphenous vein and saphenous nerve. The depression on the apex of the medial malleolus gives attachment to the apex of the deltoid ligament (medial ligament of the ankle joint).
- The **fibular notch** gives attachment to the interosseous tibiofibular ligament in the inferior (distal) tibiofibular joint (fibrous joint or syndesmosis).

Ossification of the Tibia

The tibia ossifies in cartilage from one primary and two secondary centres (fig. 53): *Primary centre:* appears in the middle of the shaft in the seventh week of intrauterine life.

Secondary centres

1- A centre for the upper end which appears at the end of the ninth month of intrauterine life, i.e. shortly before birth.

2- A centre for the lower end which appears in the first or second year.

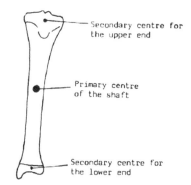

Fig. 53: Ossification of the tibia.

FIBULA

Upper End (Head)

- The head of the fibula is easily felt on the posterolateral aspect of the knee, 2 cm below the line of the knee joint. It articulates with the fibular facet of the lateral condyle of the tibia to form the superior (proximal) tibiofibular joint (plane synovial joint) (figs. 54, 55, 56 and 57).

- The apex of the head (styloid process) gives attachment to the fibular collateral (lateral) ligament of the knee. It also gives insertion to the biceps femoris around the front, lateral side and back of the fibular collateral ligament.

- The front of the head gives origin to the upper fibers of the extensor digitorum longus, its lateral side to the upper fibers of peroneus longus and its back to the upper fibers of the soleus.

- The ***neck of the fibula*** is a very important surgical landmark. Its lateral side is closely related to the termination of the common peroneal nerve which lies in a dangerous position deep to the fibers of peroneus longus. Its medial side is closely related to the anterior tibial vessels as they pass to the anterior compartment of the leg through a gap in the upper part of the interosseus membrane.

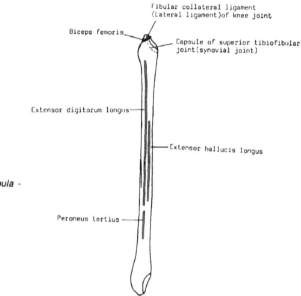

Fig. 54: Right fibula - Anterior view.

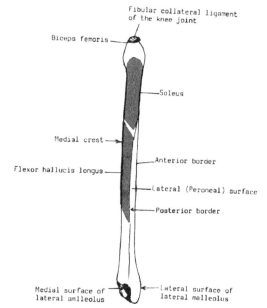

Fig. 55: Right fibula -
Posterior view.

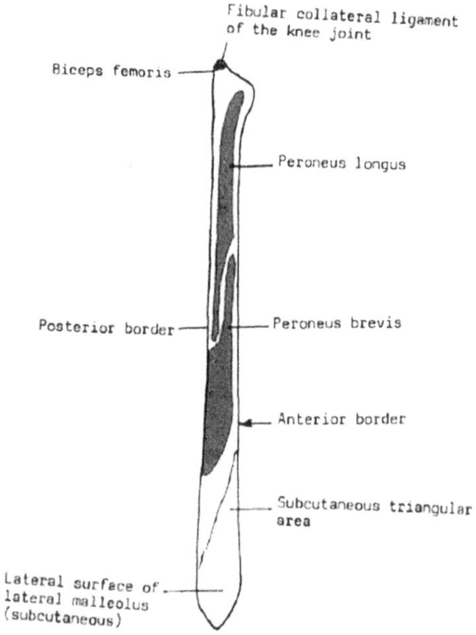

Fig. 56: Right fibula -
Lateral view.

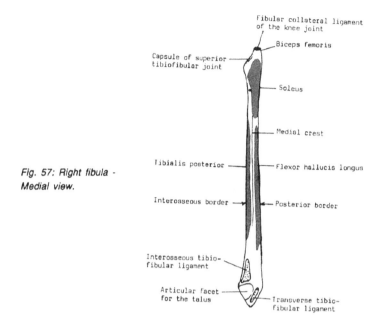

Fibular collateral ligament
of the knee joint

Biceps femoris

Capsule of superior
tibiofibular joint

Soleus

Medial crest

Tibialis posterior

Flexor hallucis longus

*Fig. 57: Right fibula -
Medial view.*

Interosseous border

Posterior border

Interosseous tibio-
fibular ligament

Articular facet
for the talus

Transverse tibio-
fibular ligament

Shaft

The shaft of the fibula is covered by muscles except the triangular subcutaneous area above the lateral malleolus. The anterior border of this triangular area gives attachment to the superior extensor retinaculum while its posterior border gives attachment to the superior peroneal retinaculum.

Anterior border: gives attachment to the anterior intermuscular septum of deep fascia of the leg.

Posterior border: gives attachment to the posterior intermuscular septum of deep fascia of the leg.

Interosseous border: gives attachment to the interossseous membrane of the leg.

Anterior (Extensor) surface: gives origin to the extensor (dorsi flexor) muscles of the foot and digits (fig. 54). The extensor digitorum longus has a linear origin from its upper three-fourths while the lower fourth gives origin to the peroneus tertius. Its middle two-fourths give origin to the extensor hallucis longus medial to the extensor digitorum longus.

Lateral (Peroneal) surface: gives origin to the peronei longus and brevis (fig. 56). Its upper two-thirds give origin to the peroneus longus while its lower two-thirds give origin to the peroneus brevis, i.e. the middle third is common for both muscles. But as it descends, the peroneus longus overlaps the brevis.

Posterior (Flexor) surface: gives origin to the flexor (plantar flexor) muscles of the foot and digits (figs. 55, 57). However, its upper third gives partial origin to the soleus muscle. Below the soleus, this surface gives origin to two muscles. The area between the interosseous border and medial crest gives partial origin to the tibialis posterior. The area between the medial crest and posterior border gives origin to the flexor hallucis longus.

The medial crest gives attachement to the second septum of deep fascia of the leg which covers the tibialis posterior. The peroneal artery descends close to the crest and gives a nutrient artery to the fibula.

The lower part of the posterior surface deviates medially where it presents a rough area which gives attachment to the interosseous tibiofibular ligament of the inferior tibiofibular joint (fibrous joint or syndesmosis) (fig. 57).

Lower End (Lateral Malleolus)

The lower end (lateral malleolus) descends to a lower level than the medial malleolus. Its lateral surface is subcutaneous. Anteriorly, it gives attachment to the anterior talofibular ligament. Posteriorly, it presents a groove for the tendon of peroneus brevis which lies under cover of peroneus longus.

The articular part of its medial surface articulates with the body of the talus in the ankle joint. The malleolar fossa gives attachment to the transverse tubiofibular ligament and posterior talofibular ligament.

The notch on the tip of the lateral malleolus gives attachment to the calcaneofibular ligament.

Ossification of the Fibula

The fibula ossifies in cartilage from one primary and two secondary centres (fig. 58):

Primary centre: appears in the middle of the shaft in the eighth week of intrauterine life.

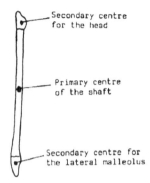

Fig. 58: Ossification of the fibula.

Secondary centres

1- A centre for the lower end which appears at the age of 1-2 years.

2- A centre for the upper end which appears at 3-4 years.

The upper end fuses with the shaft at 15-17 years in females and 17-19 years in males.

The lower end fuses with the shaft at 17-19 years in females and 19-21 years in males. Accordingly, the lower end is the growing end of the fibula.

From the above description, it is observed that the fibula is exceptional as regards its ossification, as the lower end ossifies first and fuses later with the shaft while the upper end ossifies later but fuses earlier with the shaft.

SKELETON OF THE FOOT

Tarsus

Talus

The *head* articulateswiththenavicularboneinthetalocalcaneonavicular joint (fig. 59). The plantar surface of the head carries three articular areas separated by smooth ridges. The anteromedial area articulates with the upper surface of the spring ligament. The anterolateral area articulates with the most anterior articular surface on the superior surface of the calcaneus. The posterior area articulates with the upper surface of the sustanculum tali.

The **neck** is the constriction between the head and body. It is rough and gives attachment to ligaments. Its plantar surface is grooved to form the *sulcus tali* which forms the roof of the *sinus trasi.*. The sinus is occupied by the interosseous talocalcanean ligament (fig. 62).

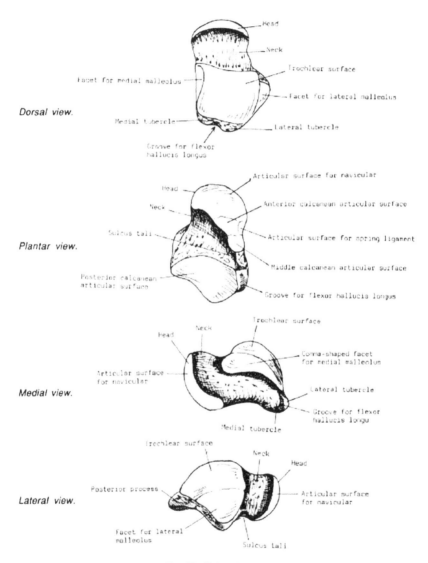

Fig. 59: Right talus.

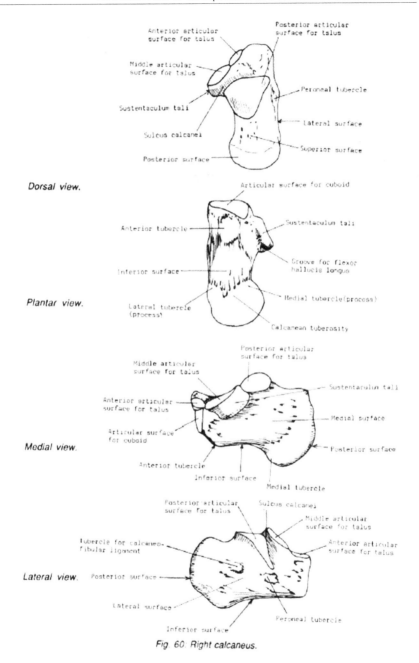

Fig. 60. Right calcaneus.

The **body** is covered dorsally by the *trochlear surface* which articulates with the lower ends of the tibia and fibula in the ankle joint. Its medial surface carries a comma-shaped articular surface for the medial malleolus in the ankle joint. Its lateral surface carries a somewhat triangular articular surface for the lateral malleolus in the ankle joint.

The posterior surface is rough and presents a *groove for the flexor hallucis longus* (figs. 59, 61). The groove is bounded by a large *lateral tubercle* and a small *medial tubercle.*

The plantar surface presents an oval concave articular surface for articulation with the posterior articular surface on the middle third of the superior surface of the calcaneous to form the subtalar (talocalcanean) joint. The talus does not give attachment to muscles; but shares in three joints: ankle, talocalcanean (talocalcaneal or subtalar) and talocalcaneonavicular joints.

Calcaneus

This is the largest of the tarsal bones. The middle third of its **superior surface** carries an articular surface for the body of the talus in the talocalcanean (talocalcaneal or subtalar) joint (fig. 60). The posterior third of this surface is rough. The anterior third carries an articular surface for the head of the talus in the talocalcaneonavicular joint.

The anterior part of the calcaneous forms a medial projection called the **sustentaculum tali.** This is so called because it carries and supports the head of the talus. The inferior surface of the sustentaculum tali is grooved by the tendon of flexor hallucis longus (fig. 61). The superior surface of the sustentaculum tali carries an articular surface for the head of the talus in the talocalcaneonavicular joint.

Fig. 61: Relation of the tendon of flexor hallucis longus to the posterior surface of the talus and the inferior surface of the sustentaculum tali.

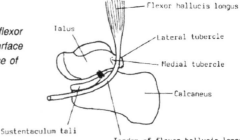

The **superior surface** of the calcaneus presents a groove between the middle and posterior articular surfaces. This groove is called the *sulcus calcanei* and forms the floor of the *sinus tarsi*. This sinus is occupied by the interosseous talocalcanean (talocalcaneal) ligament (fig. 62).

The **plantar surface** is rough. Its posterior part shows an elevation called the *calcanean tuberosity* which is divided into a large *medial tubercle (process)* and a smaller *lateral tubercle (process)*. Its anterior part shows an elevation called the *anterior tubercle*.

The **anterior surface** articulates with the cuboid bone to form the calcaneocuboid joint.

The middle part of the **posterior surface** gives insertion to the tendo calcaneus and tendon of plantaris. Its upper part is smooth and separated from the tendo calcaneus by fat and a bursa. Its lower part is subcutaneous and forms the *heel* (fig. 193).

The **lateral surface** is rough and nearly flat; its greater part is subcutaneous. Its anterior part presents an elevation called the *peroneal tubercle or trochlea*. This tubercle can be felt 2 cm below the tip of the lateral malleolus and separates the tendons of peronei longus and brevis deep to the inferior peroneal retinaculum. The calcaneofibular ligament is attached to a small elevation one cm above and behind the peroneal tubercle.

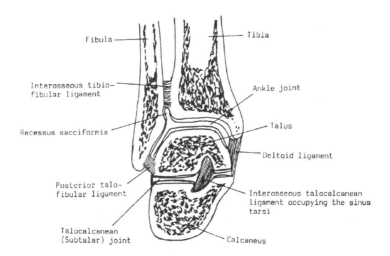

Fig. 62: *Coronal section in the tibia, fibula, talus and calcaneus showing the sinus tarsi occupied by the interosseous talocalcanean ligament.*

The *medial surface* is concave. Its anterior and superior part projects to form the *sustentaculum tali*. As previously described, the inferior surface of the sustentaculum tali is grooved by the flexor hallucis longus while its superior surface carries the middle articular surface for articulation with the head of talus in the talocalcaneonavicular joint. The medial border of the sustentaculum tali gives attachment to the deltoid ligament.

Navicular

Its *proximal (posterior) surface* presents an oval concave articular surface which articulates with the head of talus in the talocalcanveonavicular joint (fig. 63).

Its *distal (anterior) surface* is convex and divided into three aricular facets which articulate with the three cuneiform bones to form the cuneonavicular joint.

The *dorsal surface* is rough and convex. The *plantar surface* is rough and concave.

The *medial surface* forms a well defined projection called the *tuberosity of navicular bone* which receives the main insertion of the tibialis posterior.

The *lateral surface* is rough, but usually carries a small facet for articulation with the cuboid in the cuboideonavicular joint.

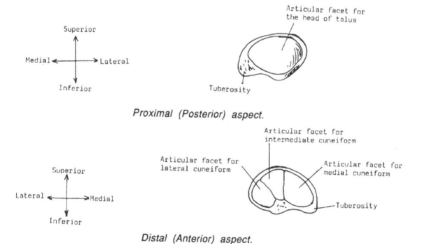

Fig. 63: Right navicular bone.

Cuboid

This is the lateral bone of the distal row of the tarsus. Its *proximal (posterior) surface* articulates with the anterior surface of the calcaneus to form the calcaneocuboid joint (fig. 64).

The *distal (anterior) surface* articulates with the bases of the fourth and fifth metalateral bones (trasometatarsal joints). The *dorsal surface* is rough.

The *plantar surface* presents an oblique *groove for the tendon of peroneus longus*. Behind the lateral end of the groove, there is an oval facet for the sesamoid bone in the tendon of peroneus longus.

The *lateral surface* is rough and shows the beginning of the groove for the tendon of peroneus longus, anterior to the tuberosity of cuboid bone.

The *medial surface* carries an articular facet for the lateral cuneiform bone (cuneocuboid joint). Behind this facet, the medial surface usually carries a small facet for articulation with the navicular bone (cuboideonavicular joint).

Cuneiform bones

These are three wedge-shaped bones arranged as medial, intermediate and lateral cuneiform bones, and forming the medial part of the distal row of the tarsus. They vary in size, the medial one being the largest while the intermediate one is the smallest (figs. 65, 66).

The three bones articulate proximally (posteriorly) with the navicular bone to form the cuneonavicular joint. Distally, the three cuneiform bones articulate with the bases of the first three metatarsal bones (Tarsometatarsal joints).

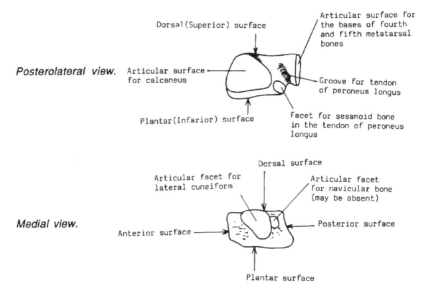

Fig. 64: Right cuboid bone.

The adjacent surfaces of the three bones partly articulate with each other to form intercuneiform joints.

The lateral cuneiform bone carries a facet on its lateral surface for articulation with the cuboid (cuneocuboid joint).

Particular features on the dorsum of the foot

- The tibialis anterior is inserted into the medial side of the medial cuneiform bone and adjacent part of the base of first metatatarsal bone (fig. 65).
- The extensor hallucis longus is inserted into the dorsum of the base of the terminal phalanx of the big toe.
- The extensor hallucis brevis (medial slip of extensor digitorum brevis) is inserted into the base of the proximal phalanx of the big toe.
- The middle slips of the dorsal digital (extensor) expansion are inserted into the bases of the middle phalanges; while the two collateral slips join together to be inserted into the bases of the terminal phalanges of the lateral four toes.
- The peroneus tertius is inseted into the dorsum of the base of the fifth metatarsal bone.

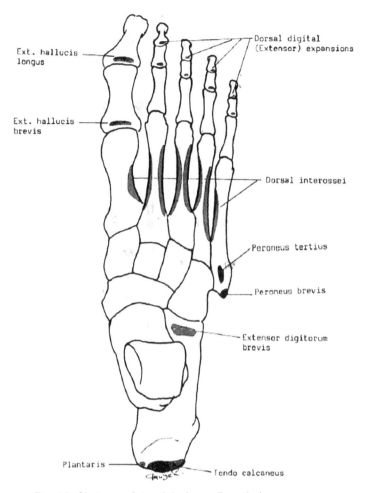

Ext. hallucis longus

Ext. hallucis brevis

Dorsal digital (Extensor) expansions

Dorsal interossei

Peroneus tertius

Peroneus brevis

Extensor digitorum brevis

Plantaris

Tendo calcaneus

Fig. 65: Skeleton of the right foot - Dorsal view.

- The perneus brevis is inserted into the tuberosity of the base of the fifth metatarsal bone.
- The extensor digitorum brevis takes partial origin from the anterior part of the superior surface of the calcaneus.

  The stem of the inferior extensor retinaculum is attached to the anterior part of the superior surface of the calcaneus. The same part gives attachment to the upper end of the inferior peroneal retinaculum.

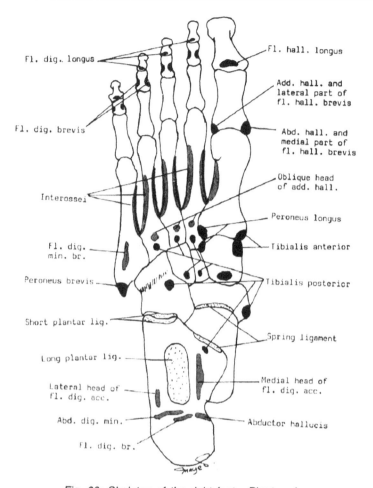

Fig. 66: Skeleton of the right foot - Plantar view.

Particular features on the sole of the foot

- The plantar aponeurosis is attached to the medial tubercle of calcaneus (fig. 66).
- The abductor hallucis takes origin from the flexor retinaculum and medial tubercle of calcaneus.
- The flexor digitorum brevis takes origin from the medial tubercle of calcaneus.
- The abductor digiti minimi takes origin from both lateral and medial tubercles of the calcaneus.
- The flexor hallucis longus is inserted into the base of the terminal phalanx of the big toe.

- The flexor digitorum brevis is inserted by slips into the margins of the middle phalanges of the lateral four toes.
- The flexor digitorum longus is inserted by slips into the bases of the terminal phalanges of the lateral four toes.
- The flexor digitorum accessorius takes origin by two heads from the calcaneus: a medial fleshy head from the medial surface of the calcaneus and a lateral tendinous head from the lateral margin of the plantar surface of the calcaneus.
- The flexor hallucis brevis takes origin from the cuboid bone and adjacent slips of the tendon of tibialis posterior. The medial part of this muscle is inserted with the abductor hallucis into the medial side of the base of the proximal phalanx of big toe. The lateral part is inserted with the adductor hallucis into the lateral side of the base of the proximal phalanx of big toe.
- The flexor digiti minimi brevis takes origin from the plantar surface of the base of the fifth metatarsal bone and the fibrous sheath of the peroneus longus tendon. It is inserted with the abductor digiti minimi into the lateral side of the base of the proximal phalanx of little toe.
- The oblique head of adductor hallucis takes origin from the bases of second, third and fourth metatarsal bones and from the fibrous sheath of peroneus longus. The transverse head takes origin from the plantar ligaments of the metatarsophalangeal joints of the lateral four toes. It is inserted with the lateral part of flexor hallucis brevis into the lateral side of the base of the proximal phalanx of big toe.
- The tendon of peroneus longus passes across the groove on the plantar surface of the cuboid bone to be inserted into the base of the first metatartasal bone and adjacent part of the medial cuneiform bone.
- The tibialis posterior is inserted by slips into all tarsal bones except the talus and to the bases of the second, third and fourth metatarsal bones. The main insertion is into the tuberosity of navicular bone.
- The plantar and dorsal interossei arise from the shafts of the metatarsal bones. Their tendons are partly inserted into the bases of the proximal phalanges and partly into the dorsal digital (extensor) expansions of the lateral four toes.
- The spring (plantar calcaneonavicular) ligament extends from the sustentaculum tali to the plantar surface of navicular bone.
- The deltoid ligament is attached to the following structures arranged anteroposteriorly: tuberosity of navicular bone, medial

border of spring ligament, neck of talus, sustentaculum tali and body of talus.
- The short plantar ligament (plantar calcaneocuboid ligament) extends from the anterior part of the plantar surface of the calcaneus to the plantar surface of the cuboid.
- The long plantar ligament is attached to the plantar surface of the calcaneus in front of the calcanean tuberosity. The deep fibers of the ligament are attached to the margins of the groove for peroneus longus, forming the fibrous sheath of the tendon. The superficial fibers of the ligament divide into slips which are attached to the bases of the second, third and fourth metatarsal bones.

Heel
- is formed by the lower subcutaneous part of the posterior surface of the calcaneus (fig. 193).
- The middle part of the posterior surface of calcaneus gives insertion into the tendo calcaneus and to the tendon of plantaris muscle close to the medial side of tendo calcaneus.
- The tendo calcaneus is separated from the upper smooth part of the posterior surface of the calcaneus by fat and a bursa.
- The medial border of the heel gives attachment to the lateral end of the flexor retinaculum.

Ossification of the Bones of the Foot

Ossification of the tarsus: Each tarsal bone ossifies in cartilage from a single centre (fig. 67). The only exception is the calcaneus which has an additional secondary centre for its posterior part.

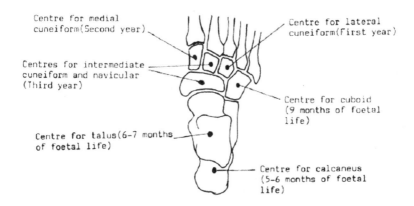

Centre for medial cuneiform(Second year)

Centres for intermediate cuneiform and navicular (Third year)

Centre for talus(6-7 months of foetal life)

Centre for lateral cuneiform(First year)

Centre for cuboid (9 months of foetal life)

Centre for calcaneus (5-6 months of foetal life)

Fig. 67: Ossification of the tarsus.

The tarsal bones begin to ossify in the following order:

Calcaneus: at 5-6 months of intrauterine life.
Talus: at 7-8 months of intrauterine life.
Cuboid: at 9 months of intrauterine life.
Lateral cuneiform: in the first year after birth.
Medial cuneiform: in the second year.
Intermediate cuneiform: in the third year.
Navicular: in the third year.

The secondary centre for calcaneus (calcanean epiphysis) appears at 6-8 years in females and 8-10 years in males. It is a scale-like epiphysis which fuses with the bone at 14 years in females and 15 years in males.

Ossification of the metatarsus: Each metatarsal bone ossifies in cartilage from one primary and one secondary centre. The *primary centre* appears in the middle of the shaft at 9-10 weeks of intrauterine life. The *secondary centre* appears in the base of the first metatarsal bone and in the heads of the other metatarsal bones at 3-4 years and fuses with the shaft at 17-20 years.

Ossification of the phalanges: Each phalanx ossifies in cartilage from one primary and one secondary centre. The *primary centre* appears in the middle of the shaft. In the distal phalanges it develops at 9-12 weeks of intrauterine life. In the proximal phalanges it develops at 11-15 weeks of intrauterine life. In the middle phalanges it develops after the fifteenth week of intrauterine life. The *secondary centre* appears in the base of each phalanx at 2-8 years and fuses with the shaft at 17-18 years.

Front of the Thigh

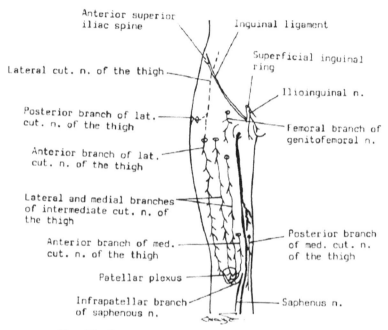

Fig. 68: Cutaneous nerves on the front of the thigh.

Cutaneous Nerves

Lateral cutaneous nerve of the thigh (L. 2, 3): branch of the lumbar It descends to the thigh by passing behind the lateral end of the inguinal ligament close to the anterior superior iliac spine (fig. 68). It divides into anterior and posterior branches which pierce the deep fascia. The anterior branch descends down to the front of the patella and shares in the patellar plexus. The posterior branch deviates backwards and supplies the skin of the anteroinferior part of the gluteal region.

Intermediate cutaneous nerve of the thigh (L. 2, 3): branch of femoral nerve. It divides into lateral and medial branches which pierce the deep fascia and descend on the front the thigh. Both branches terminate in the patellar plexus.

Medial cutaneous nerve of the thigh (L. 2, 3): branch of femoral nerve. It divides into anterior and posterior branches. The anterior branch pierces the deep fascia and reaches down to the patellar plexus. The posterior branch pierces the deep fascia lower down and descends to the upper part of the leg.

Femoral branch of genitofemoral nerve (L. 1, 2): descends through the lateral compartment of the femoral sheath with the femoral artery. It pierces the anterior wall of the femoral sheath and deep fascia to supply a small area of skin below the inguinal ligament overlying the femoral triangle.

Patellar plexus of nerves: is a plexus of cutaneous nerves in the superficial fascia covering the front of the patella and ligamentum patellae. It is formed by the anterior branches of the lateral and medial cutaneous nerves of the thigh, both branches of the intermediate cutaneous nerve of the thigh and infrapatellar branch of the saphenous nerve.

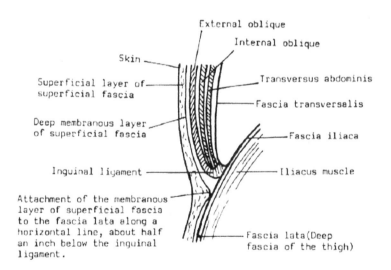

Fig. 69: Longitudinal section showing the arrangement of the two layers of superficial fascia in the lower part of anterior abdominal wall and upper part of the front of the thigh.

Superficial Fascia of the Thigh

The superficial fascia of the upper part of the front of the thigh, like that in the lower part of the anterior abdominal wall, is differentiated into a *superficial fatty layer* and a *deep membranous layer.* The deep membranous layer becomes adherent to the deep fascia of the thigh along a horizontal line half an inch below the inguinal ligament (figs. 69, 71).

Applied anatomy: Rupture of the male urethra may lead to extravasation of urine into the perineum and anterior abdominal wall. The urine passes through the interval between the membranous layer of superficial fascia and the aponeurosis of external oblique. Gravitation of urine into the thigh is arrested by the line of attachment of the membranous layer of superficial fascia to the deep fascia of the thigh just below the inguinal ligament.

Deep Fascia of the Thigh

This is called the *fascia lata.* It is very strong as compared with the deep fascia in other regions of the body, specially laterally where it is greatly thickened to form the *iliotibial tract* (described later).

Superiorly, the fascia lata is attached around the circumference of the thigh at its junction with the trunk. It is attached along a line to the inguinal ligament, iliac crest, back of the sacrum and coccyx, sacrotuberous ligament, ischial tuberosity and pubic arch.

Inferiorly, the fascia lata is attached to all bony prominences around the knee, i.e. to both condyles of femur, both condyles of tibia, patella and head of fibula. However, posteriorly it is continuous over the popliteal fossa where it forms the *popliteal fascia* which is continuous down with the deep fascia of the back of the leg.

Inguinal Ligament

This is the lower border of the aponeurosis of the external oblique muscle of the abdomen folded backwards upon itself, forming the boundary between the anterior abdominal wall and the front of the thigh.

The inguinal ligament is attached laterally to the anterior superior iliac spine and medially to the pubic tubercle (fig. 70). The ligament is curved with a downward convexity due to the attachment and downward pulling of the fascia lata upon the ligament.

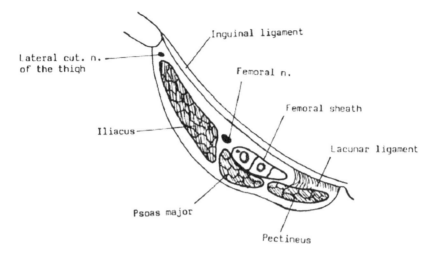

*Fig. 70: Cross section of the front of the thigh showing
the structures passing deep to the inguinal ligament.*

The medial part of the ligament spreads to form a triangular part which is called the ***lacunar ligament.*** The lacunar ligament is attached anteriorly to the inguinal ligament and posteriorly to the pectineal line. Its apex lies at the pubic tubercle. It has a free sharp crescentic base which forms the medial boundary of the femoral ring.

Fibers from the base of the lacunar ligament extend laterally along the pectineal line to form the *pectineal ligament..*

For more details of the inguinal ligament refer to the "Abdomen".

The structures passing deep to the inguinal ligament are arranged as follows:

1- Iliacus laterally and psoas major medially.

2- Femoral nerve in the groove between the psoas major and iliacus.

3- Femoral sheath with its three compartments and contents as described later.

4- Lateral cutaneous nerve of the thigh close to the anterior superior iliac spine.

5- Lymphatic vessels ascending from the deep inguinal to the external iliac lymph nodes.

Saphenous Opening

This is an oval opening in the deep fascia of the thigh one and half inches below and lateral to the pubic tubercle (fig. 71). This opening is one inch long and half an inch wide. When displayed, the opening has a margin called the *falciform margin* which is sharp superiorly, laterally and inferiorly. But medially, the margin is smooth where it is formed by the fascia covering the pectineus muscle.

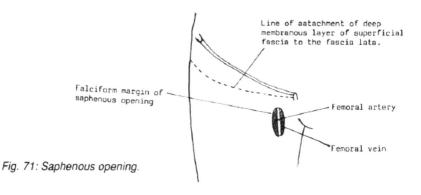

Fig. 71: Saphenous opening.

The saphenous opening is closed by a thin layer of deep fascia called the *cribriform fascia* as it is pierced by the great saphenous vein, superfical inguinal arteries and many lymphatics.

Surface anatomy: The centre of the saphenous opening is one and half inches (4 cm) below and lateral to the pubic tubercle.

Great Saphenous Vein

This is the longest vein in the body. It begins on the dorsum of the foot by the union of the dorsal venous arch with the medial dorsal digital vein of the big toe and passes posteriorly on the medial border of the dorsum of the foot (fig. 72).

The vein ascends to the leg in front of the medial malleolus. Then it crosses the lower third of the medial surface of the tibia obliquely and continues up on the medial side of the leg and knee. Along its course on the dorsum of the foot and leg, it is closely accompanied by the saphenous nerve.

As it ascends to the thigh, the great saphenous vein deviates forwards and laterally to reach the saphenous opening. Here, it hooks on the falciform margin of the saphenous openings, piercing the cribriform fascia, to terminate in the femoral vein.

The great saphenous vein receives several superficial veins in the leg and thigh in addition to a communicating vein from the the upper part of the small saphenous vein. In addition, it receives the three superficial inguinal veins which are the superficial epigastric, superficial external pudendal and superficail circumflex iliac veins.

The great saphenous vein contains numerous valves along its course, the most important valve lying close to its termination into the femoral vein.

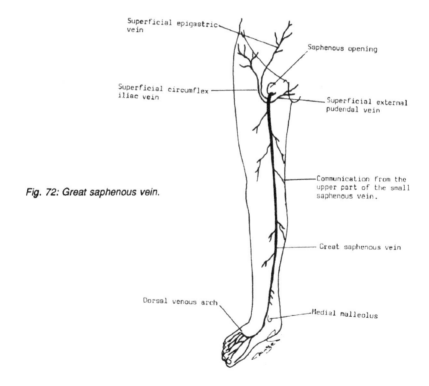

Fig. 72: Great saphenous vein.

Numerous *perforating veins* connect the great saphenous vein with the deep veins in the leg. The most important of these veins are:

A - Three perforating veins slightly above the medial malleolus, connecting the great saphenous vein with the deep veins in the posterior compartment of the leg.

B - A perforating vein at the level of the tibial tuberosity, connecting the great saphenous vein with the veins of the calf.

C - A perforating vein between the great saphenous vein and the popliteal vein at the level of the knee joint.

D - A perforating vein at the junction of the middle and lower thirds of the thigh connecting the great saphenous vein with the femoral vein in the middle of the adductor canal.

Perforating veins are also described in other sites on the dorsum of the foot, leg and thigh.

Applied anatomy: The perforating veins contain valves which allow passage of venous blood from the greater saphenous vein to the deep veins and not in the opposite direction. Affection of these valves resulting from thrombophlebitis leads to regurgitation of venous blood from the deep veins to the great saphenous vein. The resulting increase in venous pressure leads to what is known as *varicose veins of the lower limb* where the great saphenous vein and, sometimes in addition, the small saphenous vein become dilated, tortuous and engorged with venous blood.

However, varicose veins of the lower limbs may result from thrombophlebitis of the saphenous veins themselves or incomptence of their valves.

Thoracoepigastric vein: is a superficial vein in the anterolateral part of the trunk, connecting the superficial epigastric and lateral thoracic veins. This vein forms an important connection between the femoral and axillary veins, i.e. an important anastomosis between the inferior and superior venae cavae.

Superficial Inguinal Lymph Nodes

These are the main lymph nodes of the lower limb. They lie in the superficial fascia of the groin below the inguinal ligament and are arranged into two groups (fig. 73):

A - Upper (Horizontal) group: which are arranged horizontally below the inguinal ligament.

B- **Lower (Vertical) group:** which are arranged vertically around the upper part of the great saphenous vein.

The superficial inguinal lymph nodes receive afferent lymphatics from:

1- Greater part of the lower limb.

2- Superficial parts of the gluteal region.

3- Superficial part of the anterior abdominal wall below the level of the umbilicus.

4- Superficial structures in the perineum including the external genital organs and the lower part of the anal canal.

Effeerent lymphatics from the superficial inguinal lymph nodes pierce the cribriform fascia and surrounding deep fascia to drain into the deep inguinal lymph nodes.

Superficial Inguinal Arteries

These are three branches of the femoral artery just below the inguina ligament. They pierce the anterior wall of the femoral sheath and the cribriform fascia to reach the superficial fascia of the groin where they radiate into different directions (fig. 73). These arteries are:

1- *Superficial epigastric artery:* which ascends upwards and medially in the superficial fascia of the lower part of the anterior abdominal wall towards the umbilicus.

2- *Superficial external pudendal artery:* which passes medially across the front of the spermatic cord or round ligament of the uterus to supply the external genitalia.

3- *Superficial circumflex iliac artery:* which runs upwards and laterally along the lower border of the inguinal ligament and outer lip of the iliac crest.

As previously described, the three superficial inguinal veins terminate into the upper part of the great saphenous vein.

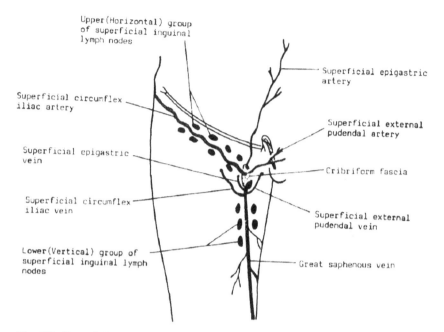

Fig. 73: Superficial inguinal vessels and superficial inguinal lymph nodes.

Compartments of the Thigh

The thight is divided into three compartments by three fascial intermuscular septa which connect the fascia lata with the linea aspera of the femur (fig. 74). These are called the *medial, posterior and lateral intermuscular septa.*

The compartments of the thigh are:

A - *Anterior compartment:* which contains the quadriceps femoris and femoral nerve.

B - *Medial compartment:* which contains the adductor muscles and obturator nerve.

C - *Posterior compartment:* which contains the hamstring muscles and sciatic nerve.

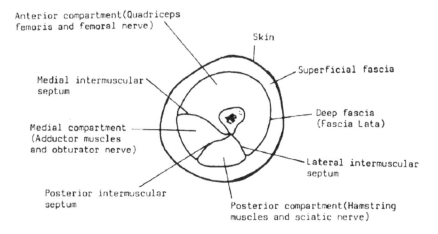

Fig. 74: Compartments of the thigh - Cross section.

Femoral Triangle

This is a triangular space on the front of the upper third of the thigh just below the inguinal ligament.

Boundaries: inguinal ligament forming the base of the triangle, medial border of satorius laterally and medial border of adductor longus medially (fig. 75).

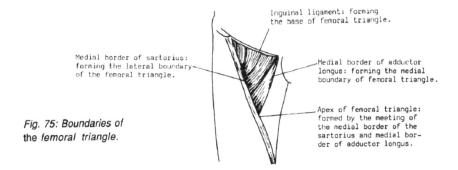

Fig. 75: Boundaries of the femoral triangle.

Roof: Skin, superficial fascia and deep fascia. The superficial fascia of the roof contains portions of the intermediate and medial cutaneous nerves of the thigh, femoral branch of genitofemoral nerve, upper part of great saphenous vein, superficial inguinal vessels and superficial inguinal lymph nodes.

Floor: is formed by four musles; arranged from the medial to the lateral side, they are: adductor longus, pectineus, psoas major and iliacus (fig. 76).

Contents: Femoral sheath, femoral artery and its branches, femoral vein and its tributaries, femoral nerve and its branches and deep inguinal lymph nodes (fig. 77).

Surface anatomy: The femoral triangle corresponds to an inverted triangle with its base formed by the inguinal groove on the front of the upper third of the thigh.

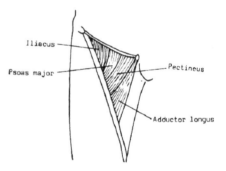

Fig. 76: Floor of the femoral triangle.

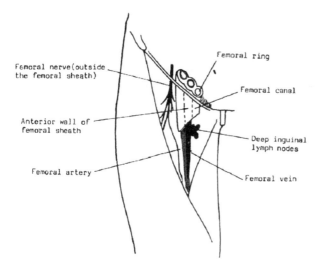

Femoral nerve(outside the femoral sheath)

Femoral ring

Femoral canal

Anterior wall of femoral sheath

Deep inguinal lymph nodes

Femoral artery

Femoral vein

Fig. 77: Contents of the femoral triangle.

Femoral Sheath

This is a funnel-shaped fascial sheath which extends down from the abdominal walls to surround the upper one and half inches of the femoral vessels (fig. 78).

The sheath has anterior and posterior walls. The ***anterior wall*** is a downward continuation of the fascia transversalis of the anterior abdominal wall while the ***posterior wall*** is a downward continuation of the fascia iliaca of the posterior abdominal wall (fig. 79).

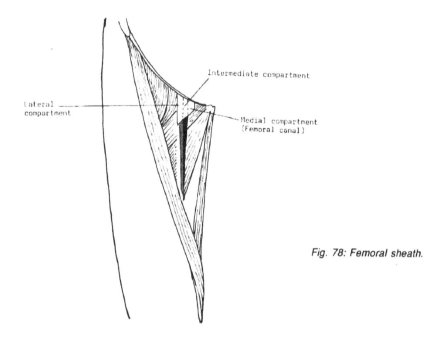

Fig. 78: Femoral sheath.

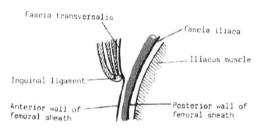

Fig. 79: Longitudinal section in the lateral compartment of the femoral sheath.

As previously described, the sheath is about one and half inches long, but its medial part is much shorter, being only half an inch long.

The sheath is divided by two anteroposterior septa into three compartments (fig. 80):

A - *Lateral compartment:* transmits the femoral artery and the femoral branch of genitofemoral nerve.

B - *Intermediate compartment:* transmits the femoral vein.

C - *Medial compartment:* is known as the *femoral canal.* It is the shortest compartment, being half an inch long and is relatively empty as it contains loose areolar fatty tissue and a small lymph node, and transmits some lymph vessels.

The femoral canal is closed inferiorly by fusion of its walls, but superiorly the canal has an abdominal opening called the *femoral ring*. The femoral ring is half an inch wide and is closed by a condensation of extraperitoneal fat called the *femoral septum*.

The femoral ring has the following boundaries:

1- *Anteriorly:* inguinal ligament.

2- *Posteriorly:* pectineal line and pectineal ligament.

3- *Laterally:* femoral vein.

4- *Medially:* the sharp cresentic base of the lacunar ligament.

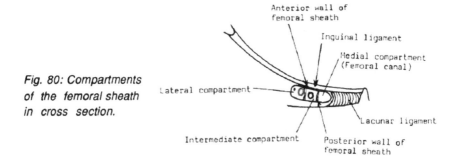

Fig. 80: Compartments of the femoral sheath in cross section.

Being relatively empty, the femoral canal accomodates the distension of the femoral vein occuring due to increased venous return from the lower limb during muscular exercise.

Surface anatomy: The femoral ring lies behind the inguinal groove, 3/4 of an inch or 2 cm medial to the midinguinal point.

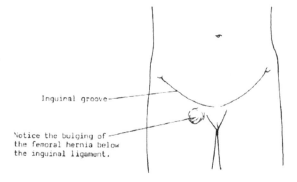

Fig. 81: Femoral hernia.

Inguinal groove

Notice the bulging of
the femoral hernia below
the inguinal ligament.

Applied anatomy: The femoral canal is surgically important as its abdominal opening (femoral ring) forms a weak part in the abdominal wall. Under an increase in the intra-abdominal pressure, the parietal peritoneum may protrodue into the femoral canal leading to a *femoral hernia*. Because the femoral ring is wider in females, femoral hernias are much more common in females than in males.

The herinal sac is formed by the parietal peritoneum and the contents of the hernia are usually the small intestine and or greater omentum.

Line of descent: The hernia first descends vertically through the femoral canal and then bulges forwards through the saphenous opening (fig. 81). If the hernia enlarges more, the hernial sac curves upwards and laterally as a result of pressure of the falciform margin of the saphenous opening on the sac.

Line of reduction: The hernia is reduced in an opposite direction to the line of descent. The thigh is flexed and medially rotated to relax the ligaments and fasciae in the groin. The hernia is first pushed downwards and backwards through the saphenous opening and finally upwards through the femoral canal.

Coverings: The coverings of femoral hernia from inside outwards are (fig. 82):
1- Stretched femoral septum.
2- Anterior wall of femoral sheath.
3- Cribriform fascia.
4- Two layers of superficial fascia. 5- Skin.

The differences between femoral and inguinal hernia are given in the "Abdomen".

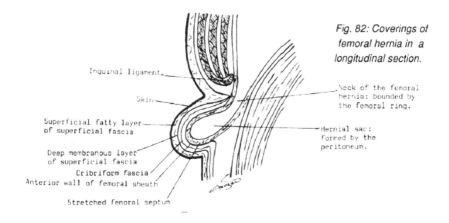

Inguinal ligament

Skin

Superficial fatty layer of superficial fascia

Deep membranous layer of superficial fascia

Cribriform fascia

Anterior wall of femoral sheath

Stretched femoral septum

Fig. 82: Coverings of femoral hernia in a longitudinal section.

Neck of the femoral hernia: bounded by the femoral ring.

Hernial sac: formed by the peritoneum.

Femoral Artery

Origin: continuation of the external iliac artery at the midinguinal point (fig. 83):

Termination: At the lower end of the adductor canal, the artery passes through the adductor opening (opening in the adductor magnus) to continue as the popliteal artery.

Relations in the femoral triangle

Anteriorly: Skin, superficial fascia with its contents as previously described and deep fascia (fascia lata) The upper part of the artery is covered by the anterior wall of the femoral sheath.

Posteriorly: The artery descends on the following muscles in order: psoas major, pectineus and adductor longus. The posterior wall of the femoral sheath lies behind the upper part of the artery. The nerve to pectineus passes medially behind the femoral sheath and femoral vessels to reach the pectineus. The psoas major separates the femoral artery from the hip joint and head of the femur. The profunda vessels descend behind the femoral artery, separating it from the pectineus. The femoral vein is posterior to the artery at the apex of the femoral triangle.

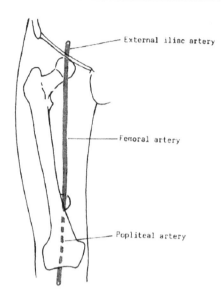

Fig. 83: Femoral artery.

Laterally: The artery is related to the femoral nerve and its branches in the upper part of the femoral triangle.

Branches
A - *Superficial inguinal arteries*
    1- Superficial epigastric artery.
    2- Superficial external pudendal artery.
    3- Superficial circumflex iliac artery.

    These three arteries were described on page 65 (figs. 73, 84).

B - *Deep external pudendal artery:* which arises from the medial side of the femoral artery one and half inches below the inguinal ligament. It passes medially deep to the spermatic cord or round ligament of the uterus to supply the external genitalia.

C - *Profunda femoris artery:* is the largest branch of femoral artery and is the main source of blood supply to the thigh. It is described later (See page 74).

D - *Descending genicular artery:* arises from the femoral artery in the adductor canal just above the adductor opening. Then, it desends through the vastus medialis in front of the tendon of adductor magnus to end by anastomosing with the superior medial genicular artery. It gives a saphenous branch which accompanies the saphenous nerve and muscular branches to the vastus medialis and adductor magnus.

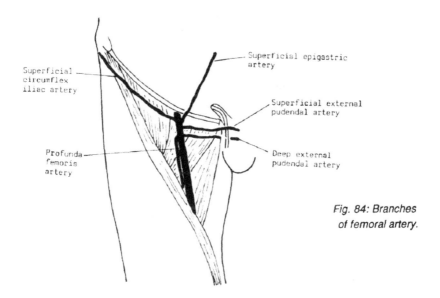

Fig. 84: Branches of femoral artery.

Surface anatomy: The thigh is slightly flexed, abducted and rotated laterally (fig. 85). The femoral artery corresponds to the upper two-thirds of a line between the midinguinal point and the adductor tubercle. The upper third of the line corresponds to the femoral artery in the femoral triangle while the middle third corresponds to the femoral artery in the adductor canal.

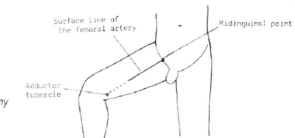

Fig. 85: Surface anatomy of the femoral artery.

Applied anatomy: To control arterial haemorrhage from the lower limb as a preliminary first aid, digital pressure can be effectively done on the uppermost part of the femoral artery against the superior pubic ramus and head of the femur. Here, the artery is only separated from the bone by the psoas major.

A torniquet can be applied at the middle of the thigh where the femoral artery can be effectively compressed against the shaft of the femur.

Profunda Femoris Artery

Origin: from the posterolateral aspect of the femoral artery one and half inches below the inguinal ligament (fig. 84).

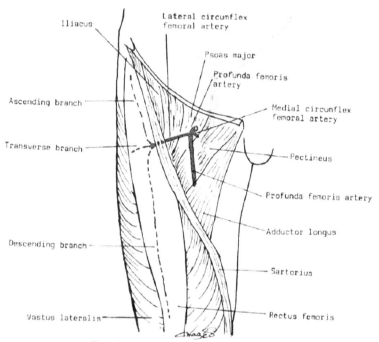

Fig. 86: Profunda femoris artery.

Course and relations: As the artery descends, it curves medially to descend behind the femoral vessels and in front of the pectineus muscle. Then it leaves the femoral triangle by passing between the pectineus and adductor longus (fig. 86).

The profunda femoris artery continues down behind the adductor longus which separates the profunda vessels from the femoral vessels. In this part of its course, the profunda artery lies in front of the adductors brevis and magnus.

In the lower part of its course, the profunda artey gives three perforating arteries and terminates as the fourth perforating artey.

Along its course, the profunda vein is closely anterior to the profunda artery. At the apex of the femoral triangle, a cross section shows that the structures are arranged as follows anteroposteriorly (fig. 87): femoral artery, femoral vein, adductor longus, profunda femoris vein and profunda femoris artery *(Artery - Vein - Muscle - Vein - Artery)*.

Branches

1- *Lateral circumflex femoral artery:* a large branch which arises from the profunda artery close to its origin and passes laterally through the branches of the femoral nerve and then deep to the satorius and rectus femoris where it divides into three branches:

   a- *Ascending branch:* which ascends along the intertrochanteric line deep to the tensor fasciae latae. It gives branches to the neck of the femur, hip joint and greater trochanter. It anastomoses with branches of the superior gluteal and deep circumflex iliac arteries.

   b- *Transverse branch:* which runs horizontally round the thigh through the vastus lateralis to reach the back of the thigh where it shares in the cruciate anastomosis.

   c- *Descending branch:* which descends deep to the rectus femoris along the anterior border of the vastus lateralis with the nerve to vastus lateralis. It supplies the adjacent muscles and its terminal part shares in the anastomoses around the knee joint.

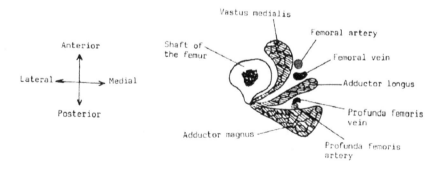

Fig. 87: Cross section showing the arrangement of the structures at the apex of the femoral triangle.

2- ***Medial circumflex femoral artery:*** arises from the profunda artery close to its origin. Immediately it passes backwards between the psoas major and pectineus and then between the obturator externus and adductor brevis (fig. 114). Then, it emerges on the back of the thigh between the quadratus femoris and upper border adductor magnus where it divides it into ascending and transverse branches. It gives the following branches:

  a- *Acetabular branch:* which passes through the acetabular foramen and then along the ligament of the head of the femur to supply the head of the femur and hip joint.

  b- *Acending branch:* which ascends along the obturator externus to the trochanteric fossa where it anastomoses with branches of the superior and inferior gluteal and lateral circumflex femoral arteries (trochanteric anastomoses).

  c- *Transverse branch:* which runs along the upper border of the adductor magnus and shares in the cruciate anastomosis.

3- ***Perforating arteries:*** four branches arranged first to fourth from above downwards; the profunda artery itself ending as the fourth perforating artery. They arise from the lower part of the profunda artery between the adductors longus and magnus; and are so called because they pass laterally across the linea aspea through the insertion of adductor magnus. They are protected by tendinous arches in the insertion of the adductor magnus as they cross the linea aspera to terminate through the vastus lateralis.

The perforating arteries share in a series of ansastomoses in the back of the thigh (fig. 138). They anastomose together; the first one shares in the cruciate anastomosis while the fourth one anastomoses with the muscular branches of the popliteal artery.

The second perforating artery usually gives a nutrient artery to the femur which passes through the bone close to the linea aspera.

From the above describtion, it is clear that the profunda femoris artery is the main source of blood supply to the thigh.

Applied anatomy

A - If the external iliac artery is ligated or obstructed just distal to the origin of its branches, i.e. close to the inguinal ligament, a collateral circulation caries arterial blood to the lower limb through:

1- Anastomosis between the pubic branches of inferior epigastric and obturator arteries.

2- Anastomosis between the deep circumflex iliac artery and both superficial circumflex iliac and lateral circumflex femoral arteries.

B - If the femoral artery is ligated or obstructed above the origin of the profunda femoris artery, a collateral circulation carries arterial blood to the lower limb through:

1- Cruciate anastomosis (described later).

2- Anastomoses between the obturator and medial circumflex femoral arteries.

3- Anastomosis between the internal and external pudendal arteries.

4- Anastomoses between the superficial and deep circumflex iliac arteries.

Profunda Femoris Vein

This vein runs close to the front of the profunda femoris artery. It is formed in the lower part of the thigh by union of the perforating veins and ascends to the femoral triangle where it joins the upper part of the femoral vein.

The lateral and medial circumflex femoral veins usually end directly into the upper part of the femoral vein.

Femoral Vein

Origin: Continuation of the popliteal vein at the adductor opening.

Course: It ascends through the adductor canal and then through the femoral triangle from its apex to its base (fig. 88). Along its course, the femoral vein contains many valves. One of these valves lies just above its junction with the great saphenous vein and another one close to its upper end.

Termination: It ascends behind the inguinal ligament to continue as the external iliac vein.

Relations: As it ascends, the femoral vein gradually changes its position in relation to the femoral artery. At its origin in the lower part of adductor canal, the femoral vein is posterolateral to the femoral artery. But, in the upper part of the canal and at the apex of femoral triangle, the vein becomes posterior to the artery. At the base of the femoral triangle, the vein becomes medial to the artery. The uppermost part of the vein lies in the intermediate compartment of the femoral sheath.

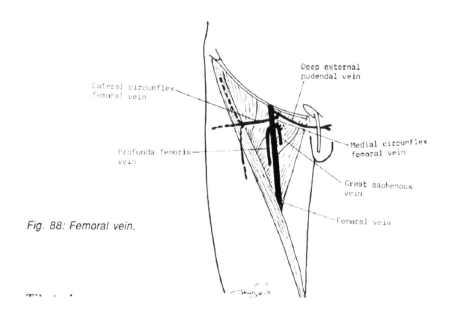

Fig. 88: Femoral vein.

Tibutaries
1- Muscular veins.
2- Descending genicular vein.
3- Profunda femoris vein.
4- Deep external pudendal vein.
5- Lateral circumflex femoral vein. 6- Medial circumflex femoral vein. 7- Great saphenous vein.

Deep Inguinal Lymph Nodes

These are few but large lymph nodes close to the upper part of the femoral vein (fig. 77). They receive afferent lymphatics from the superficial inguinal lymph nodes and the deep lymphatics of the lower limb which are relatively few and run along the main deep blood vessels of the lower limb. In addition, they receive lymphatics from the popliteal lymph nodes and some of the deep lymphatics of the perineum. Their efferent lymphatics ascend behind the inguinal ligament to end in the external iliac lymph nodes.

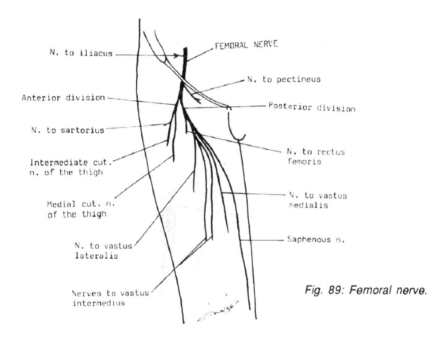

Fig. 89: Femoral nerve.

Femoral Nerve

Origin: The femoral nerve (L. 2, 3, 4) is a branch of the lumbar plexus. It takes origin from the *dorsal divisions* of the *ventral rami* of the second, third and fourth lumbar nerves.

Course and relations in the thigh: The nerve reaches the thigh by passing behind the midpoint of the inguinal ligament. One inch below the inguinal ligament, it ends by two *divisions* which break into a number of branches (fig. 89).

In the thigh the femoral nerve lies in the groove between the psoas major and iliacus, lateral to the femoral artery and *outside* the femoral sheath.

Branches

1- ***Nerve to iliacus:*** which arises from the femoral nerve in the abdomen, above the inguinal ligament and supplies the iliacus in the abdomen.

2- ***Nerve to pectineus:*** which arises from the femoral nerve just below the inguinal ligament and passes medially behind the femoral sheath and femoral vessels to supply the pectineus.

3- ***Anterior division:*** gives the following branches:

    1- *Intermediate cutaneous nerve of the thigh:* described on page 60.
    2- *Medial cutaneous nerve of the thigh:* described on page 60.
    3- *Muscular branch:* to the sartorius.

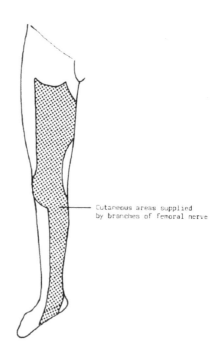

Fig. 90: Cutaneous areas supplied by the femoral nerve.

Cutaneous areas supplied by branches of femoral nerve

4- ***Posterior division:***

a- *Muscular branches* to the quadriceps femoris which are arranged as follows:

- A branch to the rectus femoris. This branch sends an articular filament to the hip joint.
- A branch to the vastus lateralis which descends along the anterior border of the muscle with the descending branch of the lateral circumflex femoral artery. This branch sends an articular filament to the knee joint.
- A branch to the vastus medialis which descends to the adductor canal to enter the muscle about the middle of the adductor canal. It also gives an articular filament to the knee joint.
- Two or three branches which supply the vastus intermedius. From these branches a muscular filament supplies the articularis genu muscle and an articular filament descends to the knee joint.
b- *Saphenous nerve:* is the longest cutaneous nerve in the body. It descends lateral to the femoral artery in the femoral triangle to reach the adductor canal where it crosses in front of the femoral artery from its lateral to medial side.

In the adductor canal, it gives a branch to the subsartorial plexus (described later). At the lower end of the canal, it pierces the fibrous roof of the canal and emerges behind the sartorius where it pierces the deep fascia to become subcutaneous on the medial side of the knee.

The nerve then descends on the medial side of the leg with the great saphenous vein along the medial border of the tibia. In the lower third of the leg, it crosses the medial surface of the tibia obliquely and descnds in front of the medial malleolus to the dorsum of the foot.

On the dorsum of the foot, it runs close to its medial border and ends opposite the metatarsophalangeal joint of the big toe, i.e. short of the big toe. The saphenous nerve gives an *infrapatellar branch* which shares in the patellar plexus (See page 61). It gives cutaneous branches along its course in the leg and dorsum of the foot which supply the skin of the medial side of the leg and medial part of the dorsum of the foot (fig. 90).

N.B.: The femoral nerve gives vascular branches to the femoral artery and its branches. These are postgangionic sympathetic fibers from the lumbar ganglia of the sympathetic trunk which join the lumbar plexus. These fibers are vasoconstrictor to the femoral artery and its branches.

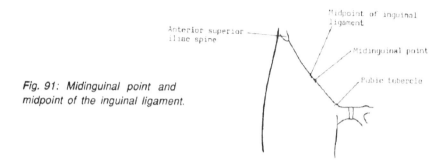

*Fig. 91: Midinguinal point and
midpoint of the inguinal ligament.*

Subsartorial plexus of nerves: is a plexus of fine nerves deep to the sartorius and overlying the fibrous roof of the adductor canal. It is formed by branches from the saphenous nerve in the adductor canal, posterior branch of medial cutaneous nerve of the thigh and a cutaneous branch from the anterior branch of obturator nerve. This plexus supplies the skin on the medial side of the middle third of the thigh.

Surface anatomy: The femoral nerve reaches the thigh by passing behind the midpoint of the inguinal ligament and corresponds to a line which descends for one inch from the point.

Applied anatomy: Injury of the femoral nerve may result from wounds in the groin. This leas to:

1- Paralysis of the quadriceps femoris which leads to the loss of extension of the knee.

2- Diminished cutaneous sensations on the front and medial aspects of the thigh which are the areas supplied by the intermediate and medial cutaneous nerves of the thigh (fig. 90).

3- Diminished cutaneous sensations on the medial side of the leg and medial part of the dorsum of the foot which are the areas supplied by the saphenous nerve.

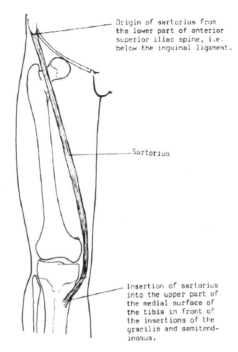

Origin of sartorius from
the lower part of anterior
superior iliac spine, i.e.
below the inguinal ligament.

Sartorius

Fig. 92: Sartorius muscle.

Insertion of sartorius
into the upper part of
the medial surface of
the tibia in front of
the insertions of the
gracilis and semitend-
inosus.

Important Surface Markings on the Front of the Thigh

Inguinal groove: is the furrow at the junction of the anterior abdominal wall with the front of the thigh. This groove corresponds to the inguinal ligament.

Midinguinal point: is a point on the inguinal groove or ligament midway between the anterior superior iliac spine and the pubic *symphysis* (fig. 91). Accordingly, this point is not the midpoint of the inguinal ligament.

Midpoint of inguinal ligament: is a point on the inguinal groove or ligament midway between the anterior superior iliac spine and pubic *tubercle*. This means that this point corresponds to the middle of the inguinal ligament.

Anterior superior iliac spine: is the bony prominence felt at the lateral end of the inguinal groove.

Pubic tubercle: Abduct the thigh. The tendon of origin of adductor longus is seen and felt as a cord-like ridge on the uppermost part of the medial side of the thigh. Follow the tendon up to its origin. The small bony projection felt just above the origin of adductor longus is the pubic tubercle.

Sartorius

Origin: from the lower part of the anterior superior iliac spine, i.e. below the inguinal ligament (fig. 92).

Insertion: into the upper part of the medial surface of the tibia (fig. 93).

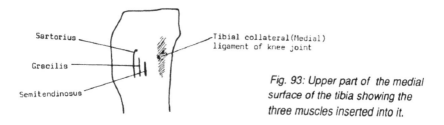

Fig. 93: Upper part of the medial surface of the tibia showing the three muscles inserted into it.

Nerve supply: femoral nerve.

Actions: flexion and abduction of the thigh. It also helps in flexion of the knee joint.

Relations: In the upper third of the thigh, it forms the lateral boundary of the femoral triangle. In the middle third, it covers the roof of the adductor canal. In the lower third, it shares in the upper medial boundary of the popliteal fossa.

Pectineus

Origin: from the pectineal surface of the superior pubic ramus (fig. 94).

Insertion: into the back of the femur along the upper part of a line between the lesser trochanter and linea aspera.

Nerve supply: femoral nerve.

Actions: adduction of the thigh. It helps in flexion of the hip joint. It also steadies the head of the femur during movements of the hip joint.

Relations: Anteriorly, it forms a part of the floor of femoral triangle and is related to the femoral sheath and femoral vessels. Posteriorly, it is related to the anterior branch of obturator nerve and adductor brevis. The medial circumflex femoral vessels leave the femoral triangle by passing through the interval between the psoas major and pectineus. The profunda femoris vessels leave the femoral triangle by passing through the interval between the pectineus and adductor longus.

Iliopsoas

This term refers to the fused lower parts of the psoas major and iliacus muscles as they reach the front of the thigh.

The *psoas major* arises mainly from the lumbar vertebrae and descends to the thigh by passing behind the inguinal ligament (fig. 95). In the thigh, it lies close to the front of the capsule of hip joint with a bursa called the *psoas (iliac) bursa* intervening. It is inserted by a strong tendon into the lesser trochanter.

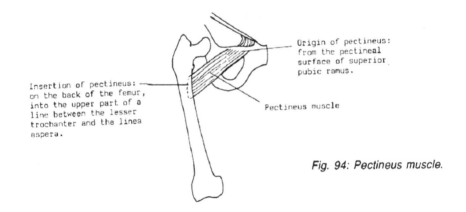

Origin of pectineus: from the pectineal surface of superior pubic ramus.

Insertion of pectineus: on the back of the femur, into the upper part of a line between the lesser trochanter and the linea aspera.

Pectineus muscle

Fig. 94: Pectineus muscle.

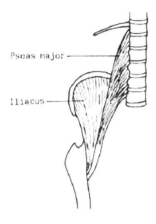

Fig. 95: Iliopsoas muscles.

The *iliacus* takes origin from the iliac fossa and descends behind the inguinal ligament lateral to the psoas major. The fibers of the iliacus converge into a tendon which mostly joins that of the psoas major into the lesser trochanter. But, some fibers of the iliacus are inserted directly into the back of the femur for one inch below the lesser trochanter.

The psoas major and iliacus are the main flexors of the hip joint. For more details refer to the "Abdomen".

Applied anatomy: The iliopsoas have no role in lateral or medial rotation of the thigh. But, in cases of fractures of the upper part of the shaft of the femur, the upper bony fragment is flexed and rotated laterally by the iliopsoas (fig. 96).

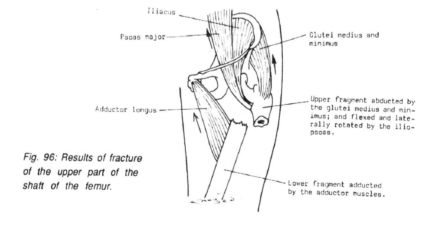

Fig. 96: Results of fracture of the upper part of the shaft of the femur.

Quadriceps Femoris

This is a large muscle on the front of the thigh which is formed of four heads that have a common insertion into the patella (figs. 97, 98).

The four heads of the quadriceps are:

1- **Rectus femoris:** is a fusiform muscle which arises by two tendinous heads from the hip bone: a straight head from the upper part of the anterior inferior iliac spine and a reflected head from an impression just above the acetabulum.

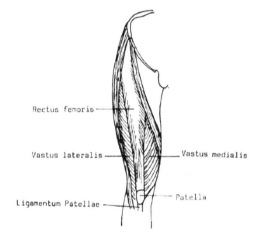

Fig. 97: Quadriceps femoris.

Rectus femoris

Vastus lateralis

Vastus medialis

Ligamentum Patellae

Patella

2- **Vastus lateralis:** arises by a linear origin from the upper part of the intertrochanteric line, root of the greater trochanter, lateral margin of the gluteal tuberosity and lateral lip of the linea aspera (fig. 99). Some fibers take origin from the lateral intermuscular septum of deep fascia.

3- **Vastus medialis:** also arises by a linear origin from the lower part of the intertrochanteric line, spiral line and medial lip of the linea aspera. Some of its lower fibers take origin from the tendon of the ischial part of adductor magnus.

4- **Vastus intermedius:** arises by a wide origin from the anterior and lateral surfaces of the upper three-fourths of the shaft of the femur.

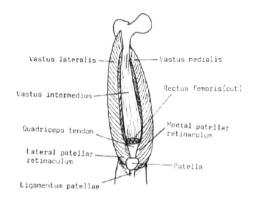

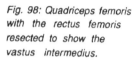

Fig. 98: Quadriceps femoris
with the rectus femoris
resected to show the
vastus intermedius.

Insertion: The four heads fuse into a common tendon called the *quadriceps tendon* which is inserted into the base, lateral and medial borders of the patella. The vastus lateralis gives a tendinous expansion called the *lateral patellar retinaculum* along the lateral side of the patella to be attched to the front of the upper end of the tibia. The vastus medialis gives a similar tendinous expansion called the *medial patellar retinaculum* along the medial side of the patella to be attached to the front of the upper end of the tibia.

Through the ligamentum patellae, the insertion of the quadriceps is carried into the tibial tuberosity.

The quadriceps tendon, patella, patellar retinacula and ligamentum patellae replace the capsule of knee joint anteriorly.

Nerve supply: The four heads of the quadriceps are supplied by the femoral nerve. For details refer to page 79.

Actions: The quadriceps is the extensor of the knee joint. The rectus femoris also helps in flexion of the hip joint.

Ligamentum patellae: is a thick and strong ligament which carries the insertion of the quadriceps femoris into the tibial tuberosity. Superiorly, it is attached to the apex and the lower nonarticular part of the posterior surface of the patella. Inferiorly, it is attached to the smooth upper part of the tibial tuberosity.

The superficial fibers of the quadriceps tendon descend close to the front of the patella to continue directly into the ligamentum patellae down to the tibial tuberosity, the patella thus acting as a sesamoid bone in the insertion of quadriceps.

Suprapatellar bursa: is a bursa which lies between the quadriceps tendon and the front of the lower part of the shaft of the femur. This bursa is an upward continuation of the synovial membrane of the knee joint. When the knee is extended, this bursa extends for about three fingers breadth above the patella.

Subcutaneous prepatellar bursa: is a bursa between the skin and the lower part of the patella and upper part of the ligamentum patellae.

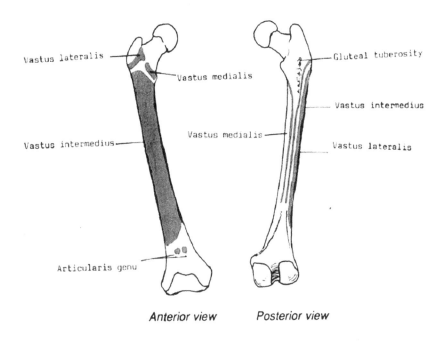

Anterior view   Posterior view

Fig. 99: Origins of vasti muscles from the right femur.

Applied anatomy: Inflamatation and enlargement of the subcutaneous prepatellar bursa may result from traumatic pressure on the bursa. This condition usually affects persons who kneel over the knees during work. That is why this condition is known as *"Housemaid's knee"*.

Articularis genu: is formed of small muscle bundles which arise from the front of the lower part of the shaft of the femur below the level of and under cover of the vastus intermedius (fig. 99). Its fibers are inserted into the upper extension of the synovial membrane of the knee joint deep to the quadriceps tendon (suprapatellar bursa).

It receives twigs from the nerves supplying the vastus intermedius. Its fibers pull up the synovial membrane of the suprapatellar bursa during extension of the knee joint to prevent it from damage between the patella and trochlear (patellar) surface of the femur.

Adductor Canal

The adductor (Subsartorial or Hunter's) canal is a fascial-lined intermuscular tunnel in the anteromedial part of the middle third of the thigh. Its upper end lies at the apex of the femoral triangle while its lower end is formed by the adductor opening (opening in the adductor magnus).

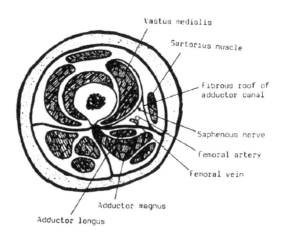

Fig. 100: Boundaries of the adductor canal in cross section of the middle of the thigh.

Boundaries: The canal is triangular in cross section and has three boundaries (fig. 100):

1- **Anterolateral wall:** is formed by the vastus medialis and its covering deep fascia.

2- **Posterior wall (floor):** is formed by the adductor longus above and adductor magnus below together with their covering deep fascia.

3- *Anteromedial wall (roof):* is formed by a thicknening of deep fascia forming the fibrous roof of the canal. This roof stretches from the fascia covering the vastus medialis to the fascia covering the adductors longus and magnus, and is covered by the sartorius muscle.

Contents

1- *Femoral artery:* reaches the canal by passing through its upper end (fig. 101). It leaves the canal at its lower end by passing through the adductor opening where it continues as the popliteal artery.

2- *Femoral vein:* reaches the canal through its lower end by passing through the adductor opening as a continuation of the popliteal vein. It leaves the canal through its upper end where it ascends into the femoral triangle.

As previously described, the femoral vein is posterolateral to the artery in the lower part of the adductor canal and gradually becomes posterior to the artery in the upper part of the canal.

3- *Saphenous nerve:* enters the canal through its upper end and crosses in front of the femoral artery from its lateral to medial side. It leaves the canal at its lower end by piercing the fibrous roof of the canal.

4- *Nerve to vastus medialis:* enters the canal through its upper end. In the middle of the canal, it enters into the substance of the vastus medialis.

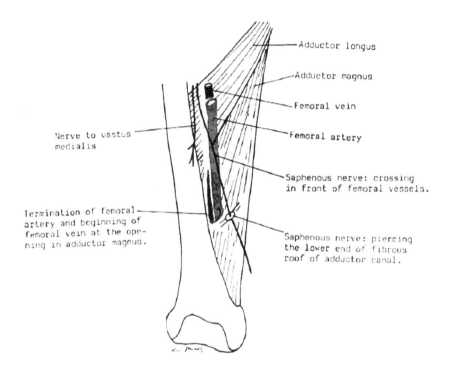

Adductor longus

Adductor magnus

Femoral vein

Femoral artery

Saphenous nerve: crossing
in front of femoral vessels.

Saphenous nerve: piercing
the lower end of fibrous
roof of adductor canal.

Nerve to vastus
medialis

Termination of femoral
artery and beginning of
femoral vein at the ope-
ning in adductor magnus.

Fig. 101: Content of the adductor canal after
removal of the fibrous roof of the canal.

MEDIAL SIDE OF THE THIGH

Cutaneous Nerves

Ilioinguinal nerve (L.1): branch of the lumbar plexus. It reaches the thigh by passing through the superficial inguinal ring with the spermatic cord or round ligament of the uterus. It gives branches to the scrotum in male or labium majus in female and skin of the upper part of the medial side of the thigh (fig. 68).

Cutaneous branch of obturator nerve (L. 2, 3, 4): branch of the anterior branch of obturator nerve. It shares in the subsartorial plexus of nerves and supplies the skin of the middle third of the medial side of the thigh, i.e. the region overlying the adductor canal (See page 80).

Posterior branch of the medial cutaneous nerve of the thigh (L. 2, 3): supplies the area of skin on the lower part of the medial side of the thigh, extending down to the upper part of the medial side of the leg.

Adductor Muscles

The adductor muscles are three: adductor longus, brevis and mangus. They are arranged into three strata. The adductor longus forms an anterior stratum; the adductor brevis forms a middle stratum while the adductor magnus forms a posterior stratum.

The gracilis muscle runs a relatively superficial course on the medial side of the three adductors just beneath the deep fascia of the thigh.

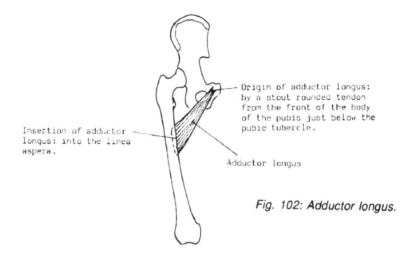

Origin of adductor longus:
by a stout rounded tendon
from the front of the body
of the pubis just below the
pubic tubercle.

Insertion of adductor
longus: into the linea
aspera.

Adductor longus

Fig. 102: Adductor longus.

Adductor Longus

Origin: by a stout rounded tendon from the front of the body of the pubis just below the pubic tubercle (fig. 102, 104).

Insertion: into the linea aspera (fig. 105).

Nerve supply: anterior branch of obturator nerve.

Actions: adduction of the thigh. It helps in flexion and lateral rotation of the thigh.

Relations: It forms parts of the floor of the femoral triangle and adductor canal. The femoral vessels descend anterior to the muscle while the profunda femoris vessels descend posterior to the muscle (fig. 100).

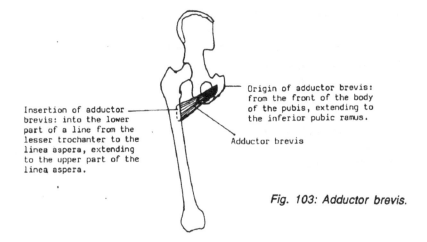

Insertion of adductor
brevis: into the lower
part of a line from the
lesser trochanter to the
linea aspera, extending
to the upper part of the
linea aspera.

Origin of adductor brevis:
from the front of the body
of the pubis, extending to
the inferior pubic ramus.

Adductor brevis

Fig. 103: Adductor brevis.

Adductor Brevis

Origin: from the body of the pubis and inferior pubic ramus (figs. 103, 104).

Insertion: into the back of the femur along the lower part of a line between the lesser trochanter and linea aspera, extending to the upper part of the linea aspera (fig. 105).

Nerve supply: anterior branch of obturator nerve.
Actions: adduction of the thigh. It helps in flexion and lateral rotation of the thigh.

Relations: Anteriorly, it is covered by the pectineus and adductor longus with the anterior branch of obturator nerve intervening. Posteriorly, it is related to the adductor magnus with the posterior branch of obturator nerve intervening.

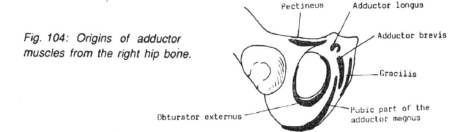

Fig. 104: Origins of adductor muscles from the right hip bone.

Pectineus

Adductor longus

Adductor brevis

Gracilis

Obturator externus

Pubic part of the adductor magnus

Adductor Magnus

It is a composite muscle which is formed of a *pubic part* belonging to the adductor muscles and an *ischial part* belonging to the hamstring muscles (figs. 106, 107).

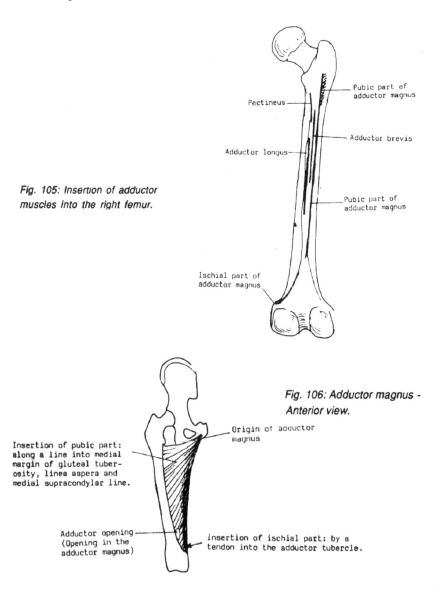

Pectineus

Adductor longus

Pubic part of adductor magnus

Adductor brevis

Pubic part of adductor magnus

Ischial part of adductor magnus

Fig. 105: Insertion of adductor muscles into the right femur.

Fig. 106: Adductor magnus - Anterior view.

Origin of adductor magnus

Insertion of pubic part: along a line into medial margin of gluteal tuberosity, linea aspera and medial supracondylar line.

Adductor opening (Opening in the adductor magnus)

Insertion of ischial part: by a tendon into the adductor tubercle.

Origin: The pubic part arises from the conjoined pubic and ischial rami lateral to the adductor brevis and gracilis. The ischial part arises from the lateral part of the lower area of ischial tuberosity (fig. 104).

Insertion: The pubic part spreads to gain a linear insertion into the medial margin of the gluteal tuberosity, linea aspera and upper part of the medial supracondylar line. The insertion is interrupted by tendinous arches over the perforating branches of the profunda femoris artery and a large tendinous arch which bounds the adductor opening (fig. 107). The ischial part, like the hamstrings, forms a tendon which descends vertically to be inserted into the adductor tubercle of the femur.

Fig. 107: Adductor magnus - Posterior view.

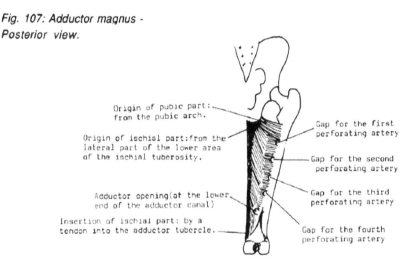

Origin of pubic part: from the pubic arch.

Origin of ischial part: from the lateral part of the lower area of the ischial tuberosity.

Adductor opening (at the lower end of the adductor canal)

Insertion of ischial part: by a tendon into the adductor tubercle.

Gap for the first perforating artery

Gap for the second perforating artery

Gap for the third perforating artery

Gap for the fourth perforating artery

Nerve supply: The pubic part is supplied by the posterior branch of obturator nerve. The ischial part is supplied by the sciatic nerve.

Actions: The pubic part adducts the thigh and helps in its flexion and lateral rotation. The ischial part is an extensor of the hip joint like the hamstrings.

Relations

Anteriorly: The adductor magnus is related to the adductors longus and brevis and obturator nerve. The profunda femoris vessels descend between it and the adductor longus. It forms part of the floor of the adductor canal where it is related to the femoral vessels.

Posteriorly: sciatic nerve and hamstring muscles.

Gracilis

Origin: from the medial margin of the pubic arch (conjoined rami) (fig. 108).

Insertion: into the upper part of the medial surface of the shaft of the tibia behind the sartorius (fig. 109). A bursa separates the insertions of both muscles.

Nerve supply: anterior branch of obturator nerve.

Actions: adduction of the thigh. It is also a flexor of the knee joint.

Relations: The muscle is covered medially by the skin, superficial fascia and deep fascia. Its deep surface is related to the three adductor muscles.

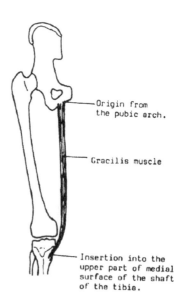

Fig. 108: Gracilis muscle.

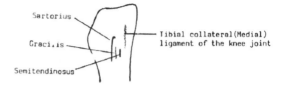

Fig. 109: Upper part of the medial surface of the right tibia showing the insertions of sartorius, gracilis and semitendinosus.

Obturator Nerve

Origin: The obturator nerve (L. 2, 3, 4) is a branch of the lumbar plexus (figs. 110, 111). It arises from the *ventral divisions* of the *ventral rami* of the second, third and fourth lumbar nerves (fig. 111).

Course and relations in the thigh: It reaches the thigh by passing through the obturator canal. Immediately it divides into anterior and posterior branches. The *anterior branch* descends in front of the adductor brevis and behind the pectineus and adductor longus. The *posterior branch* passes through the obturator externus and then descends behind the adductor brevis and in front of the adductor magnus (fig. 111).

Anterior branch: gives the following branches: 1- An articular branch to the hip joint.

1- A muscular branch to the adductor longus.

2- A muscular branch to the adductor brevis. However, the adductor brevis may be supplied by the posterior branch of obturator nerve.

3- Cutaneous branch which supplies the skin on the middle third of the medial side of the thigh through the subsartorial plexus (See pages 80 and 89) (fig. 112).

4- A muscular branch to the gracilis; the anterior branch of obturator nerve ending by supplying the gracilis muscle.

5- A muscular branch to the gracilis; the anterior branch of obturator nerve ending by supplying the gracilis muscle.

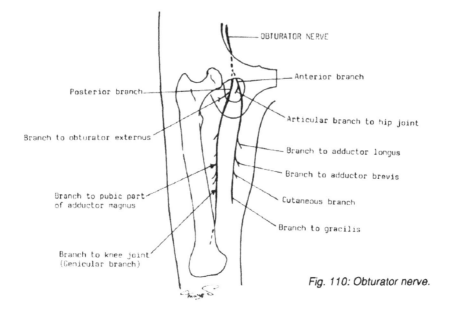

Fig. 110: Obturator nerve.

Posterior branch: gives the following branches:

1- Muscular branch to the obturator externus.

2- Muscular branch to the pubic part of adductor magnus.

3- Genicular branch: which is an articular twig to the knee joint. It is a long slender nerve which descends through the adductor magnus. Then it pierces the lower part of adductor magnus or passes through the adductor opening and follows the popliteal artery to the back of the knee joint.

N.B.: Similar to the femoral nerve, the obturator nerve carries vasoconstrictor postganglionic sympathetic fibers from the lumbar part of the sympathetic trunk to the obturator artery and its branches.

Accessory obturator nerve: an occasional branch of the lumbar plexus which is only found in about 12% of subjects. When present, it descends close to the medial side of the psoas major across the front of the superior pubic ramus, i.e. behind the inguinal ligament. Deep to the pectineus, it breaks into branches for the pectineus and hip joint.

Applied anatomy: Injury of obturator nerve leads to marked weakness of adduction of the thigh. A slight degree of adduction can be done by the pectineus.

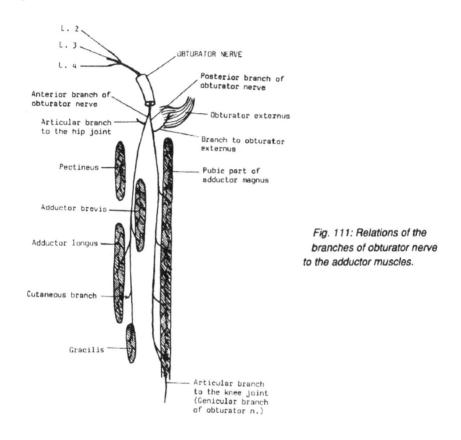

Fig. 111: Relations of the branches of obturator nerve to the adductor muscles.

Fig. 112: Cutaneous area supplied by the obturator nerve.

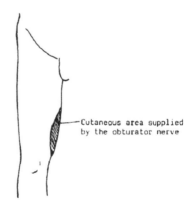

Obturator Artery

Origin: is a branch of the anterior division of the internal iliac artery in the pelvis.

Course and relations in the thigh: The artery reaches the thigh by passing through the obturator canal and immediately divides into *anterior and posterior branches* (fig. 113). The two branches diverge and run on the outer surface of the obturator membrane along the margin of the obturator foramen and under cover of the obturator externus.

Distribution: The two branches of the obturator artery anastomose together to form an arterial circle from which the following branches are given:

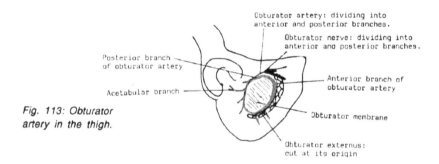

Fig. 113: Obturator artery in the thigh.

1- *Muscular branches* to the obturator externus, adductors, pectineus and gracilis.

2- *Acetabular branch* to the hip joint. This artery passes through the acetabular foramen and then along the ligament of the head of the femur to supply the hip joint and head of the femur.

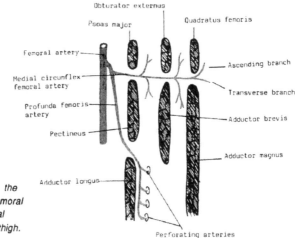

Fig. 114: Course of the medial circumflex femoral artery in the medial compartment of the thigh.

3- *Anastomotic twigs* with the medial circumflex femoral and inferior gluteal arteries.

Medial Circumflex Femoral Artery

This is a branch of the profunda femoris artery. Its origin, course and distribution were previously described (See page 75). But during dissection of the medial side of the thigh, the course of the artery is clearly displayed. It leaves the femoral triangle by passing between the psoas major and pectineus (fig. 114). Then, it passes, between the obturator externus and adductor brevis. Finally, the artery reaches the back of the thigh by passing between the quadratus femoris and upper border of adductor magnus where it terminates by giving ascending and transverse branches as previously described.

GLUTEAL REGION

Cutaneous Nerves

Lateral branch of subcostal nerve (T.12): crosses the iliac crest to supply the anterosuperior part of the gluteal region (fig. 115).

Lateral branch of iliohypogastric nerve (L.1): also crosses the iliac crest to supply the anterosuperior part of the gluteal region.

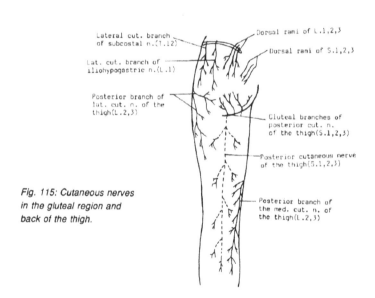

Lateral cut. branch
of subcostal n.(T.12)

Lat. cut. branch of
iliohypogastric n.(L.1)

Posterior branch of
lat. cut. n. of the
thigh(L.2,3)

Dorsal rami of L.1,2,3

Dorsal rami of S.1,2,3

Gluteal branches of
posterior cut. n.
of the thigh(S.1,2,3)

Posterior cutaneous nerve
of the thigh(S.1,2,3)

Posterior branch of
the med. cut. n. of
the thigh(L.2,3)

Fig. 115: Cutaneous nerves in the gluteal region and back of the thigh.

Cutaneous branches of the upper three lumbar dorsal rami: supply the posterosuperior part of the gluteal region.

Cutaneous branches of the upper three sacral dorsal rami: supply the posterosuperior part of the gluteal region.

Posterior branch of the lateral cutaneous nerve of the thigh (L. 2, 3):
deviates backwards to supply the anteroinferior part of the gluteal region.

Gluteal branches of the posterior cutaneous nerve of the thigh (S. 1, 2, 3): curve round the lower border of the gluteus maximus to supply the posteroinferior part of the gluteal region.

Gluteus Maximus

Origin: from the upper part of the area behind the posterior gluteal line, back of the sacrum and coccyx and back of the sacrotuberous ligament (figs. 116, 117).

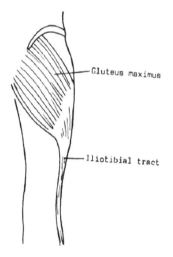

Fig. 116: Gluteus maximus.

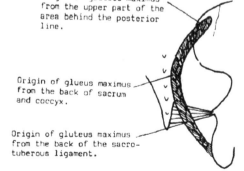

Fig. 117: Origin of gluteus maximus.

Insertion: Three quarters of the muscle are inserted into the iliotibial tract; while the lower deep quarter is inserted into the gluteal tuberosity of the femur (figs. 118, 119).

Nerve supply: inferior gluteal nerve.

Actions: The gluteus maximus is the main extensor of the hip joint. Its upper fibers abduct the thigh. Through the iliotibial tract, it stabilizes the femur on the tibia during standing when the quadriceps is relaxed.

Structures under cover of the gluteus maximus:

1- **Bones:** Extracapsular part of the neck of the femur, greater trochanter, sciatic notches, ischial spine and ischial tuberosity.

2- **Muscles:** Posterior part of gluteus medius, piriformis, tendon of obturator internus, gemilli, quadratus femoris, origin of hamstrings and upper part of adductor magnus (figs. 120, 121).

3- **Nerves:** Sciatic, superior and inferior gluteal, posterior cutaneous of thigh, nerve to quadratus femoris, pudendal and nerve to abturator internus.

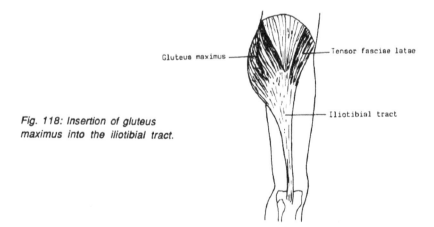

Gluteus maximus — Tensor fasciae latae

Iliotibial tract

Fig. 118: Insertion of gluteus maximus into the iliotibial tract.

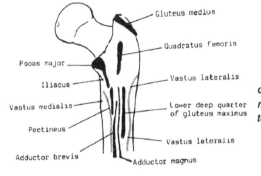

Fig. 119: Insertion of the lower deep quarter of the gluteus maximus into the gluteal tuberosity of the femur.

4- **Vessels:** Superficial division of superior gluteal, inferior gluteal and a very short course of the internal pudendal vessels.

5- **Joints:** Hip and sacroiliac joints.

6- **Ligaments:** Sacrotuberous, lateral part of the sacrospinous and posterior sacroiliac ligaments.

7- **Bursae:**

   a- Trochanteric bursa: between the muscle and greater trochanter.

   b- A bursa between the muscle and origin of vastus lateralis from the root of the greater trochanter.

   c- A bursa between the muscle and origins of hamstring muscles from the ischial tuberosity.

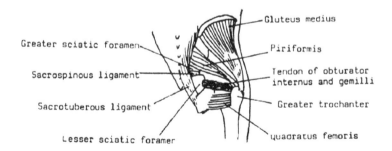

Fig. 120: Muscles under cover of the gluteus maximus.

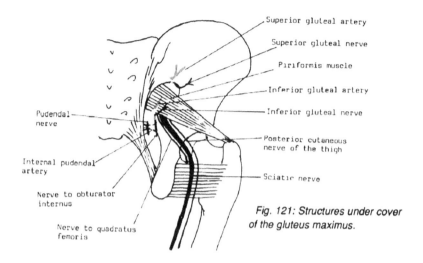

Fig. 121: Structures under cover of the gluteus maximus.

Gluteus Medius

Origin: from the gluteal surface of the ilium, in the area limited by the iliac crest and the posterior and middle gluteal lines (fig. 122).

Insertion: into the posterosuperior angle and the oblique ridge on the lateral surface of the greater trochanter (fig. 123).

Nerve supply: superior gluteal nerve.

Actions: The glutei medius and minimus are the main abductors of the thigh. Their anterior fibers are medial rotators of the thigh. The muscles of both sides contract reflexly during walking in an alternating manner to prevent tilting of the pelvis to the unsupported side when the leg is raised from the ground.

Relations: The anterior part of the muscle is only covered by the skin, superficial fascia and deep fascia while its posterior part is covered by the gluteus maximus. The deep surface of the muscle is related to the gluteus minimus, superior gluteal nerve and deep division of the superior gluteal artery (and accompanying veins).

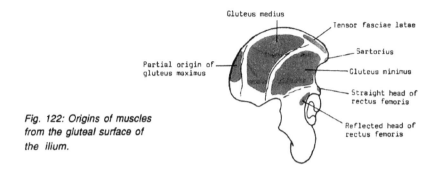

Fig. 122: Origins of muscles from the gluteal surface of the ilium.

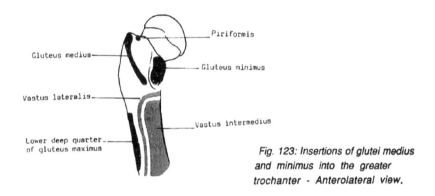

Fig. 123: Insertions of glutei medius and minimus into the greater trochanter - Anterolateral view.

Gluteus Minimus

Origin: from the gluteal surface of the ilium in the area bounded by the middle and inferior gluteal lines (figs. 122, 124).

Insertion: into an impression on the anterior surface of the greater trochanter (fig. 123).

Nerve supply: superior gluteal nerve.

Actions: The same as those of the gluteus medius.

Relations: It is covered completely by the gluteus medius with the superior gluteal nerve and deep division of superior gluteal artery (and veins) intervening. Deeply, it is related to the reflected head of rectus femoris and capsule of hip joint.

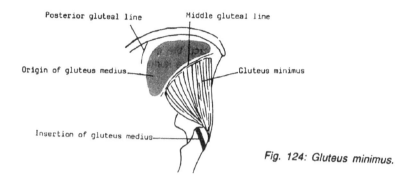

Fig. 124: Gluteus minimus.

Tensor Fasciae Latae

Origin: from the anterior part of the outer lip of the iliac crest (figs. 122, 125).

Insertion: into the iliotibial tract.

Nerve supply: superior gluteal nerve.

Actions: It helps in abduction and medial rotation of the thigh. But, its role in abduction of the thigh is doubtful. Through the iliotibial tract, it helps in extension of the knee and lateral rotation of the leg. With the gluteus maximus, it also helps in stabilizing the femur on the tibia during standing when the quadriceps is relaxed. With the glutei medius and minimus, it also plays a role in stabilizing the pelvis during walking.

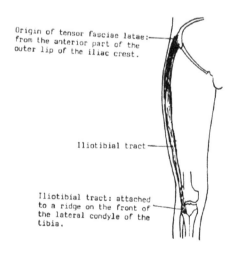

Fig. 125: Tensor fasciae latae and iliotibial tract.

Iliotibial Tract

This is the thickened lateral part of the fascia lata (deep fascia of the thigh). Its upper part splits to receive the insertions of the tensor fasciae latae and superficial three-fourths of the gluteus maximus (figs. 118, 125). The tract gradually narrows inferiorly to be attched to an oblique ridge on the front of the lateral condyle of the tibia.

Through their insertions into the tract, the gluteus maximus and tensor fasciae latae help in stabilizing the femur on the tibia during standing when the quadriceps is relaxed.

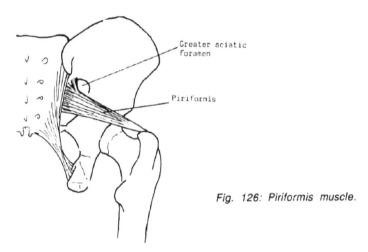

Fig. 126: Piriformis muscle.

Piriformis

Origin: from the pelvic (ventral) surface of the middle three pieces of the sacrum. Few fibers arise from the gluteal surface of the ilium just above the greater sciatic foramen (fig. 126).

Insertion: The muscle passes out through the greater sciatic foramen and converges into a tendon which is inserted into the upper border of the greater trochanter (fig. 131).

Nerve supply: Twigs from the ventral rami of the first and second sacral nerves in the pelvis.

Action: When the hip joint is extended, it rotates the thigh laterally. When the hip joint is flexed, it abducts the thigh. It also helps in controlling of other movements at the hip joint.

Obturator Internus

Origin: from the front and lateral wall of the pelvic cavity. This origin includes the inner surface of the obturator membrane, inner margin of obturator foramen and the wide area above and behind the obturator foramen (fig. 127).

Insertion: The fibers of the muscle converge into a tendon which passes out of the lesser sciatic foramen and changes its direction on the bone with a bursa intervening. The tendon passes laterally and forwards to be inserted into the medial surface of the greater trochanter (figs. 128, 131).

Nerve supply: nerve to obturator internus from the sacral plexus.

Actions: lateral rotation of the thigh. It helps in controlling of other movements at the hip point.

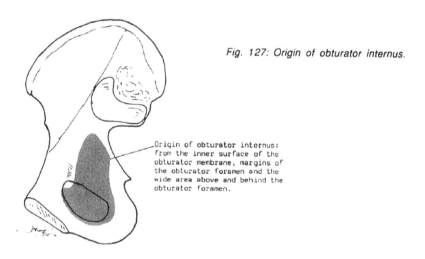

Fig. 127: Origin of obturator internus.

Origin of obturator internus: from the inner surface of the obturator membrane, margins of the obturator foramen and the wide area above and behind the obturator foramen.

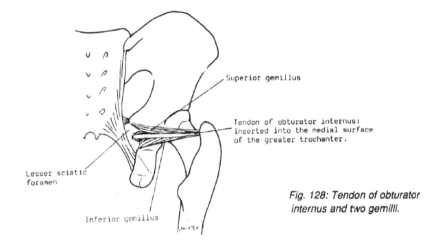

Fig. 128: Tendon of obturator internus and two gemilli.

Gemilli Muscles

These are two small muscles which surround the tendon of obturator internus (fig. 128). The *superior gemillus* arises from the upper margin of the lesser sciatic notch while the *inferior gemillus* arises from the lower margin of the notch. The two muscles pass laterally to be inserted into the tendon of obturator internus.

The superior gemillus receives a twig from the nerve to obturator internus while the inferior gemillus receives a twig from the nerve to quadratus femoris.

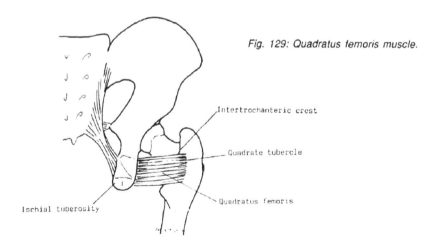

Fig. 129: Quadratus femoris muscle.

Quadratus Femoris

Origin: from the lateral border of the ischial tuberosity (fig. 129).

Insertion: into the quadrate tubercle and lower part of the intertrochanteric crest (fig. 131).

Nerve supply: Nerve to quadratus femoris from the sacral plexus.

Action: lateral rotation of the thigh.

Relations: Superficially, it is covered by the gluteus maximus and is crossed by the sciatic nerve. Deeply, it is related to the capsule of hip joint and obturator externus. The nerve to quadratus femoris supplies the muscle through its deep surface.

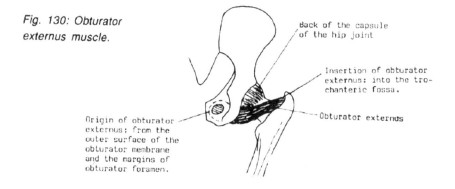

Fig. 130: Obturator externus muscle.

Back of the capsule of the hip joint

Insertion of obturator externus: into the trochanteric fossa.

Obturator externus

Origin of obturator externus: from the outer surface of the obturator membrane and the margins of obturator foramen.

Obturator Externus

Origin: from the outer margin of the obturator foramen and the outer surface of the obturator membrane (fig. 130).

Insertion: into the trochanteric fossa of the greater trochanter (fig. 131).

Nerve supply: posterior branch of obturator nerve.

Actions: lateral rotation of the thigh. It also helps in controlling of other movements at the hip joint.

Relations: From its origin to insertion, the muscle has a close relation to the capsule of hip joint and neck of the femur. The muscle lies first below and then behind the capsule of hip joint and neck of the femur. Superficially, it is covered by the quadratus femoris which separates the obturator externus from the sciatic nerve and gluteus maximus.

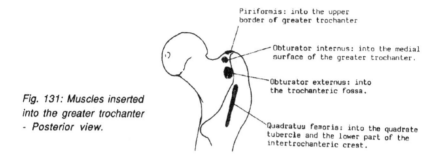

Fig. 131: Muscles inserted into the greater trochanter - Posterior view.

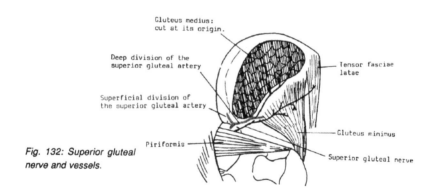

Fig. 132: Superior gluteal nerve and vessels.

Superior Gluteal Nerve

Origin: The superior gluteal nerve (L. 4, 5, S. 1) is a branch of the sacral plexus (fig. 139).

Course, relations and distribution: The nerve passes out through the greater sciatic foramen above the piriformis. Then, it passes between the glutei medius and minimus where it divides into superior and inferior branches.

The *superior branch* supplies the gluteus medius; while the *inferior branch* supplies the glutei medius and minimus and tensor fascia latae. The inferior branch also gives an articular twig to the hip joint.

Applied anatomy: In normal walking, the body weight is transmitted through one lower limb when the other limb is raised up from the ground. As a result the pelvis tilts towards the weight bearing lower limb by the action of the glutei medius and minimus, pulling from insertion to origin.

If the superior gluteal nerve is injured on one side, ask the patient to stand on the normal lower limb (fig. 133). The pelvis tilts towards the normal side to transmit the body weight.

Ask the patient to stand on the affected lower limb. The pelvis tilts to the opposite (normal) side, denoting a poisitive *Trendlenberg's sign* (fig. 134). This is due to paralysis of the glutei medius and minimus on the affected side.

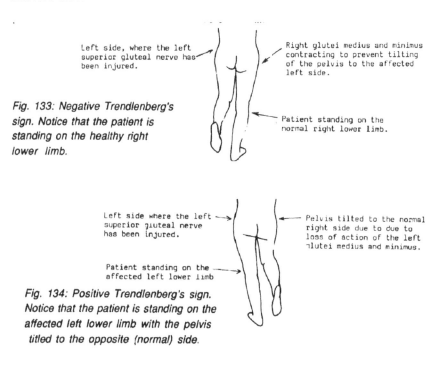

Left side, where the left superior gluteal nerve has been injured.

Right glutei medius and minimus contracting to prevent tilting of the pelvis to the affected left side.

Patient standing on the normal right lower limb.

Fig. 133: Negative Trendlenberg's sign. Notice that the patient is standing on the healthy right lower limb.

Left side where the left superior gluteal nerve has been injured.

Pelvis tilted to the normal right side due to due to loss of action of the left glutei medius and minimus.

Patient standing on the affected left lower limb

Fig. 134: Positive Trendlenberg's sign. Notice that the patient is standing on the affected left lower limb with the pelvis titled to the opposite (normal) side.

A lesion of the superior gluteal nerve leads to a *lurching gait*, as the pelvis tilts to the opposite side when the normal lower limb is raised from the ground. This denotes the important role of the glutei medius and minimus in stabilizing the pelvis during walking.

Inferior Gluteal Nerve

Origin: The inferior gluteal nerve (L. 5, S. 1, 2) is a branch of the sacral plexus.

Course, relations and distribution: It comes out of the greater sciatic foramen below the piriformis (fig. 136). Immediately, the nerve breaks into a number of branches which supply the gluteus maximus through its deep surface.

Superior Gluteal Artery

Origin: It is continuation of the posterior division of internal iliac artery.

Course, relations and distribution: The artery leaves the pelvis by passing out of the greater sciatic foramen above the piriformis (fig. 131). Immediately, it divides into superficial and deep divisions:

The *superficial division* breaks into branches which supply the gluteus maximus through its deep surface.

The *deep division* passes between the glutei medius and minimus

where it divides into superior and inferior branches which run close to the superior and inferior branches of the superior gluteal nerve. Both branches supply the glutei medius and minimus.

Close to the anterior superior iliac spine, the superior branch anastomoses with the ascending branch of the lateral circumflex femoral artery and the deep circumflex iliac artery.

The inferior branch shares in the *trochanteric anastomoses* in the

region of the trochanteric fossa with the inferior gluteal artery and the ascending branch of medial circumflex femoral artery.

The superior gluteal artery and its branches are accompanied by two venae comitantes which drain into the internal iliac vein.

Inferior Gluteal Artery

Origin: It is one of the two terminal branches of the anterior division of internal iliac artery.

Course, relations and distribution: The artery leaves the pelvis by passing out of the greater sciatic foramen below the piriformis (fig. 136). The artery immediately breaks into a number of branches which supply the gluteus maximus and adjacent muscles.

It gives the *companion artery of the sciatic nerve* which sinks into the substance of the sciatic nerve and runs through the nerve down to its termination in the middle of the thigh.

One of the branches of the inferior gluteal artery anastomoses with a branch of the superior gluteal artery. Another branch shares in the *cruciate anastomosis* at the upper border of adductor magnus (fig. 138).

The inferior gluteal artery and its branches are accompanied by two venae comitantes which drain into the internal iliac vein.

Applied anatomy: Because of the rich vascularity of the glutei muscles (both arterial and venous), it is advisable to do a short aspiration before an intramuscular gluteal injection as the tip of the needle may unfortunately lie in the lumen of a blood vessel.

Cruciate Anastomosis

This is an arterial anastomosis at the upper border of the adductor magnus where four arteries join each other in a cross-like arrangement (fig. 138).

The *horizontal limb* is formed laterally by the transverse branch of the lateral circumflex femoral artery and medially by the transverse branch of the medial circumflex femoral artery.

The *vertical limb* is formed superiorly by a branch of the inferior gluteal artery and inferiorly by a branch of the first perforating artery.

The cruciate anastomoses forms an important collateral circulation between the internal iliac and femoral arteries (See page 76).

Sacrotuberous Ligament

This is a strong ligament which connects the sacrum and coccyx to the ischial tuberosity. Superiorly, it has a wide attachment to the margins of the sacrum and coccyx and the two posterior iliac spines (fig. 135). Inferiorly, it narrows to be attached to the medial border of the ischial tuberosity. The lower end of the ligament extends as a sickle-shaped band along the ischial ramus. This band is called the *falciform process* of the sacrotuberous ligament.

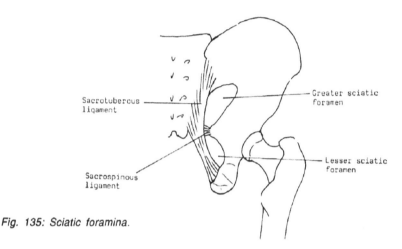

Fig. 135: Sciatic foramina.

The sacrotuberous ligament shares in the boundaries of both sciatic foramina. It also shares in the boundaries of the perineum and outlet of the pelvis. Its dorsal surface gives origin to the gluteus maximus.

Sacrospinous Ligament

This is a short fan-shaped ligament which has a wide medial attachment to the margins of the last piece of the sacrum and the coccyx. Laterally, it narrows to be attched to the tip of the ischial spine (fig. 135).

The ligament also shares in bounding the two sciatic foramina. Dorsally, it is partly covered by the sacrotuberous ligament and is crossed by the pudendal nerve. Its ventral (pelvic) surface is closely adherent to the *coccygeus muscle*; the ligament representing a degenerated dorsal part of the coccygeus muscle.

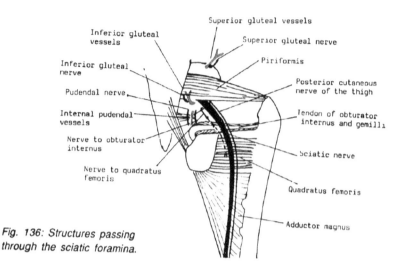

Fig. 136: Structures passing
through the sciatic foramina.

Greater Sciatic Foramen

Bounderies: greater sciatic notch and the sacrotuberous and sacrospinous ligaments (fig. 135).

Structures passing through it (fig. 136):

A - Piriformis muscle.

B - Structures above the piriformis:

    1- Superior gluteal nerve.

    2- Superior glutea

C - *Structures below the piriformis:*

    1- Sciatic nerve.

    2- Posterior cutaneous nerve of the thigh.

    3- Inferior gluteal nerve.

    4- Inferior gluteal vessels.

    5- Nerve to quadratus femoris.

    6- Nerve to obturator internus.

    7- Internal pudendal vessels.

    8- Pudendal nerve.

The last three structures have a very short course through the gluteal region as they pass from the greater to the lesser sciatic foramen.

Lesser Sciatic Foramen

Bounderies: lesser sciatic notch and the sacrotuberous and sacrospinous ligaments (fig. 135).

Structures passing through it:
1- Tendon of obturator internus.
2- Nerve to obturator internus.
3- Internal pudendal vessels.
4- Pudendal nerve.

Arrangement of structures passing from the greater to the lesser sciatic foramen (fig. 137):
1- *Nerve to obturator internus:* lateral in position, crossing the back of the base of ischial spine.
2- *Internal pudendal vessels:* intermediate in position, crossing the back of the tip of ischial spine.
3- *Pudendal nerve:* medial in position, crossing the back of the sacrospinous ligament.

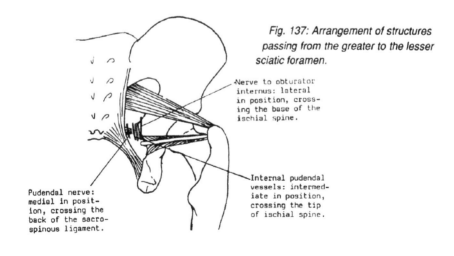

Fig. 137: Arrangement of structures passing from the greater to the lesser sciatic foramen.

Nerve to obturator internus: lateral in position, crossing the base of the ischial spine.

Internal pudendal vessels: intermediate in position, crossing the tip of ischial spine.

Pudendal nerve: medial in position, crossing the back of the sacrospinous ligament.

Posterior Cutaneous Nerve Of The Thigh

Origin: The posterior cutaneous nerve of the thigh (S. 1, 2, 3) is a combined dorsal and ventral branch of the sacral plexus.

Course and relations: The nerve comes out of the greater sciatic foramen below the piriformis. It descends in the gluteal region close to the back of the sciatic nerve under cover of the gluteus maximus (fig. 136). But, in the back of the thigh it is separated from the sciatic nerve by the hamstring muscles, and descends immediately under cover of the deep fascia in the middle line of the back of the thigh (fig. 115). It pierces the deep fascia covering the politeal fossa (popliteal fascia) and terminates by supplying the skin of the upper part of the calf (back of the leg).

Branches:
1- **Gluteal branches:** which curve round the lower border of gluteus maximus to supply the skin of the posteroinferior part of the buttock (See page 98 and figure 115).

2- **Perineal branch:** which curves forwards round the origin of the hamstring muscles from the ischial tuberosity and extends forwards into the perineum where it supplies the posterior third of the scrotum or labium majus.

3- **Other cutaneous branches:** to the back of the thigh, roof of the popliteal fossa and upper part of the calf.

Nerve To Quadratus Femoris

Origin: The nerve to quadratus femoris (L. 4, 5, S. 1) is a branch of the sacral plexus.

Course relations and distribution: The nerve passes out of the greater sciatic foramen below the piriformis (fig. 136). It descends directly on the ischium deep to the sciatic nerve and then directly on the back of the capsule of hip joint deep to the tendon of obturator internus and two gemilli which separate it from the sciatic nerve. Then, it enters into the deep surface of the quadratus femoris.

Along its course, it gives an articular branch to the hip joint and a muscular branch to the inferior gemillus.

Nerve To Obturator Internus

Origin: The nerve to obturator internus (L. 5, S. 1, 2) is a branch of the sacral plexus.

Course, relations and distribution: The nerve passes out of the greater scaitic foramen below the piriformis (fig. 137). It has a very short course in the gluteal region as it crosses the back of the ischial spine lateral to the internal pudendal vessels to enter into the lesser sciatic foramen to supply the obturator internus. Along its course it give a muscular branch to the superior gemillus.

Internal Pudendal Artery

Origin: one of the two terminal branches of the anterior division of internal iliac artery.

Course and relations in the gluteal region: The artery passes out of the greater sciatic foramen below the piriformis. It has a very short course in the gluteal region as it crosses over the tip of the ischial spine between the nerve to obturator internus laterally and the pundendal nerve medially (fig. 138). It enters into the lesser sciatic foramen to reach the pundendal canal This artery is the main source of arterial supply to the perineum.

During its very short course in the gluteal region, it gives twigs to the adjacent muscles. It is accompanied by two venae comitantes which unite to form the internal pudendal vein that drains into the internal iliac vein.

Pudendal Nerve

Origin: The pudendal nerve (S. 2, 3, 4) is the smaller of the two terminal branches of the sacral plexus.

Course and relations in the gluteal region: The nerve passes out of the greater sciatic foramen below the piriformis. It has a very short course in the gluteal region as it crosses the back of the sacrospinous ligament medial to the internal pudendal vessels (fig. 137).

It enters into the lesser sciatic foramen to reach the pundendal canal. This nerve is the main nerve of the perineum.

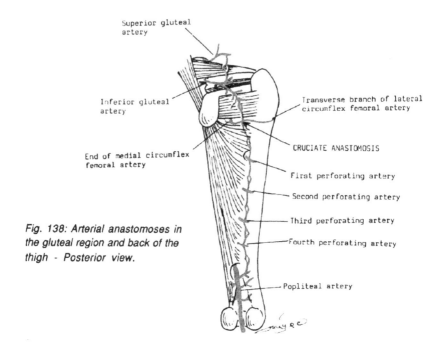

Fig. 138: Arterial anastomoses in the gluteal region and back of the thigh - Posterior view.

Applied anatomy: The chain of anastomoses extending from the gluteal region into the back of the thigh down to the popliteal fossa forms an important collateral circulation, carrying blood to the distal part of the lower limb if the femoral artery is obstructed below the origin of profunda femoris artery. These anastomoses include (fig. 138):

1- Anastomosis between the superior and inferior gluteal arteries.

2- Cruciate anastomosis (See page 110).

3- The series of anastomoses between the perforating branches of profunda femoris artery.

4- Anastomosis between the fourth perforating artery and the muscular branches of the popliteal artery.

BACK OF THE THIGH

Cutaneous Nerve Supply

Posterior cutaneous nerve of the thigh (S. 1, 2, 3): gives branches along its course which pierce the deep fascia to supply the back of the thigh, roof of popliteal fossa and upper part of the calf (fig. 115).

Medial cutaneous nerve of the thigh (L. 2, 3): Its posterior branch supplies the medial part of the back of the thigh, extending to the upper part of the back of the leg.

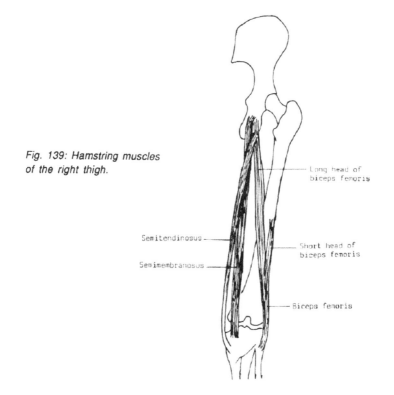

Fig. 139: Hamstring muscles of the right thigh.

Long head of biceps femoris

Semitendinosus

Short head of biceps femoris

Semimembranosus

Biceps femoris

Hamstring Muscles

The muscles of the posterior compartment of the thigh are referred to as *hamstrings* because they have a long course from origin to insertion, descending down to the popliteal region or ham.

The hamstring muscles are three: biceps femoris, semitendinosus and semimembranosus. They take origin from the ischial tuberosity and are innervated by the sciatic nerve (figs. 139, 140).

The ischial part of the adductor magnus may be included in the hamstring muscles as it has all characteristics of the hamstring muscles. It takes origin from the ischial tuberosity. Its fibers descend vertically, forming a tendon which is inserted into the adductor tubercle. It takes innervation from the sciatic nerve and is an extensor of the hip joint.

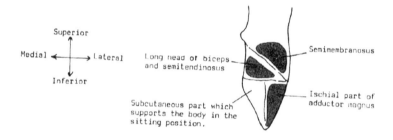

Fig. 140: Origins of the hamstring muscles from the right ischial tuberosity.

Biceps Femoris

Origin: As its name denotes, this muscle takes origin by two heads (fig. 141):

1- *Long (Medial) head:* which arises in common with the semitendinosus from the lower medial part of the upper area of the ischial tuberosity.

2- *Short (Lateral) head:* which has a linear origin from the lower part of the linea aspera and upper part of the lateral supracondylar line.

Insertion: The two heads unite in the lower part of the thigh to form the biceps femoris muscle. The muscle gives a strong tendon which is inserted into the apex of the head (styloid process) of the fibula around the attachment of the fibular collateral (lateral) ligament of the knee joint.

Nerve supply: The sciatic nerve gives a branch to each head. The branch to the long head arises from the tibial part of the sciatic nerve while the branch to the short head arises from the common peroneal part of the sciatic nerve.

Actions: flexion of the knee joint. The long head also helps in extension of the hip joint. It forms an amount of lateral rotation of the leg or medial rotation of the femur on the tibia at the end of extension of the knee leading to what is known as *"locking"* of the knee joint. This movement is so called because in such position the whole lower limb forms a rigid column from the pelvis to the ground.

Relations: The biceps femoris alone forms the upper lateral boundary of the popliteal fossa where it is closely related medially to the common peroneal nerve.

Surface anatomy: On contraction of the hamstring muscles with the knee flexed, the biceps femoris is easily seen and felt as it is the only muscle forming the upper lateral boundary of the popliteal fossa (fig. 144).

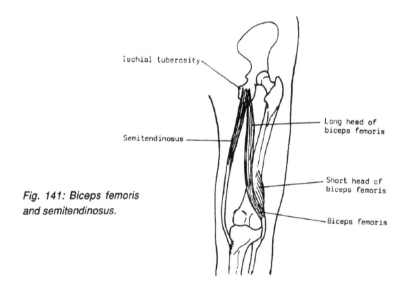

Fig. 141: Biceps femoris and semitendinosus.

Semitendinosus

Origin: in common with the long head of biceps femoris from the lower medial part of the upper area of the ischial tuberosity (figs. 140, 141).

Insertion: As its name denotes, this is a rounded muscle, the lower half of which is converted into a long tendon which descends to be inserted into the upper part of the medial surface of the tibia behind the sartorius and gracilis (fig. 142). A bursa separates the insertion from that of the gracilis.

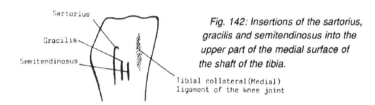

Fig. 142: Insertions of the sartorius, gracilis and semitendinosus into the upper part of the medial surface of the shaft of the tibia.

Nerve supply: sciatic nerve (a branch from tibial part of the sciatic nerve).

Actions: flexion of the knee. It also helps in extension of the hip joint and medial rotation of the thigh.

Relations: As it descends, it lies superficial (posterior) to the semimembranosus, the two muscles together forming the upper medial boundary of the popliteal fossa.

Surface anatomy: On contraction of the hamstring muscles with the knee flexed, the tendon of semitendinosus can be easily felt as a strong cord-like structure in the upper medial boundary of the popliteal fossa (fig. 144).

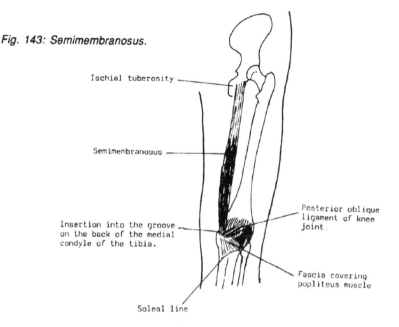

Fig. 143: Semimembranosus.

Ischial tuberosity

Semimembranosus

Insertion into the groove
on the back of the medial
condyle of the tibia.

Posterior oblique
ligament of knee
joint

Fascia covering
popliteus muscle

Soleal line

Semimembranosus

Origin: from the upper lateral part of the upper area of the ischial tuberosity (figs. 139, 140 and 143).

Insertion: As its name denotes, the upper half of this muscle is thin and flattened. But, its lower half becomes fleshy and bulky, forming the main bulk of the upper medial boundary of the popliteal fossa.

The muscle is inserted by a short strong tendon into the groove on the back of the medial condyle of the tibia. Some fibers of the tendon are reflected upwards and laterally to form the posterior oblique ligament of the knee joint. Additional fibers from the tendon spread to form the fascia covering the popliteus muscle, gaining attachment to the soleal line.

Nerve supply: sciatic nerve (a branch from the tibial part of the sciatic nerve).

Actions: flexion of the knee joint. It also helps in extension of the hip joint and medial rotation of the thigh.

Relations: It is related superficially (posteriorly) to the semitendinosus and deeply (anteriorly) to the adductor magnus. Its lower part forms the main bulk of the upper medial boundary of the polpliteal fossa. Its tendon of insertion is separated from the medial head of gastrocnemius by the *semimembranosus bursa.*

Surface anatomy: On contraction of the hamstring muscles with the thigh flexed, the semimembranosus is felt as a bulky muscle deep to the semitendinosus in the upper medial boundary of the popliteal fossa (fig. 144).

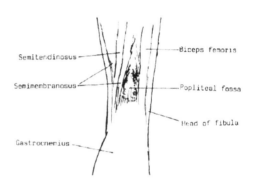

Fig. 144: Lower part of the back of the thigh in a living subject with the hamstrings contracted to show the arrangement of the hamstring muscles in relation to the popliteal fossa.

Sciatic Nerve

Origin: The sciatic nerve (L. 4, 5, S. 1, 2, 3) is the larger of the two terminal branches of the sacral plexus.

Course: The nerve leaves the pelvis into the gluteal region through the greater sciatic foramen below the piriformis (fig. 145). Then, it descends in the middle line of the back of the thigh. About the middle of the thigh, it terminates by dividing into the *tibial* (medial popliteal) and *common peroneal* (lateral popliteal) nerves.

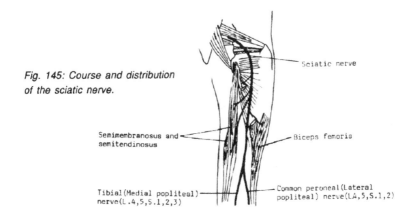

Fig. 145: Course and distribution of the sciatic nerve.

Sciatic nerve

Semimembranosus and semitendinosus

Biceps femoris

Tibial(Medial popliteal) nerve(L.4,5,S.1,2,3)

Common peroneal(Lateral popliteal) nerve(L4,5,S.1,2)

Relations: In the gluteal region, the sciatic nerve is covered by the gluteus maximus. In the back of the thigh, it is covered by the long head of biceps, semitendinosus and semimembranosus (fig. 146). In the gluteal region, it is closely related posteriorly to the posterior cutaneous nerve of the thigh. As the sciatic nerve descends, it first lies on the ischium (fig. 136). Then,

it crosses the tendon of obturator internus and two gemilli, quadratus femoris and adductor magnus from above downwards.

The upper part of the sciatic nerve is related deeply to the nerve to quadratus femoris. But, as it descends, it becomes separated from the nerve to quadratus femoris by the tendon of obturator internus and two gemilli. The obturator internus, gemilli and quadratus femoris separate the sciatic nerve from the hip joint. The quadratus femoris also separates the sciatic nerve from the obturator externus.

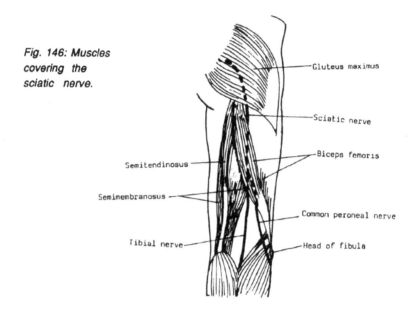

Fig. 146: Muscles covering the sciatic nerve.

Labels: Gluteus maximus, Sciatic nerve, Biceps femoris, Common peroneal nerve, Head of fibula, Tibial nerve, Semimembranosus, Semitendinosus

Fibers of the tibial part of the sciatic nerve arise from the ventral divisions of the ventral rami forming the sacral plexus while fibers of the common peroneal part of the sciatic nerve arise from the dorsal divisions of the ventral rami forming the sacral plexus. The tibial and common peroneal nerves are enclosed in the common sheath of the sciatic nerve down to the middle of the thigh where both terminal branches are separated.

However, the sciatic nerve may terminate at higher levels. Occasionally, the sciatic nerve is absent as both tibial and common peroneal nerves arise separately from the sacral plexus. In such condition, the tibial nerve passes out below the piriformis while the common peroneal nerve pierces the piriformis to reach the gluteal region.

Branches: Apart from the *two terminal branches,* the sciatic nerve gives *muscular branches* to the hamstring muscles in the upper part of the thigh (fig. 145). Nerves are given to both heads of the biceps femoris, semitendinosus, semimembranosus and ischial part of adductor magnus. The branch given to the short head of biceps arises from the common peroneal part while the branches to the other hamstrings arise from the tibial part of the sciatic nerve.

Surface anatomy: In the gluteal region, the sciatic nerve emerges from the greater sciatic foramen opposite a point at the junction of the upper and middle thirds of a line between the posterior superior iliac spine and ischial tuberosity (fig. 147).

In the gluteal region, the nerve is represented by a curved line extending from the point of exit of the nerve to a point midway between the greater trochanter and ischial tuberosity.

In the thigh, it is marked by the upper two-thirds of a line extending in the middle of the back of the thigh to the mid point of the popliteal fossa.

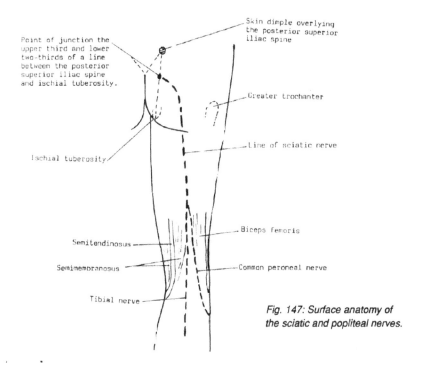

Fig. 147: Surface anatomy of the sciatic and popliteal nerves.

Applied anatomy

A - *Injury of the sciatic nerve* commonly occurs due to fractures in the middle of the shaft to the femur (fig. 148). In such conditions, the lower fragment is pulled up by the muscles descending from the hip bone and femur to the lower part of the thigh and upper part of the leg, resulting in overriding of the two bony fragments, thus exposing the sciatic nerve to injury in the middle of the thigh.

However, the sciatic nerve may be injured high up in the gluteal region due to an erroneous intragluteal injection or due to a deep wound in the gluteal region.

An injury of the sciatic nerve results in:

1- Paralysis of the hamstring muscles when the injury is in the gluteal region. But, if the injury is in the middle of the thigh, the hamstrings escape paralysis as they receive innervation high up in the thigh. Paralysis of the hamstrings leads to weakness of flexion of the knee, as some flexion can be done by the sartorius and gracilis.

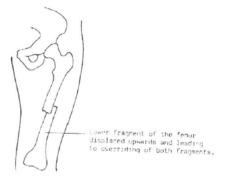

Fig. 148: Fracture of the middle of the shaft of the femur - Notice the upward displacement of the lower fragment of the femur.

Lower fragment of the femur displaced upwards and leading to overriding of both fragments.

2- Complete paralysis of all muscles of the leg and foot, leading to a condition of *flail foot.* However, there is *foot drop* resulting from the effect of gravity.

3- Loss of cutaneous sensations on the leg and foot except the area supplied by the saphenous nerve which includes the medial side of the leg and medial border of the foot to the root of the big toe (fig. 149).

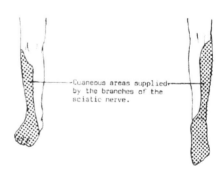

Fig. 149: Cutaneous areas supplied by the sciatic nerve.

Cutaneous areas supplied by the branches of the sciatic nerve.

Injury of the sciatic nerve is tested by:

a- Failure of dorsiflexion and plantar flexion of the foot. However, plantar flexion may result from the effect of gravity.

b- Failure of extension and flexion of the toes.

B - *Intramuscular injections* through the gluteal region *(Intragluteal injections)* are done in the upper outer quadrant of the gluteal region to be sure that the needle is inserted away from the sciatic nerve and to avoid injection of an irritant drug in the vicinity of the sciatic nerve.

POPLITEAL FOSSA

This is an important intermuscular space which occupies the back of the lower part of the thigh, knee and upper part of the leg. After dissection and displaying its contents, the fossa appears as a diamond-shaped space having four boundaries. But in nondissected specimens, the muscles greatly overlap each other and the contents of the fossa are not clearly shown, being embedded in a large amount of fat (popliteal fat).

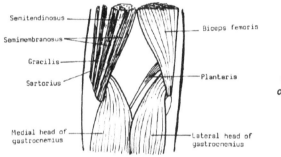

Fig. 150: Boundaries of popliteal fossa.

Boundaries

Upper lateral boundary: is only formed by the biceps femoris (fig. 150).

Upper medial boundary: is formed by the semimembranosus and semitendinosus supplimented by the sartorius, gracilis and tendon of the ischial part of adductor magnus.

Lower lateral boundary: is formed by the lateral head of gastrocnemius supplimented by the plantaris.

Lower medial boundary: is only formed by the medial head of gastrocnemius.

Roof: This forms the posterior (superficial) boundary of the fossa and is formed by the skin, superficial fascia and deep fascia. The superficial fascia contains the upper part of the small saphenous vein and branches of the posterior cutaneous nerve of the thigh. The deep fascia *(popliteal fascia)* is a downward continuation of the deep fascia of the thigh (fascia lata). About the middle of the fossa, it is pierced by the small saphenous vein to terminate into the popliteal vein. The vein is accompanied by few lymphatics which also pierce the popliteal fascia to terminate in the popliteal lymph nodes. The lower part of the popliteal fascia is also pierced by the posterior cutaneous nerve of the thigh which terminates in the upper part of the calf.

Floor: This forms the anterior (deep) boundary of the fossa (fig. 151. The upper part of the floor is formed by the popliteal surface of the femur, its middle part by the back of the capsule of knee joint and its lower part by the fascia covering the popliteus muscle. The distal border of the popliteus forms the lower limit of the fossa where it becomes continuous with the posterior compartment of the leg.

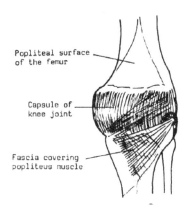

Popliteal surface of the femur

Capsule of knee joint

Fascia covering popliteus muscle

Fig. 151: Floor of popliteal fossa.

Contents

1- Common peroneal (Lateral popliteal) nerve (fig. 152.)

2- Tibial (Medial popliteal) nerve.

3- Popliteal artery.

4- Popliteal vein.

5- Terminal part of the posterior cutaneous nerve of the thigh.

6- Popliteal lymph nodes.

7- Popliteal fat through which all other contents of the fossa are embedded.

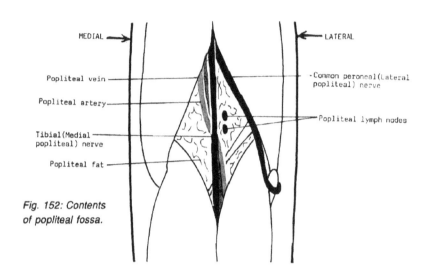

MEDIAL ➡   ⬅ LATERAL

Popliteal vein ———

Popliteal artery———

Tibial (Medial ———
popliteal) nerve

Popliteal fat ———

·Common peroneal(Lateral
popliteal) nerve

Popliteal lymph nodes

*Fig. 152: Contents
of popliteal fossa.*

Common Peroneal Nerve

Origin: The common peroneal (lateral popliteal) nerve (L. 4, 5, S. 1, 2) is the smaller of the two terminal branches of the sciatic nerve.

Course and relations: The nerve takes origin about the middle of the thigh, but as previously described its level of origin is variable. It enters the popliteal fossa at its upper angle and descends downwards and laterally close to the medial side of the biceps femoris (fig. 153). Then it leaves the fossa through its lateral angle where it crosses the plantaris and lateral head of gastrocnemius. Then, the nerve descends behind the head of the fibula and curves forwards to end on the lateral side of the neck of the fibula deep to the peroneus longus muscle. Here, the nerve gives two terminal branches which are the deep and superficial peroneal nerves.

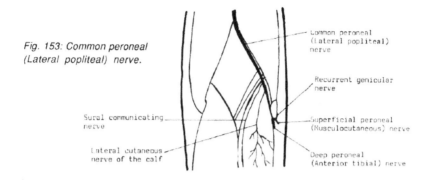

Fig. 153: Common peroneal
(Lateral popliteal) nerve.

Branches

A - *Cutaneous branches*

1- *Lateral cutaneous nerve of the calf:* which runs over the lateral part of the calf and supplies the skin of the superolateral part of the calf and anterolateral aspect of the leg (figs. 154, 163).

2- *Sural communicating nerve:* which descends to join the sural nerve in the lower part of the back of the leg and supplies the lateral part of the calf (figs. 154, 163).

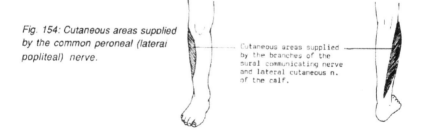

Fig. 154: Cutaneous areas supplied by the common peroneal (lateral popliteal) nerve.

B - *Muscular branches:* The common peroneal nerve does not give muscular branches in the fossa. But, as a part of the sciatic nerve, it gives a muscular branch to the short head of biceps femoris in the thigh, i.e. before reaching the fossa.

C - *Articular branches:* which supply the knee joint (fig. 155). These are:

1- *Superior lateral genicular nerve:* which runs along the superior lateral genicular artery to the knee joint.

2- *Inferior lateral genicular nerve:* which runs along the inferior lateral genicular artery to the knee joint.

3- *Recurrent genicular nerve:* which arises from the end of the common peroneal nerve and recurs up to reach the knee joint. It passes upwards and medially through the extensor digitorum longus and then through the upper part of the tibialis anterior to reach the anterior aspect of the knee joint. It gives muscular twigs to the upper part of the tibialis anterior and is accompanied by the anterior tibial recurrent artery.

D - *Terminal branches*

1- *Deep peroneal (Anterior tibial) nerve:* described later.

2- *Superficial peroneal (Musculocutaneous) nerve:* described later.

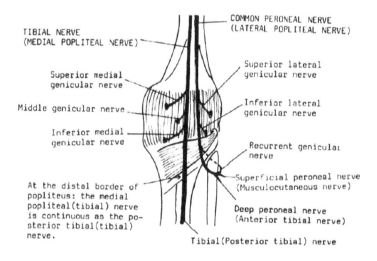

Fig. 155: Genicular branches of the common peroneal and tibial nerves.

Surface anatomy: The common peroneal nerve corresponds to a line beginning from a point on the middle line of the back of the thigh at the junction of its middle and lower thirds, and extending downwards and laterally close to the medial side of the biceps femoris, to a point on the lateral side of the neck of the fibula (fig. 147).

If you contract the biceps femoris, the nerve can be compressed and felt as a cord-like structure close to the medial side of the biceps femoris.

The termination of the nerve can be also compressed and felt in its dangerous position close to the lateral side of the neck of the fibula.

Applied anatomy: The common peroneal nerve is commonly injured at its termination on the lateral side of the neck of the fibula. Such injury leads to:

1- Paralysis of the muscles of the anterior and lateral compartments of the leg. This leads to paralysis of the dorsiflexors and evertors of the foot. This results in *"Foot drop"* which is manifested by plantar flexion and inversion of the foot.

2- Loss of cutaneous sensations on the lower part of the front of the leg, intermediate part of the dorsum of the foot and dorsum of all toes except the lateral side of little toe (supplied by sural nerve) (fig. 154).

Injury of common peroneal nerve can be tested by:

a- Inability to dorsiflex the foot.

b- Inability to extend the toes.

c- Inability to evert the foot.

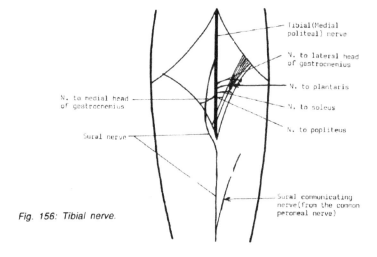

Fig. 156: Tibial nerve.

Tibial Nerve

Origin: The tibial (medial popliteal) nerve (L. 4, 5, S. 1, 2, 3) is the larger of the two terminal branches of the sciatic nerve.

Course and relations: This nerve takes origin in the middle of the thigh, but its level of origin may be variable as previously described. It bisects the popliteal fossa, i.e. it enters the fossa at its upper angle and leaves the fossa at its lower angle (fig. 156).

In the upper part of the fossa, the tibial nerve is lateral to the popliteal vessels but at a more superficial plane (fig. 158). In the middle of the fossa, it crosses behind (superficial to) the vessels. In the lower part of the fossa, it becomes medial to the vessels. Throughout its whole course the nerve is superficial to the vessels, being the most superficial of the main structures in the fossa. Throughout its whole course the nerve is separated from the popliteal artery by the popliteal vein (figs, 152, 158).

At the distal border of popliteus, the tibial nerve continues into the posterior compartment of the leg carrying the same name or may be known as the ***posterior tibial nerve.***

Branches in the popliteal fossa

A - *Cutaneous branch*

Sural nerve: is the only cutaneous branch of the tibial nerve in the popliteal fossa. This nerve descends between the two heads of gastrocnemius, pierces the deep fascia and descends to the lower part of the back of the leg where it is joined by the sural communicating nerve (fig. 163).

Then, it curves behind and below the lateral malleolus to continues forwards along the lateral border of the dorsum of the foot to end in the lateral side of the little toe (fig. 164).

Throughout its course, the sural nerve is closely accompanied by the small saphenous vein. The sural nerve supplies the back of the leg, lateral border of the foot and lateral side of the little toe (fig. 157).

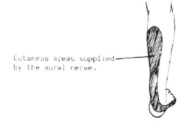

Cutaneous areas supplied
by the sural nerve.

Fig. 157: Cutaneous areas supplied
by the sural nerve.

B - *Muscular branches:* to the following muscles (fig. 156):

1- Medial head of gastrocnemius.

2- Lateral head of gastrocnemius.

3- Plantaris.

4- Popliteus.

5- Superficial part of the soleus.

The muscular branches arise from tibial nerve in the lower part of the popliteal fossa. Four of the five branches cross behind (superficial to) the popliteal vessels to reach the muscles; these are the nerves to lateral head of gastrocnemius, plantaris, popliteus and soleus (fig. 156).

The nerve to popliteus descends over the muscle and then hooks on its distal border to supply the popliteus through its deep surface (fig. 201).

The nerve to soleus passes between the plantaris and lateral head of gastocnemius and supplies the soleus through its superficial surface.

C - *Articular branches:* which supply the knee joint. These are (fig. 155):

1- *Superior medial genicular nerve:* which runs with the superior medial genicular artery to the knee joint.

2- *Middle genicular nerve:* which runs with the middle genicular artery and pierces the posterior oblique ligament of the knee joint.

3- *Inferior medial genicular nerve:* which runs along the inferior medial genicular artery to the knee joint.

NB.: The course, relations and distribution of the tibial nerve in the posterior compartment of the leg are described later (See page 168).

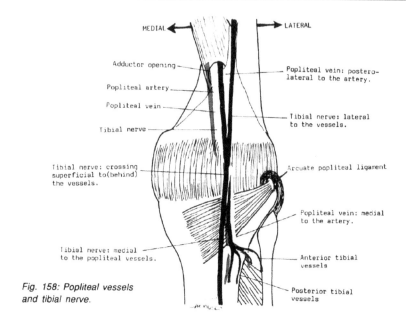

MEDIAL ◄   ► LATERAL

Adductor opening

Popliteal artery

Popliteal vein

Tibial nerve

Tibial nerve: crossing
superficial to(behind)
the vessels.

Tibial nerve: medial
to the popliteal vessels.

Popliteal vein: postero-
lateral to the artery.

Tibial nerve: lateral
to the vessels.

Arcuate popliteal ligament

Popliteal vein: medial
to the artery.

Anterior tibial
vessels

Posterior tibial
vessels

Fig. 158: Popliteal vessels
and tibial nerve.

Surface anatomy: The tibial nerve in the popliteal fossa corresponds to a vertical line which extends from a point on the middle line of the back of the thigh at the junction of its middle and lower thirds to a point on the middle line of the back of the leg at a level with the tibial tuberosity (fig. 147).

Applied anatomy: The tibial nerve is less frequently injured. Its injury in the popliteal fossa leads to:

1- Paralysis of muscles of the posterior compartment of the leg. This leads to weakness of plantar flexion as some plantar flexion can be done by the peronei longus and brevis. There is also weakness of inversion as some inversion can be done by the tibialis anterior.

As a result of paralysis of muscles of the posterior compartment of the leg, the foot is kept in a position of dorsiflexion and eversion.

2- Paralysis of the intrinsic muscles of the sole of the foot leading to atrophy of these muscles.

3- Loss of cutaneous sensations on the back of the leg, lateral border of the foot and lateral side of little toe which are the areas supplied by the sural nerve (fig. 157).

4- Loss of cutaneous sensations on the sole of the foot and plantar aspect of all digits which are supplied by the medial and lateral plantar nerves (fig. 205).

Injury of the tibial nerve in the popliteal fossa is tested by:
a- Marked limping during walking due to paralysis of the plantar flexors.

b- Inability to stand on the tips of the toes due to paralysis of the plantar and digital flexors.

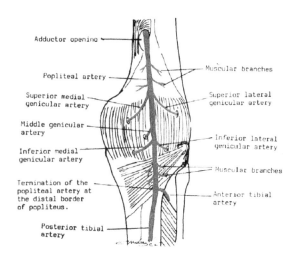

Adductor opening

Popliteal artery

Superior medial genicular artery

Middle genicular artery

Inferior medial genicular artery

Termination of the popliteal artery at the distal border of popliteus.

Muscular branches

Superior lateral genicular artery

Inferior lateral genicular artery

Muscular branches

Anterior tibial artery

Posterior tibial artery

Fig. 159: Branches of popliteal artery

Popliteal Artery

Origin: continuation of the femoral artery at the adductor opening (fig. 158).

Course and relations: It is the deepest structure in the popliteal fossa, descending on the floor. It descends first on the popliteal surface of the femur with some fat intervening. Then, it crosses the back of the capsule of the knee joint and descends on the fascia covering the popliteus muscle.

In the upper part of the fossa it is overlaped by the semimembranosus and in the lower part of the fossa it is overlapped by the two heads of gastrocnemius. In the upper part of the fossa, the popliteal vein and tibial nerve are posterolateral to the artery (fig. 158). In the middle of the fossa, the popliteal vein and tibial nerve cross posterior (superficial) to the artery.

In the lower part of the fossa, the popliteal vein and tibial nerve become medial to the artery. Throughout its whole course, the popliteal artery is separated from the tibial nerve by the popliteal vein.

The lower part of the artery is crossed superficially by the muscular branches of the tibial nerve to the lateral head of gastrocnemius, plantaris, popliteus and soleus.

At the distal border of popliteus, the popliteal artery ends by dividing into anterior and posterior tibial arteries.

Branches (fig. 159)

A - *Muscular branches*: to the adjacent hamstring and calf muscles.

B - *Cutaneous branches*: twigs to the skin from the muscular branches.

C - *Articular branches*: five genicular arteries which are the main source of arterial blood to the knee joint. According to their position, they are:

1- Superior lateral genicular artery.

2- Superior medial genicular artery.

3- Middle genicular artery.

4- Inferior lateral genicular artery.

5- Inferior medial genicular artery.

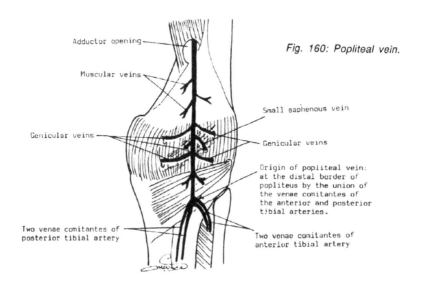

Fig. 160: Popliteal vein.

Each of these arteries is accompanied by the corresponding genicular vein and nerve. The middle genicular artery passes through the posterior oblique ligament and is the main source of arterial blood to the cruciate ligaments. The genicular arteries ansatomose together and with other arteries, forming the anastomoses around the knee joint which are described later (fig. 247).

Surface anatomy: The popliteal artery is represented by a line which begins from a point one inch medial to the middle line of the back of the thigh at the junction of its middle and lower thirds. This line is extended downwards and laterally to the midpoint of the popliteal fossa and is then extended vertically downwards to the level of the tibial tuberosity.

Popliteal vein

Origin: by the union of the venae comitantes of the anterior and posterior tibial arteries at the distal border of popliteus (fig. 160).

Course and relations: In the lower part of the popliteal fossa, the vein is medial to the artery; in the middle of the fossa the vein crosses superficial (posterior) to the artery and in the upper part of the fossa the vein becomes posterolateral to the artery. Along its whole course, the vein intervenes between the popliteal artery and the tibial nerve.

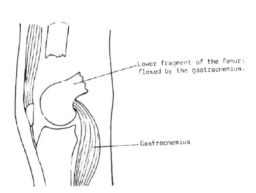

Fig. 161: Fracture of the lower part of the shaft of the femur. Notice that the lower fragment is flexed by the gastrocnemius.

Lower fragment of the femur; flexed by the gastrocnemius.

Gastrocnemius

Termination: At the adductor opening, the popliteal vein continues up into the adductor canal as the femoral vein.

Tributaries: Along its course, the popliteal vein receives the following tributaries:

1- Muscular veins from the adjacent muscles.

2- Five genicular veins corresponding to the five genicular branches of the popliteal artery.

3- Small saphenous vein.

Applied anatomy: Injury of the popliteal vessels frequently occurs in complete fractures of the lower part of the shaft of the femur (fig. 161). The lower bony fragment is flexed by the gastrocnemius, exposing the popliteal artery to be torn. The popliteal nerves are less liable to injury as they are relatively superficial to the vessels.

Popliteal Lymph Nodes

These are two small lymph nodes which lie close to the popliteal vessels in the middle of the popliteal fossa (fig. 126). They receive few deep lymphatics which run along the anterior and posterior tibial vessels. They also receive few superficial lymphatics which run along the small saphenous vein. Their efferent lymphatics ascend along the femoral vessels to drain into the deep inguinal lymph nodes.

LEG

Cutaneous Nerve Supply

Saphenous nerve: previously described on page 80. Its infrapatellar branch supplies the uppermost part of the front of the leg (fig. 162). Along its course in the leg, it supplies the medial side of the leg encroaching on its front and back.

Lateral cutaneous nerve of the calf: supplies the upper lateral part of the calf and adjacent parts of the lateral side and front of the leg (See page 127).

Posterior branch of medial cutaneous nerve of the thigh: supplies the upper part of the medial side and back of the leg (See page 60).

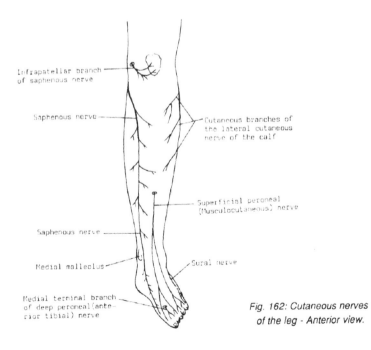

Infrapatellar branch of saphenous nerve

Saphenous nerve

Cutaneous branches of the lateral cutaneous nerve of the calf

Superficial peroneal (Musculocutaneous) nerve

Saphenous nerve

Medial malleolus

Sural nerve

Medial terminal branch of deep peroneal (anterior tibial) nerve

Fig. 162: Cutaneous nerves of the leg - Anterior view.

Posterior cutaneous nerve of the thigh: Its terminal part supplies the upper part of the calf (fig. 163) (See page 112).

Sural communicating nerve: supplies the lower lateral part of the calf (See page 127).

Sural nerve: Supplies the lower part of the back of the leg (See page 130).

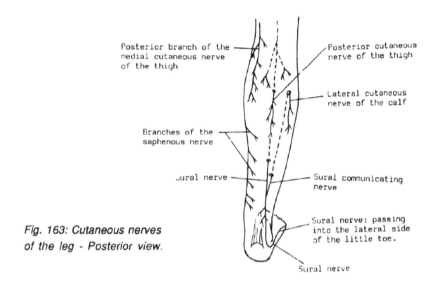

Fig. 163: Cutaneous nerves of the leg - Posterior view.

Small Saphenous Vein

Origin: on the dorsum of the foot by the union of the lateral end of the dorsal venous arch with the lateral dorsal digital vein of the little toe (fig. 164).

Course and relations: The vein is superficial throughout its whole extent. It passes backwards along the lateral border of the dorsum of the foot. Then, it curves up, passing below and then behind the lateral malleolus and ascends on the back of the leg. About the middle of the popliteal fossa, it pierces the popliteal fascia to end in the popliteal vein.

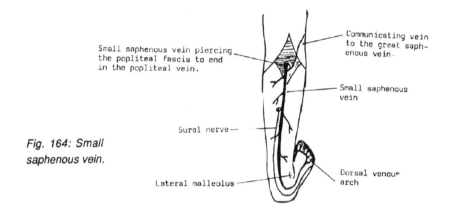

Small saphenous vein piercing the popliteal fascia to end in the popliteal vein.

Communicating vein to the great saphenous vein.

Small saphenous vein

Sural nerve —

Fig. 164: Small
saphenous vein.

Lateral malleolus —

Dorsal venous arch

Along its course it is closely accompanied by the sural nerve. It receives tributaries from the dorsum of the foot and leg. It is joined to the deep veins of the calf by a number of perforating veins. Its upper part is connected to the great saphenous vein by a communicating vein which ascends in the back of the thigh and then deviates medially to join the great saphenous vein in the middle of the thigh.

Deep Fascia of the Leg

The deep fascia of the leg does **not** completely encircle the leg (fig. 165). It extends from the anterior border (shin) of the tibia round the leg to be attached to the medial border of the tibia, leaving the medial surface of the tibia subcutaneous.

In addition, the deep fascia does not cover the triangular area on the lateral side of the lower part of the shaft of the fibula above the lateral malleolus, leaving this area subcutaneous.

At the ankle, the deep fascia forms thickened bands which are called *retinacula* as they keep the tendons in position around the ankle joint.

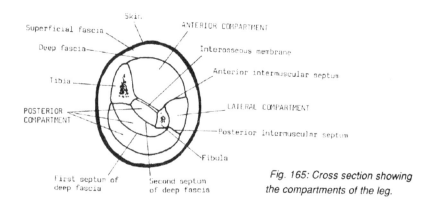

Fig. 165: Cross section showing the compartments of the leg.

Intermuscular Septa

Two septa of deep fascia connect the deep fascia with the fibula (fig. 165). The *anterior intermuscular septum* connects the deep fascia with the anterior border of the fibula. The *posterior intermuscular septum* connects the deep fascia with the posterior border of the fibula.

Compartments Of The Leg

The deep fascia, tibia, fibula, interosseus membrane and the two intermuscular septa divide the leg into three osseofascial compartments (fig. 165):

A - *Anterior compartment:* contains the extensor muscles, anterior tibial vessels and deep peroneal (anterior tibial) nerve.

B - *Lateral compartment:* contains the peroniei longus and brevis and the superficial peroneal (musculocutaneous) nerve.

C - *Posterior compartment:* contains the flexor muscles, posterior tibial vessels and tibial (posterior tibial) nerve.

ANTERIOR COMPARTMENT OF THE LEG

Contents

1- Tibialis anterior (fig. 166).

2- Extensor hallucis longus.

3- Extensor digitorum longus.

4- Peroneus tertius.

5- Anterior tibial vessels.

6- Deep peroneal (Anterior tibial) nerve.

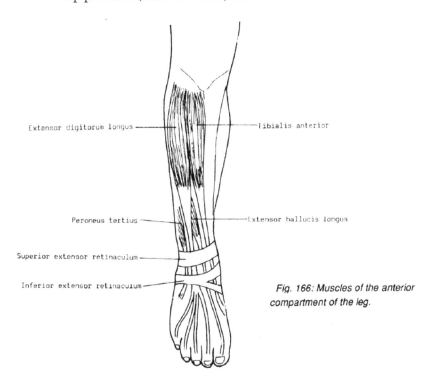

Extensor digitorum longus

Tibialis anterior

Peroneus tertius

Extensor hallucis longus

Superior extensor retinaculum

Inferior extensor retinaculum

Fig. 166: Muscles of the anterior compartment of the leg.

Tibialis Anterior

Origin: from the upper two-thirds of the lateral surface of the tibia (fig. 167).

Insertion: into the medial surface of the medial cuneiform bone and adjacent part of the base of the first metatarsal bone.

Nerve supply: deep peroneal (anterior tibial) nerve. The upper fibers of the muscle are supplied by the recurrent genicular nerve.

Actions: dorsiflexion and inversion of the foot.

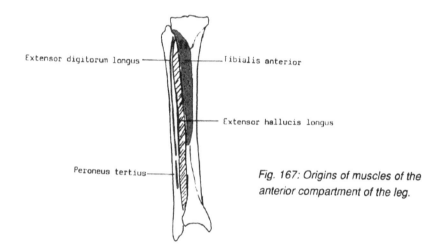

Fig. 167: Origins of muscles of the anterior compartment of the leg.

Extensor Hallucis Longus

Origin: from the middle two-fourths of the anterior (extensor) surface of the fibula and adjacent part of the interosseous membrane of the leg (fig. 167).

Insertion: The upper part of the muscle is overlaped by the tibialis anterior and extensor digitorum longus (fig. 166). But, its tendon appears between the two muscles in the lower part of the leg where it crosses in front of the deep peroneal (anterior tibial) nerve and anterior tibial vessels from the lateral to the medial side (fig. 171).

The tendon passes deep to both superior and inferior extensor retinacula to the dorsum of the foot, reaching to its insertion into the dorsum of the base of the terminal phalanx of the big toe.

Nerve supply: deep peroneal nerve.

Actions: extension of the interphalangeal and metatarsophalangeal joints of the big toe. It is also a dorsiflexor of the foot.

Extensor Digitorum Longus

Origin: from the upper three-fourths of the anterior (extensor) surface of the fibula lateral to the extensor hallucis longus and partly from the interosseous membrane of the leg (fig. 167).

Insertion: The muscle gives four tendons which descend deep to both extensor retinacula to the dorsum of the foot where they join the dorsal digital (extensor) expansions of the lateral four toes. Through the dorsal digital (extensor) expansions they gain an insertion into the middle and terminal phalanges.

Nerve supply: deep peroneal nerve.

Actions: extension of the interphalangeal and metatarsophalangeal joints of the lateral four toes. It is also a dorsiflexor of the foot.

Peroneus Tertius

Origin: from the distal fourth of the anterior (extensor) surface of the fibula in line with the extensor digitorum longus (fig. 167). At its origin it appears to be a part of the extensor digitorum longus.

Insertion: In the lower part of the leg it appears as a separate muscle giving a tendon which descends deep to both extensor retinacula to reach an insertion into the dorsum of the base of the fifth metatarsal bone.

Nerve supply: deep peroneal nerve.

Actions: dorsiflexion and eversion of the foot.

N.B.:

1- *Dorsiflexion* and *plantar flexion* of the foot are two movements which occur in the ankle joint. Dorsiflexion is done by the muscles of the anterior compartment. Plantar flexion is done by the muscles of the lateral and posterior compartments (fig. 168).

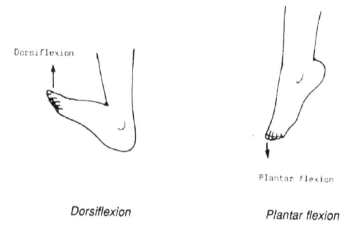

Dorsiflexion   Plantar flexion

Fig. 168: Dorsiflexion and plantar flexion of the foot. The two movements occur in the ankle joint.

2- *Inversion* and *eversion* of the foot are two movements which occur in the talocalcaneonavicular joint. Inversion is the movement which directs the sole of the foot inwards. Eversion is the movement which directs the sole of the foot outwards (fig. 169). Inversion is done mainly by the two tibialis: anterior and posterior. Eversion is done by the three peronei: longus, brevis and tertius.

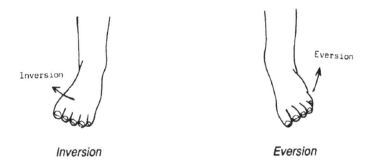

Inversion   Eversion

Fig. 169: Inversion and eversion of the foot. The two
movements occur in the talocalcaneonavicular joint.

Anterior Tibial Artery

Origin: is the smaller of the two terminal branches of the popliteal artery
at distal border of popliteus (fig. 159).

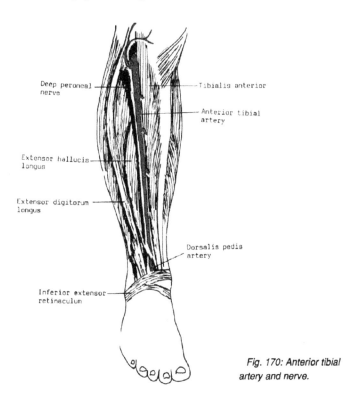

Fig. 170: Anterior tibial
artery and nerve.

Course and relations: Throughout its course the artery is closely accompanied by two venae comitantes. It leaves the posterior to the anterior compartment of the leg by passing through the upper part of the interosseous membrane close to the medial side of te neck of the fibula (fig. 170). Then, it descends close to the front of the interosseous membrane between the tibialis anterior and extensor digitorum longus and then between the tibialis anterior and extensor hallucis longus.

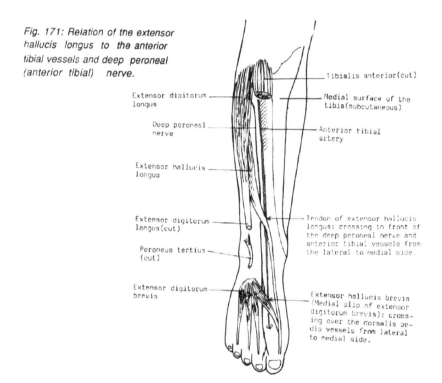

Fig. 171: Relation of the extensor hallucis longus to the anterior tibial vessels and deep peroneal (anterior tibial) nerve.

Extensor digitorum longus

Deep peroneal nerve

Extensor hallucis longus

Extensor digitorum longus(cut)

Peroneus tertius (cut)

Extensor digitorum brevis

Tibialis anterior(cut)

Medial surface of the tibia(subcutaneous)

Anterior tibial artery

Tendon of extensor hallucis longus: crossing in front of the deep peroneal nerve and anterior tibial vessels from the lateral to medial side.

Extensor hallucis brevis (Medial slip of extensor digitorum brevis): crossing over the dorsalis pedis vessels from lateral to medial side.

In the lower part of the leg, it is crossed by the extensor hallucis longus from the lateral to medial side (fig. 171) and then becomes superficial where it lies on the lower part of the tibia between the tendons of extensor hallucis longus medially and extensor digitorum longus laterally deep to the superior extensor retinaculum.

In the upper third of the leg, the deep peroneal (anterior tibial) nerve is lateral to the artery (fig. 170). In the middle third of the leg, the nerve becomes anterior to the artery. In the lower third of the leg, the nerve returns lateral to the artery once more.

Termination: As it crosses in front of the ankle joint, the anterior tibial aretry continues into the dorsum of the foot as the *dorsalis pedis artery.*

Branches (fig. 172)

1- ***Posterior tibial recurrent artery:*** which arises from the anterior tibial artery at its origin in the posterior compartment and ascends up to share in the anastomoses around the knee joint.

2- ***Anterior tibial recurrent artery:*** which arises from the anterior tibial artery just after reaching the anterior compartment. It also ascends up to share in the anastomoses around the knee joint. It accompanies the recurrent genicular nerve.

3- ***Muscular branches:*** to the muscles of the anterior compartment.

4- ***Anterior medial malleolar artery:*** which descends to the medial side of the ankle joint, sharing in the anastomoses around the ankle.

5- ***Anterior lateral malleolar artery:*** which descends to the lateral side of the ankle joint. This artery anastomoses with the perforating branch of peroneal artery and shares in the anastomoses around the ankle.

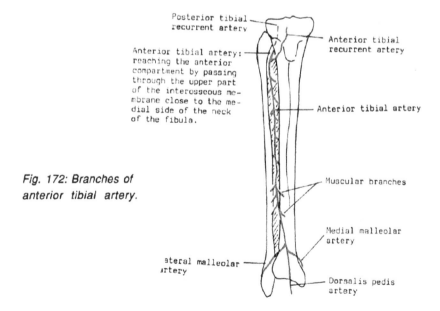

Fig. 172: Branches of anterior tibial artery.

Surface anatomy: The anterior tibial artery corresponds to a line which begins one inch below and medial to the head of the fibula to a point in front of the ankle joint midway between the two malleoli.

Deep Peroneal Nerve

Origin: The deep peroneal (anterior tibial) nerve is the larger of the two terminal branches of the common peroneal (lateral popliteal) nerve. It takes origin close to the lateral side of the neck of the fibula deep to the peroneus longus muscle.

Courseandrelations intheleg: Thenervepiercestheanteriorintermuscular septum to reach the anterior compartment. It passes through the extensor digitorum longus and then descends deeply in front of the interosseous membrane close to the anterior tibial vessels. At first it lies between the extensor digitorum longus and tibialis anterior and then between the extensor hallucis longus and tibialis anterior.

In the lower part of the leg, the nerve and vessels are crossed by the extensor hallucis longus from the lateral to medial side (fig. 171). As previously described, the nerve is lateral to the vessels in the upper third of the leg and anterior to the vessels in the middle third of the leg (fig. 170). In the lower third of the leg, the nerve returns lateral to the vessels once more. Rarely, the nerve crosses in front of the vessels to descend on their medial side.

In the lower part of the leg, the nerve becomes superficial where it lies deep to the superior extensor retinaculum between the tibialis anterior, extensor hallucis longus and anterior tibial vessels medially and the extensor digitorum longus and peroneus tertius laterally (fig. 174).

The nerve crosses the front of the ankle joint to continue into the dorsum of the foot. Its further course and distribution on the dorsum of the foot are described later.

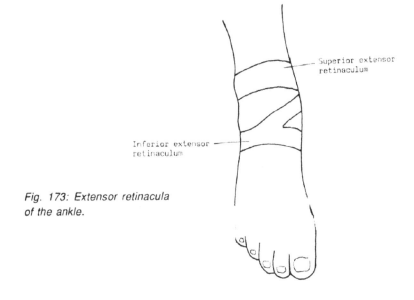

Fig. 173: Extensor retinacula
of the ankle.

Branches in the leg (fig. 179)

1- *Muscular branches:* to the muscles of the anterior compartment: tibialis anterior, extensor hallucis longus, extensor digitorum longus and peroneus tertius.

2- *Articular branches:* to the ankle joint.

Surface anatomy: The deep peroneal nerve corresponds nearly to the line of the anterior tibial artery (See page 144).

Superior Extensor Retinaculum

This is a thickened band of the deep fascia on the lower part of the front of the leg (fig. 173). It is one inch or more in breadth with its medial end attached to the lower part of the anterior border of the tibia and its lateral end attached to the anterior margin of the triangular subcutaneous area on the lateral side of the lower part of the shaft of the fibula.

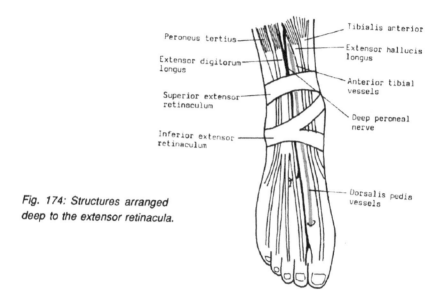

Fig. 174: Structures arranged deep to the extensor retinacula.

The structures passing deep to the superior extensor retinaculum are arranged from the medial to the lateral side as follows (fig. 174):

1- Tibialis anterior.

2- Extensor hallucis longus. 3- Anterior tibial vessels.

3- Deep peroneal (Anterior tibial) nerve.

4- Extensor digitorum longus and peroneus tertius.

The tendon of tibialis anterior and its synovial sheath actually pass through a tunnel formed by splitting of the retinaculum and not deep to the retinaculum.

DORSUM OF THE FOOT

Cutaneous Nerve Supply

Saphenous nerve: supplies the medial part of the dorsum of the foot and the medial border of the foot. This nerve stops short of the big toe (fig. 175).

Medial branch of deep peroneal (anterior tibial) nerve: Its terminal part pierces the deep fascia at the first interdigital cleft and divides to supply the adjacent sides of the big toe and second toe.

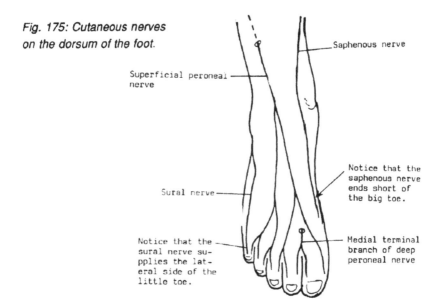

Fig. 175: Cutaneous nerves on the dorsum of the foot.

Saphenous nerve

Superficial peroneal nerve

Notice that the saphenous nerve ends short of the big toe.

Sural nerve

Notice that the sural nerve supplies the lateral side of the little toe.

Medial terminal branch of deep peroneal nerve

Superficial peroneal (Musculocutaneous) nerve: Supplies the greater intermediate part of the dorsum of the foot. Its terminal branches give dorsal digital nerves to all toes except the adjacent sides of the big toe and second toe and the lateral side of the little toe.

Sural nerve: supplies the lateral part of the dorsum of the foot, lateral border of the foot and lateral side of the little toe.

Dorsal Venous arch

This is an irregular transverse venous channel in the superficial fascia across the distal part of the dorsum of the foot, superficial to the terminal branches of the superficial peroneal nerve (fig. 72).

It receives dorsal digital veins from the toes. Its medial end joins the dorsal digital vein of the medial side of big toe to form the *great saphenous vein*. Its lateral end joins the dorsal digital vein of the lateral side of little toe to form the *small saphenous vein*.

Deep Fascia

On the dorsum of the foot, the deep fascia is characteristically very thin; but just distal to the ankle joint, it is thickened to form the *inferior extensor retinaculum*.

Inferior Extensor Retinaculum

This is a thickening of deep fascia forming a Y-shaped band across the dorsum of the foot just distal to the ankle joint (fig. 173).

The lateral end of the retinaculum (stem of the Y) is attached to the anterior part of the superior surface of the calcaneus. Medially the retinaculum diverges into upper and lower bands. The upper band is attached to the anterior border of the medial malleolus. The lower band fuses with the deep fascia on the medial border of the foot.

The retinaculum is adherent to underlying tarsal bones; but the dorsalis pedis vessels and deep peroneal nerve pass deep to it. However, the retinaculum is split to form three tunnels for the tendons of the muscles of the anterior compartment and their synovial sheaths. The medial tunnel gives passage to the tendon of tibialis anterior and its synovial sheath through the two bands of the retinaculum. The intermediate tunnel gives passage to the tendon of extensor hallucis longus and its synovial sheath through the two bands of the retinaculum. The lateral tunnel gives passage to the tendons of extensor digitorum longus and peroneus tertius through the stem of the retinaculum.

The structures passing through and deep to the inferior extensor retinaculum are arranged from the medial to the lateral side as follows (fig. 174):

1- Tibialis anterior.

2- Extensor hallucis longus. 3- Doralis pedis vessels.

3- Deep peroneal (anterior tibial) nerve.

4- Extensor digitorum longus and peroneus tertius.

Extensor Digitorum Brevis

Origin: from the anterior part of the superior surface of the calcaneus and the stem of the inferior extensor retinaculum (fig. 176).

Insertion: The muscle divides into four slips which give rise to tendons for the medial four toes. The medial slip is called the *extensor hallucis brevis* as it is inserted into the dorsum of the base of the proximal phalanx of the big toe. The tendons of the lateral three slips join the dorsal digital (extensor) expansions of the second, third and fourth toes. Through the expansions, they reach an insertion into the middle and distal phalanges.

From the above description it is clear that the tendons of extensor digitorum brevis reach to the medial four toes while those of the extensor digitorum longus reach to the lateral four toes.

Nerve supply: twigs from the lateral terminal branch of the deep peroneal (anterior tibial) nerve.

Actions: The medial slip (extensor hallucis brevis) extends the metatarsophalangeal joint of the big toe, The lateral three slips extend all joints of the second, third and fourth toes.

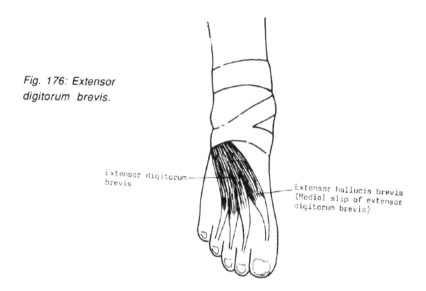

Fig. 176: Extensor digitorum brevis.

Extensor digitorum brevis

Extensor hallucis brevis (Medial slip of extensor digitorum brevis)

Dorsalis Pedis Artery

Origin: continuation of the anterior tibial artery in front of the line of the ankle joint (fig. 177).

Course and relations: It is closely accompanied by the two venae comitantes which continue along the anterior tibial artery. The dorsalis pedis artery runs forwards on the dorsum of the foot in line with the first interdigital cleft.

The artery runs closely medial to the deep peroneal nerve and its medial terminal branch. It is crossed by the inferior extensor retinaculum. The extensor hallucis brevis crosses superficial to it from the lateral to the medial side. So, the distal part of the artery is related medially to tendons of both extensors hallucis longus and brevis.

At the proximal end of the first interosseous space, the dorsalis pedis artery sinks into the sole of the foot by passing between the two heads of the first dorsal interosseous muscle. In the sole of the foot, it ends by anastomosing with the end of the plantar arch.

Branches

1- *Lateral tarsal artery:* which runs laterally on the tarsus. It anastomoses with branches of the anterior lateral malleolar, arcuate, perforating branch of peroneal and lateral plantar arteries.

2- *Medial tarsal arteries:* two or three branches which run medially to the medial border of the foot and share in the *medial malleolar network.* This network is formed by branches of the anterior medial malleolar artery, medial tarsal arteries, malleolar and calcanean branches of posterior tibial artery and medial plantar artery.

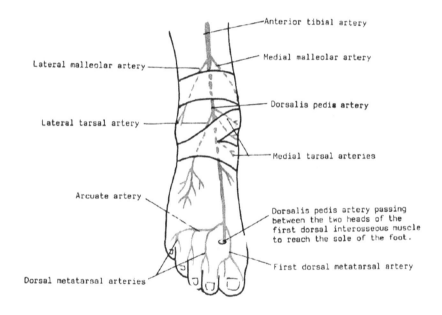

Anterior tibial artery

Medial malleolar artery

Lateral malleolar artery

Dorsalis pedis artery

Lateral tarsal artery

Medial tarsal arteries

Arcuate artery

Dorsalis pedis artery passing between the two heads of the first dorsal interosseous muscle to reach the sole of the foot.

First dorsal metatarsal artery

Dorsal metatarsal arteries

Fig. 177: Dorsalis pedis artery.

3- *Arcuate artery:* is a large branch which runs laterally, following an arched course across the dorsum of the foot on the bases of the metastarsal bones deep to the tendons of extensors digitorum longus and brevis. It gives the following branches:

a- *Second, third and fourth dorsal metatarsal arteries:* which divide into dorsal digital arteries for the adjacent sides of the second, third, fourth and little toes. In addition, the fourth dorsal metatarsal artery gives a dorsal digital branch to the lateral side of the little toe.

b- Branches to the underlying intertarsal and tarsometatarsal joints and the overlying soft tissues.

4- ***First dorsal metatarsal artery:*** which arises from the dorsalis pedis artery just before sinking into the sole of the foot. This artery runs forwards where it gives a dorsal digital artery to the medial side of the big toe and then divides into the dorsal digital arteries for the adjacent sides of the big and second toes.

5- ***First plantar metatarsal artery:*** which arises from the terminal part of the dorsalis pedis artery in the sole of the foot. It has a similar distribution to the first dorsal metatarsal artery. It gives a plantar digital branch to the medial side of the big toe and then divides into two plantar digital arteries for the adjacent sides of the big and second toes (fig. 218).

Surface anatomy: The dorsalis pedis artery corresponds to a line from a point on the front of the ankle midway between both malleoli to a point on the proximal end of the first interosseous space. This line runs along the first interdigital cleft.

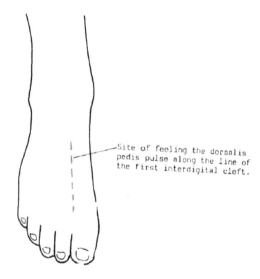

Fig. 178: Site of feeling of the dorsalis pedis pulse.

Site of feeling the dorsalis pedis pulse along the line of the first interdigital cleft.

Applied anatomy: Pulsations of the dorsalis pedis artery are easily felt on the dorsum of the foot where the artery can be effectively compressed by the tips of the fingers in the line of the first interdigital cleft (fig. 178).

Deep Peroneal Nerve

The origin, course, relations and branches of the deep peroneal (anterior tibial) nerve in the anterior compartment of the leg were described on page 144 (fig. 179).

Course and relations on the dorsum of the foot: It continues forwards on the dorsum of the foot close to the lateral side of the dorsalis pedis vessels deep to the inferior extensor retinaculum. The nerve and vessels run between the extensor hallucis longus medially and extensor digitorum longus laterally.

Just beyond the inferior extensor retinaculum, the nerve terminates by dividing into medial and lateral terminal branches (fig. 180):

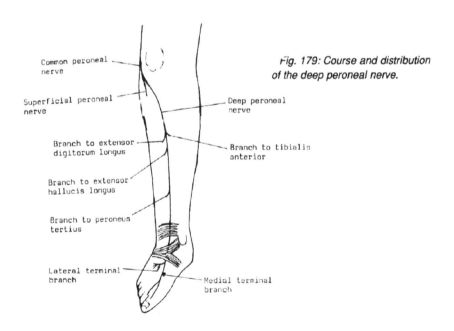

Common peroneal nerve

Superficial peroneal nerve

Branch to extensor digitorum longus

Branch to extensor hallucis longus

Branch to peroneus tertius

Lateral terminal branch

Fig. 179: Course and distribution of the deep peroneal nerve.

Deep peroneal nerve

Branch to tibialis anterior

Medial terminal branch

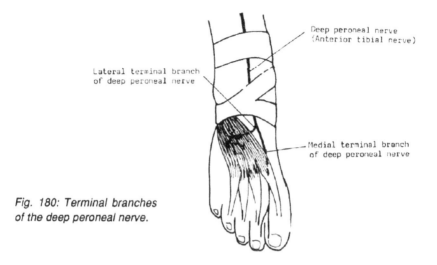

Fig. 180: Terminal branches of the deep peroneal nerve.

A - *Medial terminal branch:* is the continuation of the deep peroneal nerve. It continues forwards on the dorsum of the foot between the tendons of extensor hallucis longus and extensor digitorum longus with the dorsalis pedis artery and its first dorsal metatarsal branch close to the medial side of the nerve. It is crossed by the extensor hallucis brevis from the lateral to the medial side. Along its course, it gives articular twigs to the tarsometatarsal and metatarsophalangeal joints of the big toe. Then, it pierces the deep fascia near the first interdigital cleft and divides into two dorsal digital branches for the adjacent sides of the big and second toes. It usually gives an additional muscular twig to the first dorsal interosseous muscle.

B - *Lateral terminal branch:* deviates laterally deep to the extensor digitorum brevis where it terminates in a gangliform expansion which gives muscular twigs to the extensor digitorum brevis and articular twigs to the intertarsal and tarsometatarsal joints. It usually gives an additional muscular twig to the second dorsal interosseous muscle.

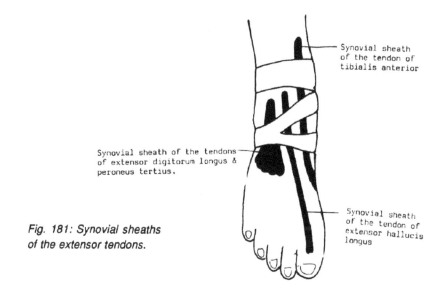

Synovial sheath
of the tendon of
tibialis anterior

Synovial sheath of the tendons
of extensor digitorum longus &
peroneus tertius.

Synovial sheath
of the tendon of
extensor hallucis
longus

*Fig. 181: Synovial sheaths
of the extensor tendons.*

Synovial Sheaths of the Extensor Tendons

The tendons of the extensor muscles, as they pass deep to and through the two extensor retinacula, are surrounded by tubular synovial sheaths to facilitate their movements. These sheaths are (fig. 181):

1- *Synovial sheath of tibialis anterior:* surrounds its tendon from the upper border of the superior extensor retinaculum to the insertion of the muscle.

2- *Synovial sheath of extensor hallucis longus:* surrounds its tendon from the lower border of the superior extensor retinaculum to the base of the big toe.

3- *Synovial sheath of extensor digitorum longus and peroneus tertius:* surrounds their tendons from the lower border of the superior extensor retinaculum to the middle of the dorsum of the foot.

Dorsal Digital (Extensor) Expansions of the Toes

The tendons of extensor digitorum longus and brevis fuse together on the dorsum of the proximal phalanges of the second, third and fourth toes to form the *dorsal digital (extensor) expansions* of the toes (fig. 182).

In addition, each expansion receives the tendons of one lumbrical and two interossei muscles from the sole of the foot, reaching the expansion by passing obliquely across the sides of the metatarsophalangeal joints.

The expansion divides into three slips. The middle slip is inserted into the base of the middle phalanx. The two collateral slips join together to be inserted into the base of the terminal phalanx.

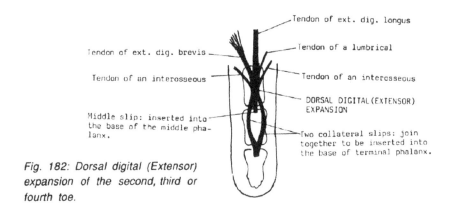

Fig. 182: Dorsal digital (Extensor) expansion of the second, third or fourth toe.

The extensor expansion of the little toe is formed only by a tendon from the extensor digitorum longus and receives the tendon of one lumbrical and only one interosseous muscle. So instead of five tendons, the extensor expansion of the little toe is formed only by three tendons. But, it divides into three slips like those of the second, third and fourth toes.

According to this pattern of insertion, the extensor expansion can extend the interphalangeal and metatarsophalangeal joints of each of the lateral four toes.

The big toe has no extensor expansion. The base of its terminal phalanx receives the insertion of the extensor hallucis longus. The base of its proximal phalanx receives the insertion of the extensor hallucis brevis.

LATERAL COMPARTMENT OF THE LEG

Contents

1- Peroneus longus (fig. 183).

2- Peroneus brevis.

3- Superficial peroneal (Musculocutaneous) nerve.

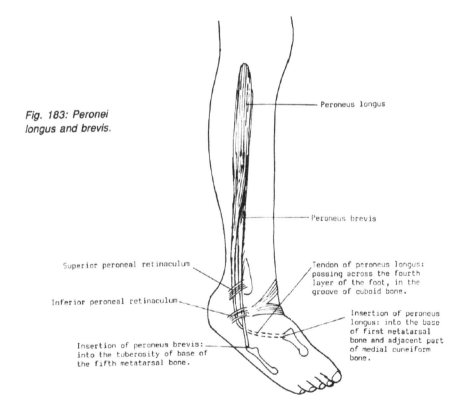

Fig. 183: Peronei longus and brevis.

Peroneus longus

Peroneus brevis

Superior peroneal retinaculum

Inferior peroneal retinaculum

Insertion of peroneus brevis: into the tuberosity of base of the fifth metatarsal bone.

Tendon of peroneus longus: passing across the fourth layer of the foot, in the groove of cuboid bone.

Insertion of peroneus longus: into the base of first metatarsal bone and adjacent part of medial cuneiform bone.

Peroneus Longus

Origin: from the upper two-thirds of the lateral (peroneal) surface of the shaft of the fibula extending up to its head (fig. 184).

Insertion: It gives rise to a tendon in the lower part of the leg. The tendon overlaps the peroneus brevis and descends behind the lateral malleolus deep to the superior peroneal retinaculum with the tendon of peroneus brevis between it and the bone (fig. 184). Then it passes below the lateral malleolus deep to the inferior peroneal retinaculum on the lateral surface of the calcaneus.

Then the tendon deviates medially to reach the sole of the foot where it runs medially and forwards in the groove on the plantar surface of the cuboid bone to reach its insertion into the lateral side of the base of the first metatarsal bone and adjacent part of the medial cuneiform bone (fig. 183). The tendon forms one of the contents of the fourth layer of the sole.

Nerve supply: superficial peroneal (musculocutaneous) nerve.

Actions: plantar flexion and eversion of the foot. It plays an important role is supporting the transverse arch of the foot.

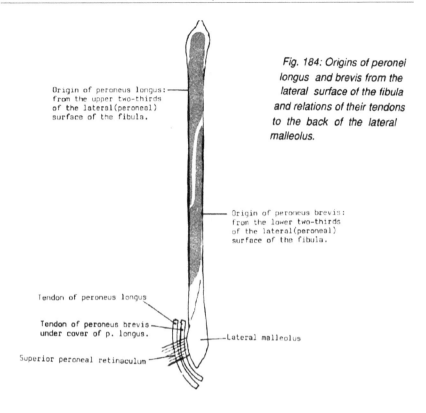

Origin of peroneus longus:
from the upper two-thirds
of the lateral(peroneal)
surface of the fibula.

Fig. 184: Origins of peronei longus and brevis from the lateral surface of the fibula and relations of their tendons to the back of the lateral malleolus.

Origin of peroneus brevis:
from the lower two-thirds
of the lateral(peroneal)
surface of the fibula.

Tendon of peroneus longus

Tendon of peroneus brevis
under cover of p. longus.

Superior peroneal retinaculum

Lateral malleolus

Peroneus Brevis

Origin: from the lower two-thirds of the lateral (peroneal) surface of the fibula. This means that the middle third of the lateral surface is common for both peronei longus and brevis (fig. 184).

Insertion: Its tendon descends closely behind the lateral malleolus grooving the bone deep to the tendon of peroneus longus and under cover of the superior peronea! retinaculum (fig. 184). Then, it passes below the lateral malleolus on the lateral surface of the calcaneus deep to the inferior peroneal retinaculum to reach an insertion into the tuberosity of the base of fifth metatarsal bone (fig. 183).

Nerve supply: superficial peroneal nerve.

Actions: plantar flexion and eversion of the foot.

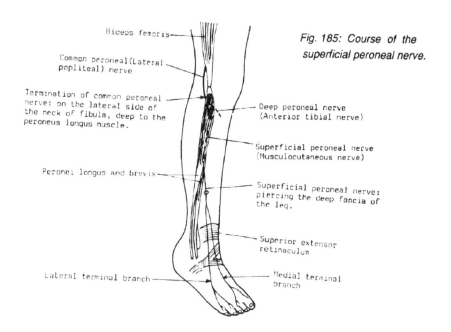

Fig. 185: Course of the superficial peroneal nerve.

Superficial Peroneal Nerve

Origin: The superficial peroneal (musculocutaneous) nerve is the smaller of the two terminal branches of the common peronea! (lateral popliteal) nerve (fig. 185). It takes origin close to the lateral side of the neck of the fibula under cover of the peroneous longus.

Course and relations: The nerve first descends through the substance of the peroneus longus and then between the peronei longus and brevis. Then, it emerges between the two muscles and descends under cover of the deep fascia. In the lower part of the leg it pierces the deep fascia where it becomes subcutaneous. It divides into medial and lateral terminal branches which descend superficial to both extensor retinacula to the dorsum of the foot where they give terminal dorsal digital branches.

Branches (figs. 185, 186)
A - *Muscular branches:* which supply the peronei longus and brevis.

B - *Cutaneous branches:* to the lower part of the front of the leg.

C - *Medial terminal branch:* with the lateral terminal branch, they give
     cutaneous branches to the lower part of the front of the leg and the

intermediate part of the dorsum of the foot. Then, it divides into two dorsal digital branches: a branch for the medial side of the big toe and a branch for the adjacent sides of the second and third toes (fig. 175).

D - *Lateral terminal branch:* with the medial terminal branch, they give cutaneous branches to the lower part of the front of the leg and the intermediate part of the dorsum of the foot. Then, it divides into two dorsal digital branches: a branch for the adjacent sides of the third and fourth toes and a branch for the adjacent sides of the fourth and little toes (fig. 175).

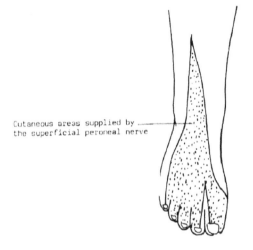

Cutaneous areas supplied by
the superficial peroneal nerve

Fig. 186: Cutaneous distribution of the superficial peroneal nerve.

Peroneal retinacula

These are two thickenings of deep fascia in the form of fibrous bands overlaping the tendons of peronei longus and brevis behind and below the lateral malleolus (fig. 187).

Superior peroneal retinaculum: lies behind the lateral malleolus and extends from the lateral malleolus to the lateral surface of the calcaneous. The tendons of both peronei longus and brevis pass deep to the retinaculum surrounded by a single synovial sheath.

Inferior peroneal retinaculum: lies below the lateral malleolus. Superiorly, it is attached to the anterior part of the superior surface of the calcaneous where it is continuous with the stem of the inferior extensor retinaculum.

Inferiorly, it is attached to the lateral surface of the calcaneus. The deep surface of the retinaculum is attached to the peroneal tubercle of calcaneus by a fibrous septum. Accordingly, the space deep to the retinaculum is divided into two compartments. The superior compartment transmits the tendon of peroneus brevis and its synovial sheath. The inferior compartment transmits the tendon of peroneus longus and its synovial sheath.

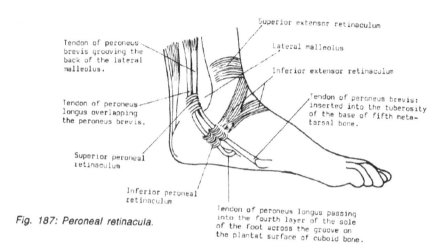

Fig. 187: Peroneal retinacula.

Synovial Sheaths of the Peronei Longus And Brevis

The tendons of peronei longus and brevis are surrounded by a single tubular synovial sheath deep to the superior peroneal retinaculum (fig. 188). This sheath begins slightly above the superior peroneal retinaculum. Just below the superior peroneal retinaculum, the synovial sheath divides into two sheaths, one surrounding each tendon separately deep to the inferior peroneal retinaculum. The two sheaths surround the tendons of peronei longus and brevis as far as their insertions (fig. 189).

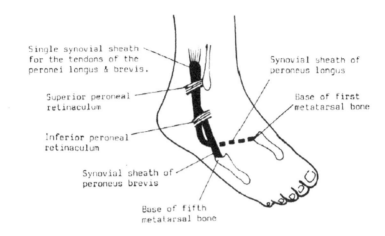

Fig. 188: Synovial sheaths of the peronei longus and brevis - Lateral view.

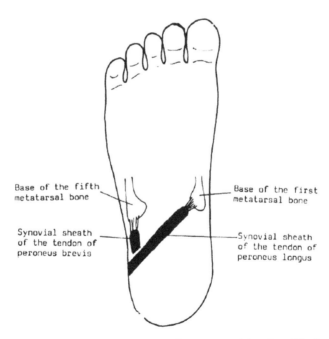

Fig. 189: Synovial sheaths of the peronei longus and brevis - Plantar view.

POSTERIOR COMPARTMENT OF THE LEG

Divisions and Contents

The posterior compartment is divided by the *first septum of deep fascia* into superficial and deep parts (fig. 165):

The **superficial part** contains three muscles:
1- Gastrocnemius.
2- Plantaris.
3- Soleus.

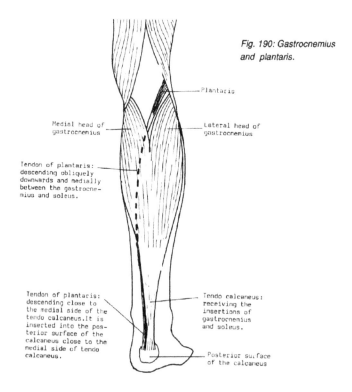

Fig. 190: Gastrocnemius and plantaris.

Plantaris

Medial head of gastrocnemius

Lateral head of gastrocnemius

Tendon of plantaris: descending obliquely downwards and medially between the gastrocnemius and soleus.

Tendon of plantaris: descending close to the medial side of the tendo calcaneus. It is inserted into the posterior surface of the calcaneus close to the medial side of tendo calcaneus.

Tendo calcaneus: receiving the insertions of gastrocnemius and soleus.

Posterior surface of the calcaneus

The ***deep part*** contains:

1- Posterior tibial vessels and their branches and tributaries.

2- Tibial (Posterior tibial) nerve.

3- Popliteus.

4- Flexor hallucis longus.

5- Flexor digitorum longus.

6- Tibialis posterior.

The *second septum of deep fascia* covers the tibialis posterior and separates it from the other deep muscles (fig. 165).

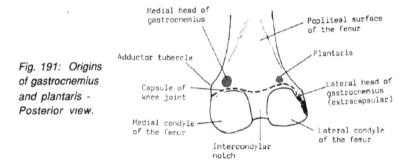

Fig. 191: Origins of gastrocnemius and plantaris - Posterior view.

Gastrocnemius

Origin: by two heads (figs. 190, 191 and 192):

1- ***Medial head:*** from the popliteal surface of the femur just above the medial condyle (fig. 191). This head is separated from the capsule of knee joint by a bursa which may communicate with the semimembranosus bursa (See page 119).

2- ***Lateral head:*** from an impression on the lateral surface of the lateral condyle of the femur just above and behind the lateral epicondyle (figs, 191, 192). This head usually contains a sesamoid bone called the fabella close to the lateral condyle of the femur.

The two heads are tendinous at their origin, but they expand into two fleshy bellies which remain separate and form aponeurotic tendons which join the tendon of soleus to form the *tendo calcaneus.*

Insertion: by the *tendo calcaneus* into the middle of the posterior surface of the calcaneus. A bursa and some fat separate the tendo calcaneus from the smooth upper part of the posterior surface of the calcaneus (fig. 193).

Nerve supply: by a branch for each head from the tibial (medial popliteal) nerve in the popliteal fossa.

Actions: Plantar flexion of the foot. It is also a flexor of the knee joint.

Plantaris

Origin: from the popliteal surface of the femur just above the lateral condyle (fig. 191).

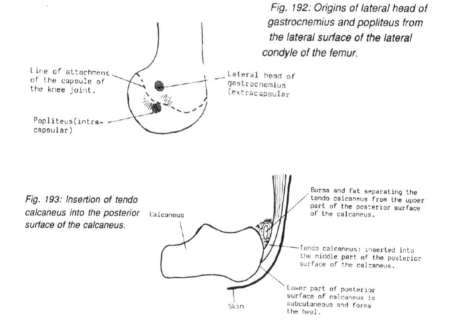

Fig. 192: Origins of lateral head of gastrocnemius and popliteus from the lateral surface of the lateral condyle of the femur.

Line of attachment of the capsule of the knee joint.

Lateral head of gastrocnemius (extracapsular

Popliteus(intra-capsular)

Fig. 193: Insertion of tendo calcaneus into the posterior surface of the calcaneus.

Calcaneus

Bursa and fat separating the tendo calcaneus from the upper part of the posterior surface of the calcaneus.

Tendo calcaneus: inserted into the middle part of the posterior surface of the calcaneus.

Lower part of posterior surface of calcaneus is subcutaneous and forms the heel.

Skin

Insertion: It is a small muscle which descends close to the medial side of the lateral head of gastrocnemius. Its small and short belly gives rise to a long slender tendon which descends obliquely downwards and medially between the gastrocnemius and soleus. The tendon then descends close to the medial side of the tendo calcaneus to be inserted into the posterior surface of the calcaneus (figs. 190, 194).

Nerve supply: by a branch from the tibial (medial popliteal) nerve in the popliteal fossa.

Actions: Plantar flexion of the foot. It also helps in flexion of the knee.

Applied anatomy: Avulsion of the tendon of plantaris may occur during running leading to a sudden and severe pain in the lower part of the calf.

Soleus

Origin: It is a strong bulky muscle which has a continuous origin from (figs. 194, 195):

1- The upper third of the posterior surface of the fibula, extending up to its head.

2- The tendinous arch between the head of the fibula and the upper end of the soleal line of the tibia. This arch bridges over the posterior tibial vessels and tibial nerve as they descend to the posterior compartment.

3- Soleal line of the tibia.

4- Middle third of the medial border of the tibia.

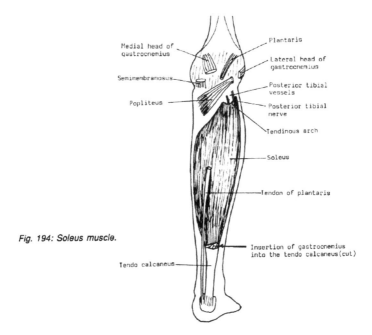

Fig. 194: Soleus muscle.

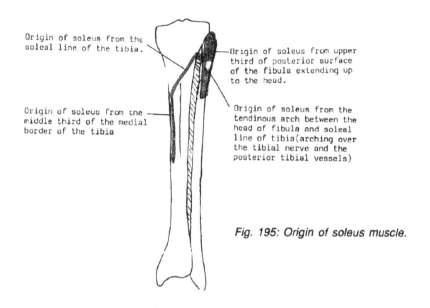

Origin of soleus from the soleal line of the tibia.

Origin of soleus from upper third of posterior surface of the fibula extending up to the head.

Origin of soleus from the middle third of the medial border of the tibia

Origin of soleus from the tendinous arch between the head of fibula and soleal line of tibia(arching over the tibial nerve and the posterior tibial vessels)

Fig. 195: Origin of soleus muscle.

Insertion: by a strong tendon with the gastrocnemius into the *tendo calcaneus.* As previously described, the tendo calcaneus is inserted into the middle of the posterior surface of the calcaneus (fig. 193).

Nerve supply: The muscle has a double nerve supply from the tibial nerve. Its superficial surface receives a branch from the tibial (medial popliteal) nerve in the popliteal fossa. Its deep surface receives a branch from the tibial (posterior tibial) nerve in the leg.

Action: It is a powerful plantar flexor of the foot.

Posterior tibial artery

Origin: is the larger of the two terminal branches of the popliteal artery at the distal border of popliteus (fig. 159).

Course and relations: The artery descends with a slight medial inclination and is closely accompanied by two venae comitantes (fig. 196). It first descends deep to the tendinous arch between the two bones and then deep to the soleus and first septum of deep fascia. In the lower part of the leg, the artery becomes superficial where it is only covered by the skin superficial fascia and deep fascia.

As it descends, the artery lies on the following structures from above downwards: tibialis posterior, flexor digitorum longus, lower part of the posterior surface of the tibia and back of ankle joint.

In the upper part of the leg, the tibial nerve descends close to the medial side of the artery. But after a short course, the nerve crosses behind the artery and descends close to the lateral side of the artery for the greater part of its course.

The posterior tibial artery terminates deep to the flexor retinaculum by dividing into medial and lateral plantar arteries.

Branches (fig. 197)

1- *Circumflex fibular artery:* a small branch which encircles the neck of the fibula deep to the soleus muscle and anastomoses the inferior lateral genicular artery. However, it may arise from the anterior tibial artery.

2- *Peroneal artery:* is the largest branch of the posterior tibial artery. It is described later (See page 168).

3- *Nutrient artery to the tibia:* which enters the tibia just below the soleal line and close to the vertical line.

4- *Muscular branches:* to the deep muscles and soleus.

5- *Communicating branch:* which runs a transverse course, connecting the posterior tibial and peroneal arteries two inches above the ankle.

6- *Malleolar branch:* which anastomoses with the anterior medial malleolar and medial tarsal arteries to form the medial malleolar network.

7- *Calcanean branches:* which ramify on the back of the tendo calcaeus and the heel. They anastomose with the calcanean branches of the peroneal artery.

8- *Terminal branches:* which are the medial and lateral plantar arteries (described later).

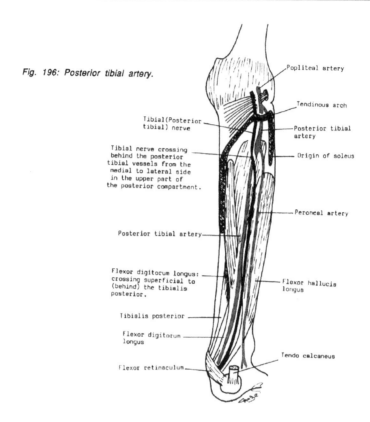

Fig. 196: Posterior tibial artery.

Surface anatomy: The posterior tibial artery corresponds to a line which extends from a point on the middle line of the calf at the level of the tibial tuberosity to a point midway between the medial malleolus and medial border of the heel.

Applied anatomy: Pulsations of the posterior tibial artery are felt by deep pressure to compress the artery by the tips of the fingers against the lower end of the tibia along a line midway between the medial malleolus and medial border of the heel (fig. 198).

Peroneal Artery

Origin: from the upper part of the posterior tibial artery, one inch below the distal border of popliteus (fig. 196). It is the largest branch of the posterior tibial artery and may be larger than its parent trunk. Sometimes, it arises from the lower end of the popliteal artery.

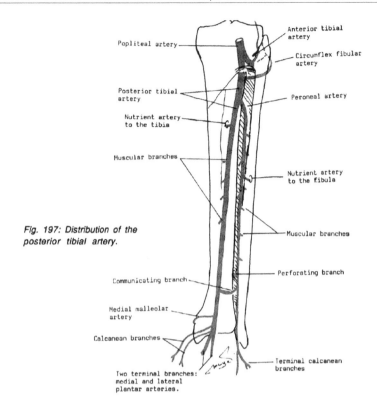

Fig. 197: Distribution of the posterior tibial artery.

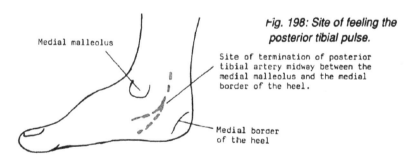

Fig. 198: Site of feeling the posterior tibial pulse.

Medial malleolus

Site of termination of posterior tibial artery midway between the medial malleolus and the medial border of the heel.

Medial border of the heel

Course and relations: It first descends downwards and laterally towards the fibula. Then, it descends vertically along the medial crest of the fibula closely accompanied by two venae comitantes.

It descends deep to the soleus and first septum of deep fascia and then deep to the flexor hallucis longus. Behind the inferior tibiofibular joint, it ends by giving terminal calcanean branches.

Branches (fig. 197)

1- *Muscular branches:* to the peronei longus and brevis, soleus, tibialis posterior and flexor hallucis longus.

2- *Nutrient aretry to the fibula:* which enters into the posterior surface of the fibula close to the medial crest.

3- *Perforating branch:* an important and large branch which passes through a hole in the interosseous membrane two inches above the ankle joint to reach the anterior compartment. It anastomoses with the anterior lateral malleolar artery and descends to the dorsum of the foot where it supplies the tarsus and intertarsal joints, and anastomoses with the lateral tarsal artery. It may be large enough to replace the dorsalis pedis artery when the latter is absent.

4- *Communicating branch:* which as previously described connects the peroneal and posterior tibial arteries two inches above the ankle.

5- *Terminal calcanean branches:* which run on the lateral surface of the calcaneus and anastomose with the anterior lateral malleolar artery. Some branches pass to the heel where they anastomose with the calcanean branches of the posterior tibial artery.

Tibial Nerve

Origin: As previously described, it is the larger of the two terminal branches of the sciatic nerve (See page 120).

Course and relations in the leg: The tibial nerve crosses the distal border of popliteus and continues into the posterior compartment of the leg (fig. 196). It descends deep to the tendinous arch between the two bones and then deep to the soleus and first septum of deep fascia close to the posterior tibial vessels. In the upper part of the leg, the nerve is medial to the vessels; but soon it crosses behind the vessels to descend lateral to the vessels for the greater part of its course (fig. 196).

As it descends, the nerve lies on the following structures in order: tibialis posterior, flexor digitorum longus, lower part of the posterior surface of the tibia and back of the ankle joint.

In the distal part of the leg, the nerve becomes relatively superficial, being only covered by the skin, superficial fascia and deep fascia. Deep to the flexor retinaculum, it terminates by dividing into medial and lateral plantar nerves.

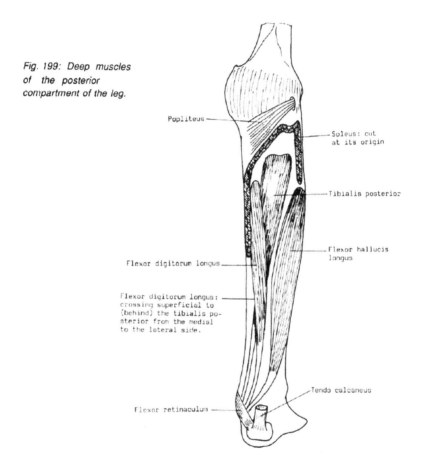

Fig. 199: Deep muscles of the posterior compartment of the leg.

Popliteus

Soleus: cut at its origin

Tibialis posterior

Flexor hallucis longus

Flexor digitorum longus

Flexor digitorum longus: crossing superficial to (behind) the tibialis posterior from the medial to the lateral side.

Tendo calcaneus

Flexor retinaculum

Branches in the posterior compartment

1- *Muscular branches:* to the soleus (through its deep surface), flexor digitorum longus, flexor hallucis longus and tibialis posterior.

2- *Medial calcanean nerves:* pierce the flexor retinaculum to supply the skin of the heel and the medial and posterior part of the sole.

3- *Vascular branches:* which are sympathetic twigs to the posterior tibial artery and its branches.

4- *Articular branch:* to the ankle joint.

5- *Terminal branches:* medial and lateral plantar nerves (described later).

Surface anatomy: The tibial nerve in the leg can be represented by a line which begins from a point on the middle line of the calf at the level of the tibial tuberosity. This line extends downwards and medially to a point midway between the medial malleolus and medial border of the heel.

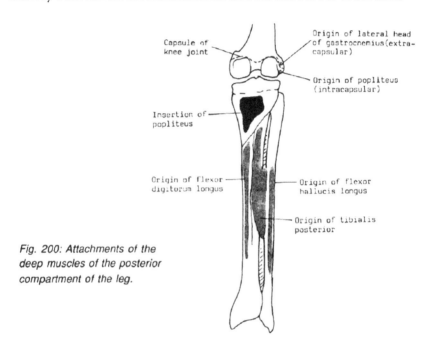

Fig. 200: Attachments of the deep muscles of the posterior compartment of the leg.

Popliteus

Origin: by a tendon from the anterior part of the groove on the lateral surface of the lateral condyle of the femur below the lateral epicondyle. This origin lies inside the capsule of knee joint (intracapsular) (figs. 192, 199 and 200).

Insertion: The tendon of origin passes out through an opening in the posterolateral aspect of the capsule of knee joint and spreads downwards and medially into a triangular fleshy muscle which is inserted into the posterior surface of the tibia above the soleal line and to the strong fascia covering the popliteus muscle.

Nerve supply: by a branch from the tibial (medial popliteal) nerve in the popliteal fossa. The nerve to popliteus descends over the fascia covering the muscle and then hooks on the distal border of popliteus to supply the muscle through its deep surface (fig. 201).

Actions: flexion of the knee joint. At the start of flexion of the extended knee, the popliteus produces a small amount of medial rotation of the leg or lateral rotation of the femur on the tibia which is referred to as *"unlocking of the knee joint".*

Fig. 201: Course of the nerve to popliteus.

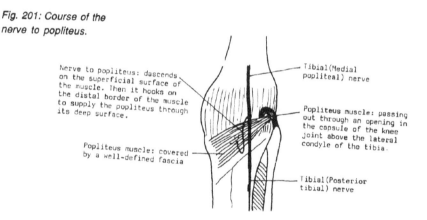

Nerve to popliteus: descends on the superficial surface of the muscle. Then it hooks on the distal border of the muscle to supply the popliteus through its deep surface.

Popliteus muscle: covered by a well-defined fascia

Tibial(Medial popliteal) nerve

Popliteus muscle: passing out through an opening in the capsule of the knee joint above the lateral condyle of the tibia.

Tibial(Posterior tibial) nerve

Flexor Digitorum Longus

Origin: from the posterior surface of the tibia below the soleal line and medial to the vertical line (fig. 200).

Insertion: It gives a tendon which descends to the lower part of the leg where it crosses superficial to (behind) the tendon of tibialis posterior from the medial to lateral side (fig. 149). Then, it descends deep to the flexor retinaculum to the sole of the foot (fig. 202). It is one of the contents of the second layer of the sole where it divides into four tendons which are inserted into the bsaes of the terminal phalanges of the lateral four toes.

Nerve supply: tibial (posterior tibial) nerve.

Actions: flexion of the interphalangeal and metatarsophalangeal joints of the lateral four toes. It is also a plantar flexor and helps in inversion of the foot. It helps in supporting the longitudinal arch of the foot.

Flexor Hallucis Longus

Origin: from the lower two-thirds of the posterior surface of the fibula below the origin of soleus and lateral to the medial crest and tibialis posterior (fig. 200).

Insertion: It is a circumpennate muscle; its fibers converging into a strong central tendon above the ankle. The tendon grooves the posterior surface of the talus (fig. 61) and then descends deep to the flexor retinaculum lateral to the tendons of tibialis posterior and flexor digitorum longus (fig. 202). The tendon passes into the sole of the foot, grooving the inferior surface of the sustentaculum tali (fig. 61). Then it continues into the second layer of the sole to be inserted into the base the terminal phalanx of the big toe.

Nerve supply: tibial (posterior tibial) nerve.

Actions: flexion of the interphalangeal and metatarsophlangeal joints of the big toe. It is a plantar flexor and helps in inversion of the foot. It also helps in supporting the longitudinal arch of the foot.

Tibialis Posterior

Origin: from the posterior surface of the tibia below the soleal line and lateral to the vertical line; from the posterior surface of the fibula medial to the medial crest and from the interosseus membrane (fig. 200).

Insertion: The muscle gives a strong tendon which descends downwards and medially where it crosses deep to the flexor digitorum longus from the lateral to medial side (fig. 199). Then, it descends close to the back of the medial malleolus grooving the bone and passing deep to the flexor retinaculum (fig. 202). It reaches the sole of the foot in the fourth layer where it divides into slips which are inserted into all tarsal bones except the talus and to the bases of the second, third and fourth metatarsal bones; the main insertion is into the tuberosity of navicular bone. Details of the insertion are described later.

Nerve supply: tibial (posterior tibial) nerve.

Actions: It is a strong plantar flexor and invertor of the foot. It plays a very important role in supporting the longitudinal arch of the foot.

NB.: As previously described plantar flexion occurs in the ankle joint while inversion occurs in the talocalcaneonavicular joint (See page 141).

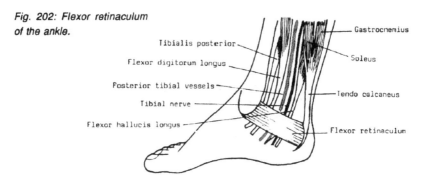

Fig. 202: Flexor retinaculum of the ankle.

Tibialis posterior
Flexor digitorum longus
Posterior tibial vessels
Tibial nerve
Flexor hallucis longus
Gastrocnemius
Soleus
Tendo calcaneus
Flexor retinaculum

Flexor Retinaculum

This is a thickening of deep fascia, forming a band behind and below the lateral malleolus (fig. 202). It extends from the posterior border of the medial malleolus to the medial tubercle of calcaneus.

The medial calcanean vessels and nerves pierce the retinaculum before their distribution.

Two septa of deep fascia divide the space deep to the retinaculum into three compartments for the tendons and their synovial sheaths.

The following structures pass deep to the flexor retinaculum arranged from the medial to the lateral side (fig. 202):

1- Tibialis posterior.

2- Flexor digitorum longus.

3- Terminal parts of the posterior tibial vessels and beginning of medial and lateral plantar vessels.

4- Terminal part of the tibial (posterior tibial) nerve and beginning of medial and lateral plantar nerves.

5- Flexor hallucis longus.

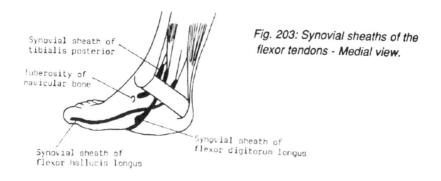

Synovial sheath of
tibialis posterior

Tuberosity of
navicular bone

Synovial sheath of
flexor hallucis longus

Synovial sheath of
flexor digitorum longus

*Fig. 203: Synovial sheaths of the
flexor tendons - Medial view.*

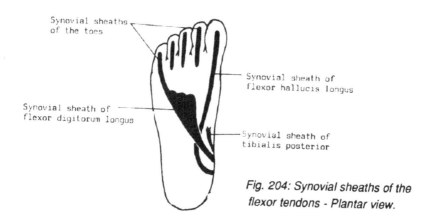

Synovial sheaths
of the toes

Synovial sheath of
flexor digitorum longus

Synovial sheath of
flexor hallucis longus

Synovial sheath of
tibialis posterior

*Fig. 204: Synovial sheaths of the
flexor tendons - Plantar view.*

Synovial Sheaths of the Flexor Tendons

There are three synovial sheaths which surround the tendons of the muscles deep to the flexor retinaculum (figs. 203, 204). The three sheaths start one inch above the flexor retinaculum.

- The *synovial sheath of tibialis posterior* extends to the navicular bone.
- The *synovial sheath of flexor digitorum longus* extends to the middle of the sole.
- The *synovial sheath of the flexor hallucis longus* extends to its insertion.

SOLE OF THE FOOT

Cutaneous Nerve Supply

Medial calcanean nerves: which are branches of the tibial (posterior tibial) nerve. They pierce the flexor retinaculum and supply the heel and posetrior part of the sole (fig. 205).

Cutaneous branches of medial plantar nerve: supply the medial two-thirds of the sole.

Plantar digital branches of medial plantar nerve: supply the medial three and half toes.

Cutaneous branches of lateral plantar nerve: supply the lateral third of the sole.

Plantar digital branches of lateral plantar nerve: supply the lateral one half toes.

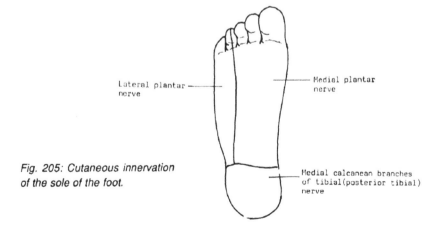

Lateral plantar nerve

Medial plantar nerve

Fig. 205: Cutaneous innervation of the sole of the foot.

Medial calcanean branches of tibial(posterior tibial) nerve

Superficial Fascia

In the sole, the superficial fascia is tough and fibrous; and contains the cutaneous nerves and vessels of the sole in addition to portions of the plantar digital nerves and vessels.

At the roots of the toes, the superficial fascia condenses into a transverse band of fibrous tissue called the *superficial transverse metatarsal ligament.*

Deep Fascia

The deep fascia of the sole is relatively thin over the medial and lateral parts of the sole. But, in the central part of the sole it is markedly thickened to form the *plantar aponeurosis.*

Over the plantar aspects of the toes, the deep fascia is also thickned to form the *fibrous flexor sheaths of the digits.*

Plantar aponeurosis: is a thick fibrous tissue sheet which is attached posteriorly to the calcanean tuberosity (fig. 206). Anteriorly, it becomes wider and divides into five slips, one for each toe.

The plantar metatarsal vessels, plantar digital nerves and lumbrical muscles pass between the slips to reach the digits.

Each slip divides into two bands which diverge on the sides of each toe to fuse with the deep fascia on the dorsal aspect of the digit. The distal borders of each two bands fuse with the fibrous flexor sheath of the digit.

Two intermuscular septa spring from the medial and lateral borders of the aponeurosis and pass on the sides of the flexor digitorum brevis into the depth of the sole.

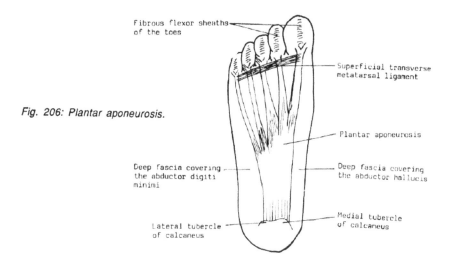

Fig. 206: Plantar aponeurosis.

Fibrous flexor sheaths of the digits: are thickenings of deep fascia overlying the flexor tendons on the plantar aspects of the digits (fig. 206). Each sheath is attached to the margins of the phalanges and interphalangeal joints, thus forming together an osseofibrous tunnel for the flexor tendons and their synovial sheath.

Layers of the Sole

The muscles and tendons in the sole are arranged into four layers which are named first to fourth in a superficial to deep direction. This means that the first layer lies under cover of the plantar aponeurosis and adjacent deep fascia while the fourth layer is close to the plantar aspect of the tarsus and metatarsus.

The plantar vessels and nerves run their course and are distributed in the fascial planes through and between the four layers.

First Layer of Muscles

This layer includes three musles. Arranged mediolaterally, they are: abductor hallucis, flexor digitorum brevis and abductor digiti minimi (fig. 207).

1- ***Abductor hallucis:*** takes origin from the medial tubercle of calcaneus and adjacent part of the flexor retinaculum. It is inserted with the medial part of the flexor hallucis brevis (third layer) into the medial side of the base of the proximal phalanx of the big toe.

It is supplied by the medial plantar nerve. It abducts the big toe from the line of the second toe. The line of the second toe is the axis on which abduction and adduction of the toes occurs.

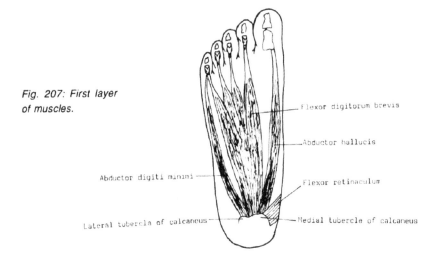

Fig. 207: First layer of muscles.

Flexor digitorum brevis

Abductor hallucis

Abductor digiti minimi

Flexor retinaculum

Lateral tubercle of calcaneus

Medial tubercle of calcaneus

2- **Flexor digitorum brevis:** takes origin from the medial tubercle of calcaneus. It divides into four slips which are inserted by tendons into the margins of the middle phalanges of the lateral four toes. Just before its insertion, each tendon splits to give passage for a tendon of the flexor digitorum longus (fig. 208).

It is supplied by the medial plantar nerve. It is flexor of the proximal interphalangeal and metatarsophalangeal joints of the lateral four toes.

3- **Abductor digiti minimi:** takes origin from both medial and lateral tubercles of the calcaneus. The medial part of its origin is covered by the flexor digitorum brevis. It is inserted with the flexor digiti minimi brevis (third layer) into the lateral side of the base of the proximal phalanx of the little toe. The deeper part of the muscle gains insertion into the base of the fifth metatartasal bone and is sometimes referred to as the *abductor of the fifth metatarsal bone.*

It is supplied by the lateral plantar nerve. It is an abductor of the little toe.

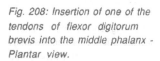

Fig. 208: Insertion of one of the tendons of flexor digitorum brevis into the middle phalanx - Plantar view.

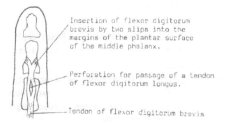

Insertion of flexor digitorum brevis by two slips into the margins of the plantar surface of the middle phalanx.

Perforation for passage of a tendon of flexor digitorum longus.

Tendon of flexor digitorum brevis

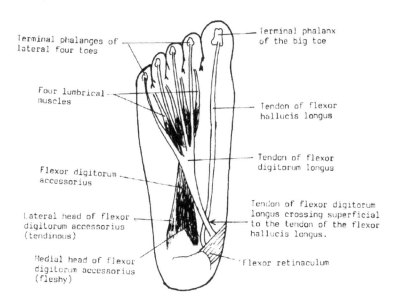

Terminal phalanges of lateral four toes

Four lumbrical muscles

Flexor digitorum accessorius

Lateral head of flexor digitorum accessorius (tendinous)

Medial head of flexor digitorum accessorius (fleshy)

Terminal phalanx of the big toe

Tendon of flexor hallucis longus

Tendon of flexor digitorum longus

Tendon of flexor digitorum longus crossing superficial to the tendon of the flexor hallucis longus.

Flexor retinaculum

Fig. 209: Second layer of muscles.

This layer includes the tendons of flexor digitorum longus and flexor hallucis longus. It also includes the flexor digitorum accessorius and four lumbrical muscles (fig. 209):

1- **Tendon of flexor digitorum longus:** reaches the sole by passing deep to the flexor retinaculum. It passes forwards and laterally, crossing superficial to the tendon of flexor hallucis longus. In the middle of the foot, it divides into four slips which are inserted into the bases of the terminal phalanges of the lateral four toes. As previously described, each slip passes through a perforation in the corresponding tendon of the flexor digitorum brevis to reach its insertion (fig. 210).

Posteriorly, the tendon of flexor digitorum longus receives the insertion of the flexor digitorum accessorius; but anteriorly the slips give origin to the four lumbrical muscles.

2- **Tendon of flexor hallucis longus:** is a thick and strong tendon which reaches the sole by passing deep to the flexor retinaculum. It passes forwards and medially, crossing deep to the tendon of flexor digitorum longus. At the site of crossing, the tendon of flexor hallucis longus gives a slip which joins the tendon of flexor digitorum longus. This lip is usually distributed through the tendon of flexor digitorum longus into the second toe. But this slip is variable in size and may reach to one or more of the other toes.

The tendon of flexor hallucis longus reaches an insertion into the plantar surface of the base of the terminal phalanx of the big toe.

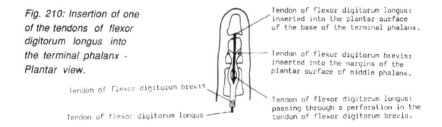

Fig. 210: Insertion of one of the tendons of flexor digitorum longus into the terminal phalanx - Plantar view.

Tendon of flexor digitorum longus: inserted into the plantar surface of the base of the terminal phalanx.

Tendon of flexor digitorum brevis: inserted into the margins of the plantar surface of middle phalanx.

Tendon of flexor digitorum brevis

Tendon of flexor digitorum longus

Tendon of flexor digitorum longus: passing through a perforation in the tendon of flexor digitorum brevis.

3- **Flexor digitorum accessorius:** takes origin by two heads: a *medial fleshy head* from the medial surface of the calcaneus and a *lateral tendinous head* from the lateral margin of the plantar surface of calcaneus. It is inserted into the tendon of flexor digitorum longus.

It is suppplied by the stem of the lateral plantar nerve. As it contracts, it brings the slips of the tendon of flexor digitorum longus more in line with the toes to obtain powerful flexion of the toes. Through its insertion into the tendon of flexor digitorum longus, it is a flexor of the interphalangeal and metatarsophalangeal joints of the lateral four toes.

4- **Lumbrical muscles:** are four slender muscles which take origin from the medial sides of the tendons of the flexor digitorum longus. They are arranged first to fourth from the medial to the lateral side, i.e. an opposite arrangement to the hand. Their tendons pass across the medial sides of the metatarsophalangeal joints to be inserted partly into the bases of the proximal phalanges and partly into the dorsal digital (extensor) expansions of the lateral four toes.

The first lumbrical (medial one) is supplied by the medial plantar nerve while the lateral three are supplied by the deep branch of the lateral plantar nerve. The lumbricals, with the interossei, flex the metatarsophalangeal joints of the lateral four toes. But, through their insertions into the dorsal digital expansions, they extend the interphalangeal joints of the lateral four toes.

Synovial sheaths in the second layer: As previously described, the *synovial sheath of flexor digitorum longus* begins one inch above the flexor retinaculum (See page 173) (figs. 203, 204). This sheath ends about the middle of the sole of the foot.

The *synovial sheath of flexor hallucis longus* also begins one inch above the flexor retinaculum and extends down to the insertion of the tendon (figs. 203, 204).

Synovial sheaths of the lateral four toes: The flexor tendons are surrounded by tubular sheaths in the toes deep to the fibrous flexor sheaths (fig. 204). The synovial sheaths of the second, third and fourth toes are separate sheaths and do not communicate with the sheath of flexor digitorum longus. On the other hand, the synovial sheath of the little toe is continuous with that of the flexor digitorum longus, a similar arrangement to that in the hand.

Fig. 211: Vincula tendinum.

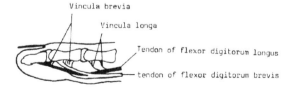

Vincula tendinum: These are small fibrous bands which connect the flexor tendons in the toes with the phalanges. They carry blood supply to the tendons and are differentiated into two types (fig. 211):

a- *Vincula longa:* relatively long and slender fibrous bands connecting the tendons with the proximal phalanges.

b- *Vincula brevia:* short and triangular fibrous bands occuping the angles between the tendons and the bones at the sites of insertion.

Third Layer of Muscles

This layer is comparable to the first layer as it includes three muscles. Arranged mediolaterally, they are: flexor hallucis brevis, adductor hallucis and flexor digiti minimi brevis (fig. 212).

1- *Flexor hallucis brevis:* takes origin from the cuboid bone and adjacent slips of the tendon of tibialis posterior. The muscle then divides into two fleshy parts.

The *medial part* gives a tendon which is inserted with the abductor hallucis (first layer) into the medial side of the base of the proximal phalanx of the big toe.

The *lateral part* gives a tendon which is inserted with the adductor hallucis into the lateral side of the base of the proximal phalanx of the big toe.

Each part contains a *sesamoid bone* which is embedded in it close to the insertion. These sesamoid bones penetrate into the metatarsophalangeal joint of the big toe where they articulate with the head of the first metatarsal bone.

The flexor hallucis brevis is supplied by the medial plantar nerve. It is a flexor of the metatarsophalangeal joint of the big toe.

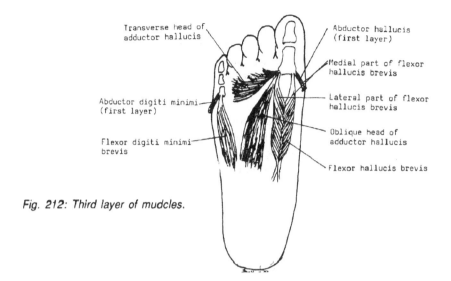

Fig. 212: Third layer of mudcles.

2- **Adductor hallucis:** takes origin by transverse and oblique heads. The *transverse head* is small and arises from the plantar ligaments of the metatarsophalangeal joints of the lateral four toes. The *oblique head* is large and arises from the bases of the second, third and fourth metatarsal bones and from the fibrous sheath covering the peroneus longus tendon. The two heads converge towards an insertion with the lateral part of flexor hallucis brevis into the lateral side of the base of the proximal phalanx of big toe.

It is supplied by the deep branch of the lateral plantar nerve. It is an adductor of the big toe. The transverse head helps in supporting the transverse arch of the foot. The oblique head also helps inflexion of the big toe.

3- **Flexor digiti minimi brevis:** is a small muscle which takes origin from the plantar surface of the base the fifth metatarsal bone and the fibrous sheath of the peroneus longus tendon. It is inserted with the abductor digiti minimi (first layer) into the lateral side of the base of the proximal phalanx of the little toe.

It is supplied by superficial branch of the lateral plantar nerve. It is a flexor of the metatarsophalangeal joint of the little toe.

Fourth Layer of Muscles

This layer is comparable to the second layer. It includes two tendons which are the tendons of peroneus longus and tibialis posterior. It also includes the plantar and dorsal interossei muscles (fig. 213).

1- ***Tendon of peroneus longus:*** passes medially and forwards across the sole of the foot where it is lodged in the groove on the plantar surface of the cuboid bone. It is inserted mainly into the lateral surface of the base of the first metatarsal bone and partly into the adjacent part of the medial cuneiform bone. As previously described, the peroneus longus tendon is surrounded by a synovial sheath which extends to its insertion (fig. 189).

A fbrous sheath bridges over the tendon and its synovial sheath in the groove of cuboid bone. This sheath is an extension of the long plantar ligament which with the groove form an osseofibrous tunnel for the tendon and its synovial sheath.

As the tendon changes its direction to reach the groove, it contains a *sesamoid bone* which plays over a facet on the lateral surface of the cuboid just behind the lateral end of the groove.

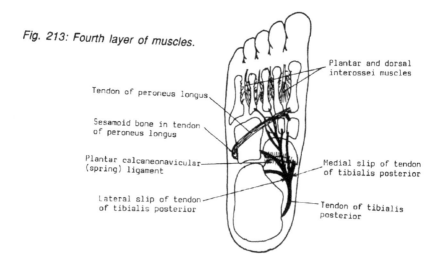

Fig. 213: Fourth layer of muscles.

Tendon of peroneus longus

Sesamoid bone in tendon of peroneus longus

Plantar calcaneonavicular (spring) ligament

Lateral slip of tendon of tibialis posterior

Plantar and dorsal interossei muscles

Medial slip of tendon of tibialis posterior

Tendon of tibialis posterior

2- **Tendon of tibialis posterior:** As it reaches the sole of the foot, it divides into a large medial part and a smaller lateral part. The *medial part* is inserted mainly into the tuberosity of navicular bone and gives a slip to the medial cuneiform bone. The *lateral part* breaks into slips which are inserted into the other tarsal bones except the talus and to the bases of the second, third and fourth metatarsal bones.

To summarize, the tendon of tibialis posterior is inserted into all tarsal bones except the talus and the bases of the second, third and fourth metatarsal bones; mainly into the tuberosity of navicular bone. As previously described, the tendon of tibialis posterior is surrounded by a synovial sheath which extends to the tuberosity of navicular bone (figs. 188, 189).

As the tendon passes to its insertion, it is closely related to the plantar (inferior) surface of the plantar calcaneonavicular (spring) ligament, thus supporting the head of the talus above the ligament in the talocalcaneonavicular joint. In this position, the tendon usually contains a sesamoid bone. The close relation of the tendon to the spring ligament and head of the talus in addition to its main insertion into the tuberosity of navicular bone make the tendon a very important factor in supporting the longitudinal arch of the foot.

3- **Plantar interossei:** are three small muscles which arise from the plantar surfaces of the shafts of the lateral three metatarsal bones (fig. 214). Each muscle arises from the metatarsal bone of the toe on which it acts. They are enumerated first to third from the medial to the lateral side.

The *first plantar interosseous* arises from the third metatarsal bone and is inserted into the base of the proximal phalanx of the third toe and partly into its dorsal digital (extensor) expansion.

The *second plantar interosseous* arises from the fourth metatarsal bone and is inserted into the base of the proximal phalanx of the fourth toe and partly into its dorsal digital expansion.

The *third plantar interosseous* arises from the fifth metatarsal bone and is inserted into the base of the proximal phalanx of the little toe and partly into its dorsal digital expansion.

The plantar interossei adduct the lateral three toes towards the line of the second toe. Through their attachment to the proximal phalanges and the dorsal digital expansions, and acting with the lumbrical muscles, they flex the metatarsophalangeal joints and extend the interphalangeal joints of the lateral three toes.

The first and second plantar interossei are supplied by the deep branch of lateral plantar nerve while the third muscle is supplied by the superficial branch of lateral plantar nerve.

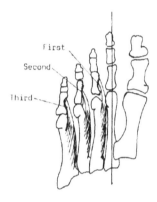

First
Second
Third

Fig. 214: Plantar interossei.

4- **Dorsal interossei:** are four small muscles, but larger than the plantar interossei and filling the interosseous spaces (fig. 215). Each muscle arises by two heads from the shafts of two adjacent metatarsal bones. They are enumerated first to fourth from the medial to the lateral side.

The *first dorsal interosseous* arise from the adjacent sides of the first and second metatarsal bones and is inserted into the base of the proximal phalanx of the second toe and partly into its dorsal digital expansion.

The *second dorsal interosseous* arises from the adjacent sides of the second and third metatarsal bones and is inserted into the base of the proximal phalanx of the second toe and partly into its dorsal digital expansion. This means that the second toe does not receive plantar interossei but receives two dorsal interossei.

The *third dorsal interosseous* arises from the adjacent sides of the third and fourth metatarsal bones and is inserted into the base of the proximal phalanx of the third toe and partly into its dorsal digital expansion.

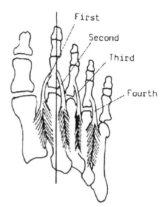

Fig. 215: Dorsal interossei.

The *fourth dorsal interosseous* arises from the adjacent sides of the fourth and fifth metatarsal bones and is inserted into the base of the proximal phalanx of the fourth toe and partly into its dorsal digital expansion.

The dorsal interossei are abductors of the toes, i.e. they produce fanning of the toes. They abduct the second, third and fourth toes away from the line of the second toe. Through their attachment to the proximal phalanges and dorsal digital expansions, and together with the plantar interossei and lumbricals, they flex the metatarsophalangeal joints and extend the interphalangeal joints of the second, third and fourth toes.

The first, second and third dorsal interossei are supplied by the deep branch of the lateral plantar nerve while the fourth muscle is supplied by the superficial branch of the lateral plantar nerve.

N.B.:

1- From the above description it is seen that all plantar and dorsal interossei are supplied by the lateral plantar nerve.

2- The first dorsal interosseus may receive an additional branch from the medial terminal branch of the deep peroneal (anterior tibial) nerve on the dorsum of the foot.

3- The second dorsal interosseous may receive an additional branch from the lateral terminal branch of the deep peroneal nerve on the dorsum of the foot.

4- From the above description, it is seen that the big toe does not receive any of the interossei muscles as the big toe has its own abdductor and adductor hallucis muscles.

5- From the above description, it is seen that the little toe receives the third plantar interosseus which is an adductor muscle; but it does not receive any of the dorsal interossei as it has its own abductor digiti minimi.

Medial Plantar Artery

Origin: is the smaller of the two terminal branches of the posterior tibial artery, taking origin deep to the flexor retinaculum (fig. 216).

Course and relations: The artery passes deep to the abductor hallucis and then continues between the abductor hallucis and flexor digitorum brevis (first layer). It is closely accompanied by two venae comitantes and runs close to the medial side of the medial plantar nerve. At the base of the first metatarsal bone, the artery is greatly reduced in size where it usually ends by anastomosing with the first plantar metatarsal artery.

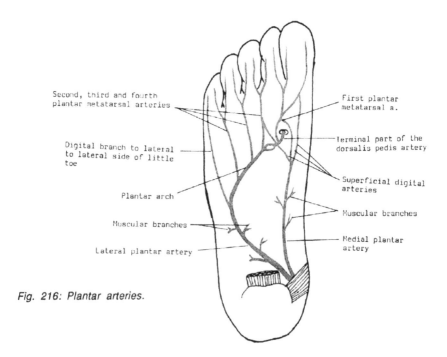

Fig. 216: Plantar arteries.

Branches

1- ***Muscular branches:*** to the abductor hallucis and flexor digitorum brevis.

2- ***Cutaneous branches:*** to the skin and fasciae of the medial part of the sole.

3- ***Superficial digital branches:*** which are three small branches that accompany the digital branches of the medial plantar nerve and end by anastomosing with the first, second and third plantar metatarsal arteries. These digital branches vary in number and size and may be absent according to the size of the medial plantar artery.

Surface anatomy: The medial plantar artery corresponds to a line which begins from a point midway between the medial malleolus and medial border of the heel. This line extends forwards in the direction of the first interdigital cleft to the level of the base of the first metatarsal bone.

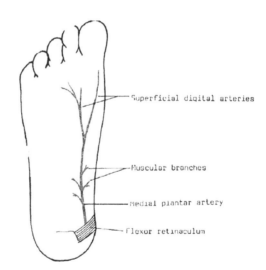

Fig. 217: Distribution of medial plantar artery.

Superficial digital arteries

Muscular branches

Medial plantar artery

Flexor retinaculum

Lateral Plantar Artery

Origin: is the larger of the two terminal branches of the posterior tibial artery, taking origin deep to the flexor retinaculum (fig. 216).

Course and relations: The artery passes obliquely forwards and laterally across the sole of the foot to the base of the fifth metatarsal bone. In this part of its course, the artery first passes deep to the abductor hallucis and then between the flexor digitorum brevis (first layer) and flexor digitorum accessorius (second layer). The artery then appears between the flexor digitorum brevis and abductor digiti minimi (first layer). It is closely accompanied by the two venae comitantes and runs close to the lateral side of the lateral plantar nerve.

Then, the artery turns medially to form the *plantar arch* (figs. 216), The arch passes across the sole from the lateral to the medial side between the third and fourth layers. The arch is curved with a slightly forward convexity and ends at the first interosseous space by anastomosing with the end of the dorsalis pedis artery. The arch is closely accompanied by the deep branch of the lateral plantar nerve which runs in the concavity of the arch, i.e. just posterior to the arch.

Branches of the first part of the artery (fig. 218):

1- *Muscular branches:* to the adjacent muscles.

2- *Cutaneous branches:* to the skin and fasciae of the lateral part of the sole of the foot.

3- *Anastomotic branches:* which run across the lateral border of the foot to anastomose with branches of the lateral tarsal and arcuate arteries.

Branches of the plantar arch (fig. 218):

1- *Muscular branches:* to the adjacent muscles.

2- *Articular branches:* to the intertarsal and tarsometatarsal joints.

3- *Posterior perforating arteries:* are three branches which ascend through the proximal parts of the second, third and fourth interosseous spaces to anastomose with the corresponding dorsal metatarsal arteries (branches of the arcuate artery).

4- *Plantar metatarsal arteries:* are three branches which run forwards along the second, third and fourth interosseous spaces, each dividing into two plantar digital arteries for the adjacent sides of the second, third, fourth and little toes. Each plantar metatarsal artery gives an *anterior perforating artery* which ascends through the corresponding interosseous space to anastomose with the corresponding dorsal metatarsal artery.

5- ***Lateral plantar digital artery of the little toe:*** arises from the beginning of the arch and pases forwards to the lateral side of the little toe. From the above description, it is seen that the plantar arch gives plantar digital arteries to the lateral three and half toes.

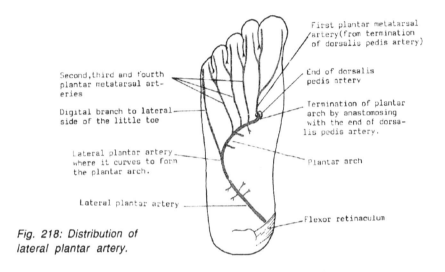

First plantar metatarsal artery(from termination of dorsalis pedis artery)

Second,third and fourth plantar metatarsal arteries

End of dorsalis pedis artery

Digital branch to lateral side of the little toe

Termination of plantar arch by anastomosing with the end of dorsalis pedis artery.

Lateral plantar artery where it curves to form the plantar arch.

Plantar arch

Lateral plantar artery

Flexor retinaculum

Fig. 218: Distribution of lateral plantar artery.

NB.: As previously described, the first plantar metatarsal artery is a branch from the end of the dorsalis pedis artery and gives plantar digital branches to the medial one and half toes (See page 151).

Surface anatomy: The lateral plantar artery corresponds to a line which begins from a point medway between the medial malleolus and medial border of the heel. This line extends obliquely forwards and laterally across the sole of the foot to a point one inch medial to the tuberosity of the base of the fifth metatarsal bone.

The plantar arch begins from the point of termination of the lateral plantar artery. It corresponds to a curved line with its convexity directed forwards extending to a point opposite the posterior end of the first interosseous space.

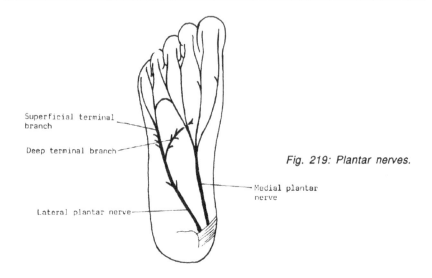

Superficial terminal branch

Deep terminal branch

Medial plantar nerve

Lateral plantar nerve

Fig. 219: Plantar nerves.

Medial Plantar Nerve

Origin: is the larger of the two terminal branches of the tibial (posterior tibial) nerve, taking origin deep to the flexor retinaculum (fig. 219).

Course and relations: The nerve passes deep to the abductor hallucis and then it extends forwards between the abductor hallucis and flexor digitorum brevis (first layer). The medial plantar vessels run close to its medial side. At the base of the first metatarsal bone, it terminates by breaking into four plantar digital nerves.

Branches (fig. 220)
1- *Cutaneous branches:* to the skin of the medial two-thirds of the sole.

2- *Muscular branches:* which supply the following muscles:

    a. Abductor hallucis: from the trunk of the nerve.

    b. Flexor digitorum brevis: from the trunk of the nerve.

    c. Flexor hallucis brevis: from the first (most medial) digital branch.

    d. First lumbrical: from the second digital branch.

3- *Articular branches:* to the adjacent intertarsal and tarsometatarsal joints.

4- *Plantar digital branches:* four branches to the plantar aspect of the medial three and half toes. The first branch supplies the medial side of the big toe. The second branch divides to supply the adjacent sides of the big and second toes. The third branch divides to supply the adjacent sides of the second and third toes. The fourth branch divides to supply the adjacent sides of the third and fourth toes.

The terminal ramifications of the plantar nerves end by supplying the skin on the dorsum of the terminal phalanges including the nail beds.

As previously described, the first digital branch gives a twig to the flexor hallucis brevis (third layer) while the second digital branch gives a twig to the first lumbrical (second layer). The fourth digital branch forms a communication with the superficial branch of the lateral plantar nerve.

NB.: From the above description, it is clear that the medial plantar nerve has a distribution in the sole of the foot which is nearly similar to that of the median nerve in the hand.

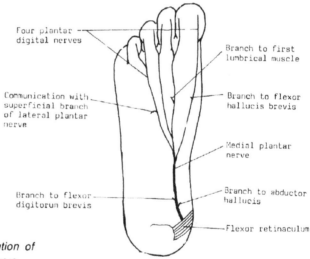

Fig. 220: Distribution of medial plantar nerve.

Surface anatomy: The medial plantar nerve corresponds to a line which begins from a point midway between the medial malleolus and medial border of the heel. This line passes forwards in the direction of the first interdigital cleft to the level of the head of first metatarsal bone.

Lateral Plantar Nerve

Origin: is the smaller of the two terminal branches of the tibial (posterior tibial) nerve, taking origin deep to the flexor retinaculum (fig. 219).

Course and relations: The nerve passes forwards and laterally deep to the abductor hallucis and then across the sole of the foot in the interval between the flexor digitorum brevis (first layer) and flexor digitorum accessorius (second layer). The lateral plantar vessels run close to its lateral side. The nerve reaches to the interval between the flexor digitorum brevis and abductor digiti minimi (first layer) where it ends by dividing into sueprficial and deep branches (figs. 219, 221).

Branches
1- *From the trunk of the nerve:* muscular branches to the flexor digitorum accessorius and abductor digiti minimi and cutaneous branches to the plantar fascia and skin of the lateral third of the sole of the foot.

2- *Superficial branch:* divides into two plantar digital branches:
   a. *Lateral plantar digital branch to the little toe:* Before reaching the little toe, this branch gives muscular twigs to the following muscles:
      • flexor digiti minimi brevis (third layer).
      • third plantar interosseous (fourth layer).
      • fourth dorsal interosseous (fourth layer).
   b. *Medial plantar digital branch:* forms a communication with the fourth digital branch of the medial plantar nerve and then divides to supply the adjacent sides of the fourth and little toes.

Like the medial plantar nerve, the plantar digital branches of the lateral plantar nerve also supply the skin on the dorsum of the terminal phalanges of the lateral one and half toes including their nail beds.

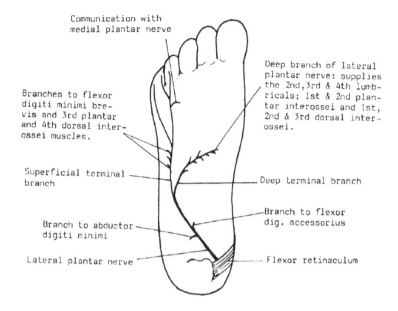

Communication with
medial plantar nerve

Deep branch of lateral
plantar nerve: supplies
the 2nd,3rd & 4th lumb-
ricals; 1st & 2nd plan-
tar interossei and 1st,
2nd & 3rd dorsal inter-
ossei.

Branches to flexor
digiti minimi bre-
vis and 3rd plantar
and 4th dorsal inter-
ossei muscles.

Superficial terminal
branch

Deep terminal branch

Branch to flexor
dig. accessorius

Branch to abductor
digiti minimi

Lateral plantar nerve

Flexor retinaculum

Fig. 221: Distribution of lateral plantar nerve.

3- **Deep branch:** passes medially in the concavity of the plantar arch, i.e. just behind the arch, between the third and fourth layers. This branch is an important nerve as it gives the following branches:

    a. *Muscular branches:* which supply the following muscles:

- Second, third and fourth (lateral three) lumbricals (second layer).
- Adductor hallucis (third layer).
- First and second plantar interossei (fourth layer).
- First, second and third dorsal interossei (fourth layer).

    b. *Articular branches:* to the adjacent intertarsal and tarsometatarsal joints.

N.B.: From the above description, it is clear that the lateral plantar nerve has a distribution in the sole of the foot which is nearly similar to that of the ulnar nerve in the hand.

Surface anatomy: The trunk of the lateral plantar nerve corresponds to a line which is similar to that of the first part of the lateral plantar artery. The deep branch corresponds to the line of the plantar arch (See pages 186 and 187).

SEGMENTAL CUTANEOUS INNERVATION OF THE LOWER LIMB

A revision of the cutaneous innervation of the different regions of the lower limb reveals that the skin of the lower limb, like that of the upper limb, is innervated in a segmental pattern by ten spinal segments which are the twelfth thoracic to the fourth sacral segments.

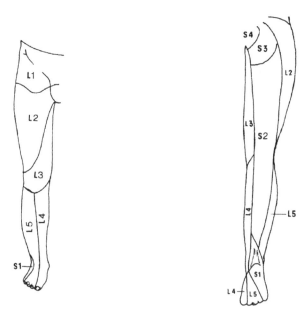

Fig. 222: Segmental cutaneous innervation of the lower limb - Anterior view.   Fig. 223: Segmental cutaneous innervation of the lower limb - Posterior view.

The segmental pattern of cutaneous innervation has a developmental basis. As the lower limb bud develops it carries with it parts of the dermatomes from the twelfth thoracic to the third sacral with their supplying spinal nerves. The preaxial border of the lower limb bud is along the line of the tibia and big toe while the postaxial border is along the fibula and little toe. Rotation of the lower limb bud occurs in a medial direction so that the preaxial border is carried medially while the postaxial border is carried laterally.

Accordingly, the segmental cutaneous innervation of the lower limb becomes arranged according to the following pattern (figs. 222, 223):

- The superior and lateral part of the gluteal region is supplied by the segments T. 12 and L. 1, 2.
- The anterior, medial and lateral aspects of the thigh are supplied by the segments L. 1, 2, 3.
- The medial part of the front of the leg, medial side of the leg and medial border of the foot are supplied by the segment L. 4.
- The lateral part of the front of the leg, lateral side of the leg and intermediate part of the dorsum of the foot are supplied by the segment L. 5.
- The lateral border of the foot is supplied by the segment S. 1.
- The sole of the foot is supplied by three successive segments: its medial part by L. 4, its intermediate part by L. 5 and its lateral part by S. 1.
- The back of the leg and thigh are supplied by the segment S. 2
- The inferior and medial part of the gluteal region is supplied by the segments S. 3, 4.

LYMPHATICS OF THE LOWER LIMB

The lymphatics of the lower limb are arranged into superficial and deep groups.

Superficial lymphatics: constitute the vast majority of the lower limb lymphatics and run through the superficial fascia, draining the skin and subcutaneous structures (figs. 224, 225).

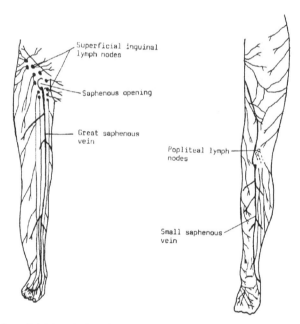

Fig. 224: Superficial lymphatics of the lower limb - Anterior view.

Fig. 225: Superficial lymphatics of the lower limb - Posterior view.

In the sole of the foot, they form a dense plexus called the *plantar plexus*. Most of the lymphatics of this plexus ascend to the dorsum of the foot and then ascend in front of the ankle joint to reach the leg. These vessels in adition to other vessels from the dorsum of the foot, leg and thigh run along the great saphenous vein to drain into the *superficial inguinal lymph nodes* (See page 65).

Few lymphatics from the lateral part of the plantar plexus, heal and back of the leg run along the small saphenous vein to drain into the *popliteal lymph nodes* (See page 135).

Lymphatics from the superficial parts of the anterior abdominal wall below the umbilicus, perineum and gluteal region drain directly into the superficial inguinal lymph nodes.

Efferent lymphatics of the superficial inguinal lymph nodes pierce the cribriform fascia and surrounding deep fascia to end in the *deep inguinal lymph nodes* (See page 78).

Deep lymphatics: are much less numerous than the superficial lymphatics. They drain the structures deep to the deep fascia and ascend along the main deep vessels of the lower limb to drain into the deep inguinal lymph nodes. Some of the vessels are interrupted in the *anterior tibial lymph node* which is a small lymph node along the upper parts of the anterior tibial vessels. Other lymphatics are interrupted in the *popliteal lymph nodes.*

Efferent lymphatics of the deep inguinal lymph nodes ascend deep to the inguinal ligament to drain into the external iliac lymph nodes.

NB.: Lymphatics from the deep parts of the gluteal region pass through the greater sciatic foramen along the superior and inferior gluteal vessels to drain into the internal iliac lymph nodes.

JOINTS OF THE LOWER LIMB

Before the study of the joints of the lower limb, the student should revise the general features of the bones of the lower limb. In addition, the bones should be always at hand during this study.

Hip Joint

This is a typical ball and socket synovial joint. The ball is formed by the head of the femur while the socket is formed by the acetabulum of the hip bone.

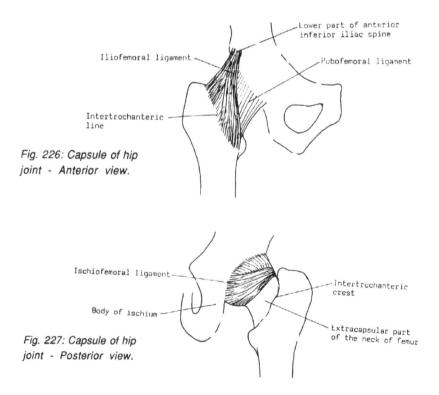

Fig. 226: Capsule of hip joint - Anterior view.

Fig. 227: Capsule of hip joint - Posterior view.

Articular surfaces

1- *Head of the femur:* forms more than half (about two-thirds) of a sphere. It is covered by hyaline cartilage which is thicker at the centre and thinner towards the periphery. Just below and behind its centre, it presents a nonarticular depression called the *fovea* of the head which gives attachment to the ligament of the head of the femur.

2- *Acetabulum:* is a cup shaped depression which carries a C-shaped articular strip called the *lunate surface.* This strip is wider above where the body weight is transmitted to the lower limb (fig. 231).

The lower margin of the acetabulum shows a large notch called the *acetabular notch* which is bridged over by a ligament called the *transverse ligament of the acetabulum* (fig. 231). By this ligament, the notch is converted into the *acetabular foramen* which gives passage to some of the vessels and nerves supplying the joint and head of the femur.

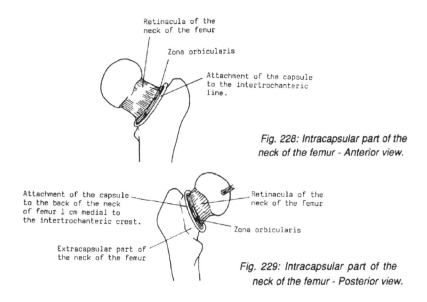

Retinacula of the neck of the femur

Zona orbicularis

Attachment of the capsule to the intertrochanteric line.

Fig. 228: Intracapsular part of the neck of the femur - Anterior view.

Attachment of the capsule to the back of the neck of femur 1 cm medial to the intertrochanteric crest.

Retinacula of the neck of the femur

Zona orbicularis

Extracapsular part of the neck of the femur

Fig. 229: Intracapsular part of the neck of the femur - Posterior view.

The acetabulum is deepened by a fibrocartilaginous rim called the *labrum acetabulare* which is attached to the margins of the acetabulum and is completed by the transverse ligament. The labrum acetabulare is triangular in cross sections, has a thin free border and is completely intracapsular (fig. 230).

The nonarticular part of the floor of the acetabulum is called the *acetabular fossa*. This fossa is filled by a pad of fat covered by synovial membrane.

Capsule

1- **Attachment to the hip bone:** The capsule is attached to the margins of the acetabulum outside the labrum acetabulare and to the lateral margin of the transverse ligament.

2- **Attachment to the femur:** Anteriorly, the capsule is attached to the intertrochanteric line. Accordingly, the neck of the femur is completely intracapsular as seen from the front (fig. 228). As the line of the capsule passes to the back of the neck, the line of attachment recedes medially, so that the capsule is attached to the back of the neck of the femur one cm medial to the intertrochanteric crest (fig. 229). Accordingly, the neck of the femur is partly intracapsular and partly extracapsular as seen from behind.

The fibers of the capsule are arranged longitudinally parallel to the neck of the femur. However, close to the neck of the femur, some of the deep fibers of the capsule are arranged circularly around the neck forming what is known as the *zona orbicularis* of the capsule (figs. 228, 229).

Some of the deep fibers of the capsule are reflected medially to cover the intracapsular part of the neck where they become closely adherent to the bone. These fibers are known as the *retinacula of the neck* as they keep the bony fragments close together in cases of fractures of the neck of the femur which is a frequent condition specially at old age.

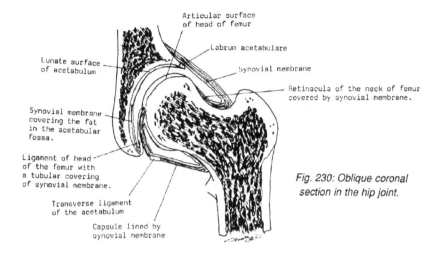

Fig. 230: Oblique coronal
section in the hip joint.

Synovial membrane: lines the inner surface of the capsule and is reflected to cover the intracapsular part of the neck of the femur (fig. 230). It also covers both surfaces of the labrum acetabulare and the fat in the acetabular fossa. It forms a sheath for the ligament of the head of the femur and accompanying blood vessels and nerves.

So, the synovial membrane of the hip joint follows the general rule for synovial joints as it covers all the structures inside the joint except the articular surfaces.

As previously described, the synovial membrane is continuous with the psoas (iliac) bursa through an opening in the front of the capsule. This opening lies between the iliofemoral and pubofemoral ligaments.

Ligaments

1- *Iliofemoral ligament:* is a very strong ligament which is closely adherent to the front of the capsule (fig. 226). It is V- or Y-shaped with its stem attached to the lower part of the anterior inferior iliac spine. Its two bands are attached to the intertrochanteric line.

In addition to strengthening the capsule, this ligament becomes very tense to prevent hyperextension of the hip joint during standing where there is a tendency of the plevis to rotate backwards under the effect of gravity.

2- **Pubofemoral ligament:** is closely adherent to the inferomedial part of the capsule (fig. 226). Medially, it is attached to the iliopubic (iliopectineal) eminence; and laterally it blends with the anterior and inferior parts of the capsule.

3- **Ischiofemoral ligament:** is closely adherent to the back of the capsule (fig. 227). Medially, it is attached to the ischium just below the acetabulum. Then, it follows a spiral course to blend with the posterior and superior parts of the capsule.

4- **Transverse ligament of the acetabulum:** previously described (See page 196).

5- **Ligament of the head of the femur:** is a triangular ligament which is intracapsular but extrasynovial. The ligament is attached by its base to the medial border of the transverse ligament and the margins of the acetabular notch, and by its apex to the fovea of the head of the femur. It is covered by a synovial sheath and carries blood vessels and nerves to the head of the femur. It has no role in the stability of the hip joint.

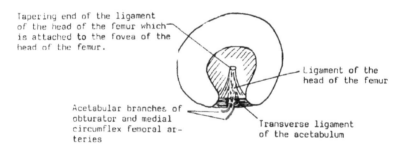

Fig. 231: Acetabulum, transverse ligament and ligament of the head of the femur - Lateral view after dislocation of the head of the femur.

Relations (fig. 232)

Anteriorly: the hip joint is related to the following muscles arranged lateromedially: straight head of rectus femoris, iliopsoas and lateral border of pectineus. The psoas (iliac) bursa separates the capsule from the iliopsoas and frequently communicates with the joint cavity. The iliopsoas separates the capsule from the femoral nerve, femoral sheath and femoral vessels.

Posteriorly: The following muscles arranged from above downwards: piriformis, tendon of obturator internus and two gemilli, quadratus femoris and obturator externus. The nerve to quadratus femoris runs close to the back of the capsule deep to the tendon of obturator internus, gemilli and quadratus femoris which separate the capsule from the sciatic nerve and gluteus maximus superficial to these muscles. The obturator externus separates the capsule from the greater part of the quadratus femoris.

Superiorly: reflected head of rectus femoris and gluteus minimus overlapped by the gluteus medius and anterior fibers of the gluteus maximus.

Inferiorly: Pectineus laterally and obturator externus medially. The intimate relation of the obturator externus to the inferior and posterior parts of the capsule was previously described (See page 107).

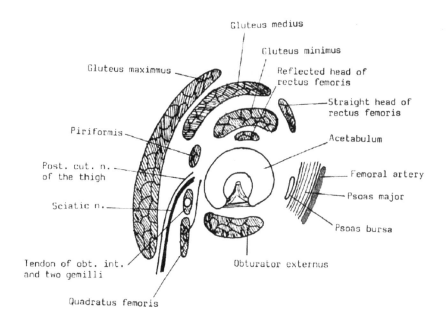

Fig. 232: Relations of the hip joint - Sagittal section.

Arterial supply: twigs from the medial circumflex femoral, obturator and superior and inferior gluteal arteries. The ascending branch of the medial circumflex femoral and the obturator arteries give *acetabular branches* which pass through the acetabular foramen and run along the ligament of the head of the femur to supply the head of the femur (fig. 231).

Nerve supply: from the following nerves:

1- Femoral nerve through the branch supplying the rectus femoris.

2- Articular branch of the anterior branch of obturator nerve.

3- Twigs from the accessory obturator nerve when the latter is present.

4- A twig from the superior gluteal nerve.

5- A twig from the nerve to quadratus femoris.

Movements

1- *Flexion:* mainly done by the iliopsoas helped by the sartorius, rectus femoris and pectineus.

2- *Extension:* mainly done by the gluteus maximus helped by the hamstrings.

3- *Abduction:* mainly done by the glutei medius and minimus helped by the tensor fasciae latae. The role of the abductors in preventing tilting of the pelvis to the unsupported side during walking was previously described (See page 108).

4- *Adduction:* mainly done by the adductors longus, brevis and magnus helped by the pectineus and gracilis.

5- *Medial rotation:* mainly done by the anterior fibers of the glutei medius and minimus helped by the tensor fasciae latae.

6- *Lateral rotation:* mainly done by the gluteus maximus and the short muscles on the back of the hip (small lateral rotators of the hip which are the piriformis, obtuartor internus, gemilli, quadratus femoris and obturator externus). These muscles are helped by the sartorius and the adductors.

7- *Circumduction:* is a combination of flexion, abduction, extension and adduction done in succession.

Stability of the hip joint: Because the body weight is transmitted through the hip joint to the lower limb, the hip joint is so constructed to be one of the very strong and stable joints in the body. This stability depends on the following factors:

1- The deep socket formed by the acetabulum which accomodates the greater part of the head of the femur.

2- The labrum acetabulare which increases the depth of the acetabulum and fits closely on the head of the femur just outside its maximum diameter. Accordingly, the labrum slightly narrows the acetabular circumference and acts as a sucker closely applied to the head of the femur, thus helping in preventing its outward displacement.

3- The strong ligaments closely surrounding the capsule specially the iliofemoral ligament.

4- The strong muscles closely related to the joint.

5- The relatively long neck of the femur which in addition to its oblique position allows the lower limb to swing easily clear of the pelvis.

6- Atmospheric pressure which plays a role in the close contact between the head of the femur and the acetabulum, resisting their separation.

Applied anatomy: Although the hip joint is a secure and strong joint, disolacation of the joint may occur as a result of car accidents or falling from height. Dislocation can be diagnosed on the outer aspect of the gluteal region by assessing the relations of some bony landmarks through Nelaton's line and Bryant's triangle.

Nelaton's line: a line drawn from the anterior superior iliac spine to the ischial tuberosity (fig. 233). This line normally passes on the top of the greater trochanter opposite the centre of the hip joint. In case of upward dislocation of the hip joint, the top of the greater trochanter is raised above the Nelaton's line.

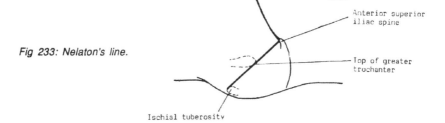

Fig 233: Nelaton's line.

Bryant's triangle: is drawn when the patient is in a recumbent position. The triangle has three boundaries (fig. 234):

1- The first line is drawn horizontally from the anterior superior iliac spine.

2- The second line is drawn from the top of the greater trochanter vertical to the first line.

3- The third line connects the anterior superior iliac spine to the top of the greater trochanter.

The two trianglse are compared on both sides. The second line is diminished in case of upward dislocation of the hip joint. The third line is prolonged in case of posterior dislocation of the hip joint.

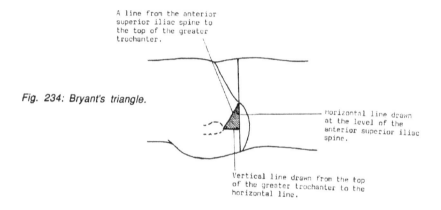

Fig. 234: Bryant's triangle.

Surface anatomy: The *buttock* is the smooth rounded and large prominence of the lower part of the gluteal region. The buttock is limited inferiorly by the *gluteal fold* (fig. 235). Both buttocks are separated by a median furrow called the natal cleft.

The gluteal fold does not correspond to the lower border of the gluteus maximus which crosses the fold obliquely downwards and laterally.

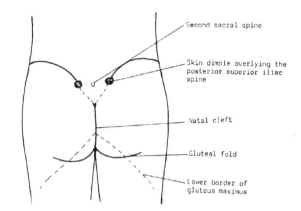

Second sacral spine

Skin dimple overlying the posterior superior iliac spine

Natal cleft

Gluteal fold

Lower border of gluteus maximus

Fig. 235: Gluteal folds.

Knee Joint

This is a condylar synovial joint; but as regards the range of movements allowed in the joint, it may be classified as a modified hinge synovial joint. It is a large and complicated joint which includes three articulations: two femorotibial and one femoropatellar articulations.

Articular surfaces

1- *Articular surface of the femur:* is a broad nearly ^- shaped strip. Its anterior part is called the *patellar surface* as it articulates with the articular surface of the patella. This surface is also called the *trochlear surface* as it is grooved longitudinally to conform with the articular surface of the patella.

The posterior parts of the articular surface extend posteriorly to cover the inferior and posterior surfaces of both condyles on both sides of the intercondylar notch. These parts articulate with the corresponding condyles of the tibia.

2- *Articular surface of the patella:* is raised about its middle by a smooth longitudinal ridge which divides it into a larger lateral part and a smaller medial part. This surface articulates with the patellar (trochlear) surface of the femur during extension of the knee joint. But, during flexion, it articulates with the articular strips of the corresponding condyles of the femur.

The medial part of the articular surface of the patella presents a small articular strip close to the medial border. This strip articulates with a crescentric part of the articular surface of the medial condyle of the femur close to the intercondylar notch during full flexion of the knee.

3- *Articular surfaces of the tibia:* These are two separate surfaces which cover the superior surfaces of both tibial condyles. The two surfaces are separated by the intercondylar area which gives attachment to the menisci and cruciate ligaments (described later). The articular surface of the medial condyle is large and oval while that of the lateral condyle is small and circular.

The two tibial condyles articulate with the corresponding femoral condyles, but the articular sufaces are largely separated by the two menisci (described later).

Capsule: As compared with that of the hip joint, the capsule of the knee joint is relatively thin. Moreover, the capsule is absent anteriorly where it is replaced by the quadriceps tendon, patellar retinacula and ligamentum patellae (fig. 236).

Attachment to the femur: As previously described, there is no anterior attachment of the capsule where it is replaced by the quadriceps tendon (fig. 236). The synovial membrane extends up deep to the quadriceps tendon, forming the suprapatellar bursa. Medially, the capsule is attached to the medial condyle of the femur close to the articular margin (fig. 237). But, laterally the capsule is attached to the lateral surface of the lateral condyle above the groove for the popliteus muscle and below the origin of the lateral head of gastrocnemius (fig. 238). Accordingly, the origin of popliteus is intracapsular (but extrasynovial) while the origin of the lateral head of gastrocnemius is extracapsular. Posteriorly, the capsule is attached to the back of both condyles of the femur close to the articular margins and to the intercondylar line. Accordingly, the intercondylar notch and its contents are intracapsular (but extrasynovial).

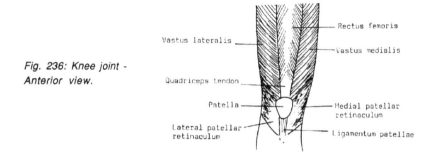

Fig. 236: Knee joint -
Anterior view.

Attachment to the tibia: As previously described, the capsule is absent anteriorly. A triangular area of the anterior surface of the upper end of the tibia lies inside the joint with its apex at the tibial tuberosity where the ligamentum patellae is attached. The sides of this triangular area give attachment to both patellar retinacula. The ligamentum patellae is separated from this triangular area by the infrapatellar pad of fat and deep infrapatellar bursa (described later). Medially and laterally, the capsule is attached to the articular margins of both tibial condyles. Posteriorly, the capsule is attached to the back of both tibial condyles close to the articular margins and to the posterior border of the intercondylar area. Accordingly, the intercondylar area with the structures attached to it are intracapsular (but extrasynovial) (fig. 245).

Just above the posterior part of the lateral condyle of the tibia, the capsule presents an opening for the passage of the tendon of origin of the popliteus muscle into the outside of the capsule (fig. 201).

The fibers of the capsule form a thickened arch over the opening for the popliteus tendon which is known as the *arcuate popliteal ligament.* (figs. 158, 239). This ligament extends from the head of the fibula to the posterior border of the intercondylar area of the tibia. The arcuate popliteal ligament may be Y-shaped with the stem of the Y-attached to the head of the fibula and the posterior limb attached to the posterior border of the intercondylar area of the tibia as described above. The anterior limb of the Y is attached to the lateral epicondyle of the femur.

Accessory ligaments: are classified into ligaments outside and ligaments inside the capsule. The ligaments outside the capsule are:
1- Ligamentum patellae.
2- Tibial collateral (Medial) ligament.

3- Fibular collateral (Lateral) ligament.

4- Posterior oblique ligament.

The ligaments inside the capsule are:
1- Anterior cruciate ligament.

2- Posterior cruciate ligament.

3- Transverse ligament.

The menisci (semilumar cartilages) also lie inside the capsule.

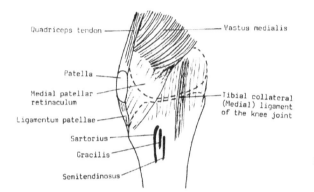

Fig. 237: Knee joint - Medial view.

Ligamentumpatellae: As previously described this is a strong ligament which extends from the apex and lower part of the posterior surface of the patella to the upper part of the tibial tuberosity (See page 85). It is a prolongation of the quadriceps insertion into the tibia, the patella being a sesamoid bone in the quadriceps insertion (fig. 240). As previously described, the ligamentum patellae is one of the structures replacing the capsule anteriorly.

Tibial collateral (Medial) ligament: is a thin broad band which extends from the medial epicondyle of the femur to the upper part of the medial surface of the tibia behind the insertions of the sartorius, gracilis and semitendinous (fig. 237). This ligament is firmly adherent to the capsule and medial meniscus.

Fibular collateral (Lateral) ligament: is a rounded cord-like ligament which extends from the lateral epicondyle of the femur to the apex of the head (styloid process) of the fibula (fig. 238). This ligament is not firmly adherent to the capsule; being separated from the capsule and lateral meniscus by the tendon of popliteus and the inferior lateral genicular nerve and vessels.

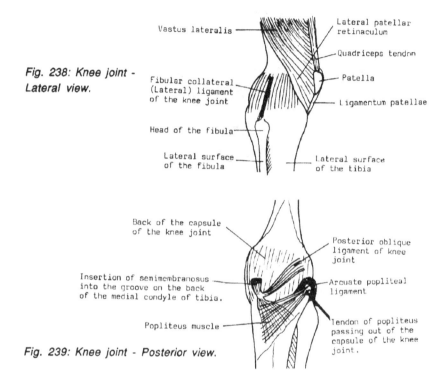

Fig. 238: Knee joint - Lateral view.

Fig. 239: Knee joint - Posterior view.

Posterior oblique ligament: is a broad oblique ligament which covers the back of the capsule (fig. 239). It extends from the medial condyle of the tibia at the insrtion of the semimembranosus upwards and laterally to be attached to the lateral condyle of the femur. It is formed by fibers reflected from the insertion of semimembranosus.

Cruciate ligaments: are so called because they form an X-shaped figure in the intercondylar notch. They are very strong fibrous cords which connect the intercondylar area of the tibia with the intercondylar notch of the femur (figs. 241, 242).

- a- *Anterior cruciate ligament:* is attached to the anterior intercondylar area of the tibia behind the anterior horn of the medial meniscus and in front of the anterior horn of the lateral meniscus (fig. 243).

It extends upwards, backwards and laterally to be attached to the posterior part of the medial surface of the lateral condyle of the femur (posterior part of the lateral wall of the intercondylar notch) (fig. 241).

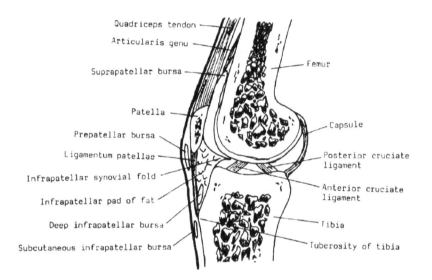

Fig. 240: Knee joint - Sagittal section.

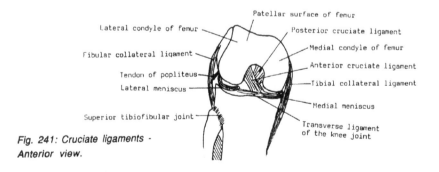

Fig. 241: Cruciate ligaments - Anterior view.

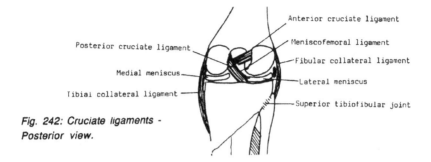

Posterior cruciate ligament

Medial meniscus

Tibial collateral ligament

Anterior cruciate ligament

Meniscofemoral ligament

Fibular collateral ligament

Lateral meniscus

Superior tibiofibular joint

*Fig. 242: Cruciate ligaments -
Posterior view.*

This ligament is lax during flexion but is tense during extension of the knee; thus playing an important role in preventing hyperextension of the knee.

b- *Posterior cruciate ligament:* is attached to the most posterior part of the posterior intercondylar area, i.e. behind the posterior horns of both menisci (fig. 243). It extends upwards, forwards and medially to be attached to the anterior part of the lateral surface of the medial condyle of the femur (anterior part of the medial wall of the intercondylar notch) (fig. 242). Contrary to the anterior cruciate, the posterior cruciate ligament is lax during extension but is tense during flexion of the knee. However, the posterior cruciate ligament does not play a role in limiting flexion of the knee, as flexion of the knee is limited by the apposition of both posterior (flexor) aspects of the leg and thigh.

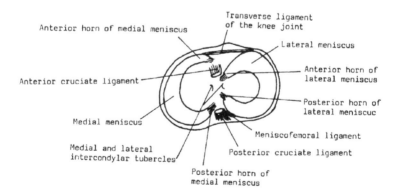

Anterior horn of medial meniscus

Transverse ligament
of the knee joint

Lateral meniscus

Anterior horn of
lateral meniscus

Anterior cruciate ligament

Posterior horn of
lateral meniscuc

Medial meniscus

Meniscofemoral ligament

Medial and lateral
intercondylar tubercles

Posterior cruciate ligament

Posterior horn of
medial meniscus

Fig. 243: Menisci and structures attached to the intercondylar area of the tibia.

Menisci (Semilunar cartilages): are two C-shaped fibrocartilage plates which partly cover the articular surfaces of both tibial condyles, intervening partly between them and the corresponding condyles of the femur (fig. 243). Their peripheral borders are thick, but they gradually become thinner towards their sharp inner borders.

The inferior surfaces of the menisci are flat and lie over the articular surfaces of both tibial condyles; but their superior surfaces are concave to conform with the articular surfaces of both femoral condyles. So the menisci help in adaptation of the femoral to the tibial condyles. In addition, they facilitate distribution of the synovial fluid over the articular surfaces during movements of the joint.

The two menisci move with the tibia during flexion and extension of the leg. But, during rotatory movements of the knee with the foot fixed on the ground, the menisci move with the femur on the fixed tibia.

Each meniscus is attached to the anterior intercondylar area by an anterior horn and to the posterior intercondylar area by a posterior horn.

1- *Medial menisus:* is wider than the lateral meniscus, but it forms the smaller part of a large circle. Its anterior horn is attached to the anterior part of the anterior intercondylar area, anterior to the anterior cruciate ligament (fig. 243). Its posterior horn is attached to the posterior intercondylar area anterior to the posterior cruciate ligament. Its outer border is firmly attached to the capsule and tibial collateral ligament which lead to a limited range of mobility of the medial meniscus.

2- *Lateral meniscus:* which is narrower than the medial meniscus, but forms the greater part of a smaller circle. Its anterior horn is attached to the anterior intercondylar area just anterior to the intercondylar eminence, i.e. posterior to the anterior cruciate ligament (fig. 243). Its posterior horn is attached to the posterior intercondylar area just behind the intercondylar eminence, i.e. anterior to the posterior horn of medial meniscus and posterior cruciate ligament.

The *meniscofemoral ligament* is a fibrous band from the posterior horn of the lateral meniscus which extends along the posterior cruciate ligament to the intercondylar notch (fig. 242, 243).

The outer border of the lateral meniscus is not firmly adherent to the capsule and fibular collateral ligament, being separated from them by the tendon of popliteus and the inferior lateral genicular nerve and vessels.

Accordingly, the lateral meniscus is more mobile than the medial meniscus during the rotatory movements of the knee.

Applied anatomy: Injury of the menisci is a common surgical problem specially in foot-ball players. It is caused by sudden rotatory movements of the partially flexed knee with the foot fixed on the ground. The lateral meniscus is less frequently injured as it is more mobile and can adapt itself to sudden rotatory movements of the knee. On the other hand, the medial meniscus is more liable to injury as it is less mobile. The injury is usually in the form of a tear in the medial meniscus or sometimes a partial detachment from the inner aspect of the capsule.

Transverse ligament: is a thin fibrous ligament lying transversely in the anterior part of the anterior intercondylar area (figs. 241, 243). It interconnects the anterior horns of both menisci.

Synovial membrane: is more extensive than that of any other joint due to the large size and complexity of the joint. It lines the inner surface of the capsule except posteriorly and covers the nonarticular parts of the femur and tibia inside the joint; but it does not cover the articular surfaces and stops close to the articular margins.

It extends deep to the quadriceps tendon for three fingers breath above the patella in the extended knee; this upward extension forming the *suprapatellar bursa* (fig. 240). The synovial membrane is reflected to cover the lower part of the front of the femur down to the articular margin. Below the patella, the synovial membrane is loose and is separated from the ligamentum patella by a fatty mass called the *infrapatellar pad of fat* (fig. 240). The loose fold of synovial membrane enclosing this pad of fat is called the *infrapatellar synovial fold* (fig. 244). This fold is triangular in shape with medial and lateral borders known as the *alar folds* and its tapering apex attached to the anterior border of the intercondylar notch of the femur.

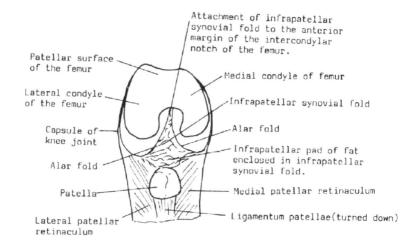

Fig. 244: Infrapatellar synovial fold, displayed after downward reflection of the quadriceps tendon, patella and patellar retinacula.

Medially, the synovial membrane lines the inner surface of the capsule, but is reflected to cover both surfaces of the medial meniscus (fig. 245).

Laterally, the synovial membrane lines the inner surface of the capsule, but is reflected to cover both surfaces of the lateral meniscus. Here, it is also forms a covering for the popliteus tendon which although intracapsular is extrasynovial. This covering extends around the tendon to the outside of the knee joint, separating the tendon from the lateral condyle of the tibia and the superior tibiofibular joint.

Posteriorly, the capsule is not lined by synovial membrane which is reflected to cover the sides and front of the cruciate ligaments which although intracapsular are extrasynovial (fig. 245). Accordingly, the cruciate ligaments are directly related to the posterior part of the capsule where they receive their blood and nerve supply through the middle genicular vessels and nerve.

As a result of continuous pressure over the menisci, their synovial covering usually disappears at adult life.

The synovial membrane of the joint may communicate with the bursa of the medial head of gastrocunemicus through an opening in the posteromedial part of the capsule.

Relations (fig. 246)

Anteriorly: structures replacing the capsule which are the quadriceps tendon and ligamentum patellae.

Anteromedially: medial patellar retinaculum, replacing the capsule.

Anterolaterally: lateral patellar retinaculum, replacing the capsule.

Posteriorly: popliteal artery, vein, lymph nodes and tibial (medial popliteal) nerve arranged from the floor to the roof of the popliteal fossa. These structures are overlapped by the semimembranosus, semitendinosus, plantaris and two heads of gastrocnemius.

Posteromedially: gracilis and sartorius.

Posterolaterally: biceps femoris and common peroneal (lateral popliteal) nerve.

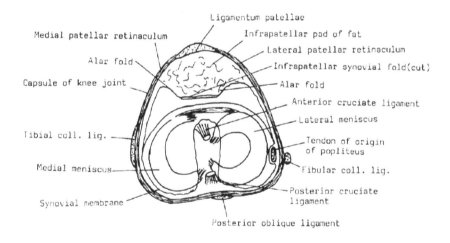

Fig. 245: Synovial membrane of the knee joint - Transverse section.

Bursae related to the joint

1- ***Suprapatellar bursa:*** which as previously described is an upward extension of the synovial membrane of the joint deep to the quadriceps tendon for three fingers breadth above the patella in the extended knee (fig. 240). This bursa separates the quadriceps tendon from the lower part of the shaft of the femur. Fibers of the articularis genu are inserted into the upper margin of the synovial membrane of the bursa.

2- **Deep infrapatellar bursa:** between the deep surface of the ligamentum patellae and the upper end of the tibia (fig. 240).

3- A bursa between the medial head of gastrocnemius and the capsule This bursa may communicate with the joint cavity.

4- A bursa between the tendon of biceps femoris and the fibular collateral (lateral) ligament.

5- A bursa between the lateral head of gastrocnemius and the capsule.

6- **Semimembranosus bursa:** which separates the semimembranosus at its insertion from the medial head of gastrocnemius at its origin.

7- **Subcutaneous prepatellar bursa:** between the skin and lower part of the patella (fig. 240) (See page 86).

8- **Subcutaneous infrapatellar bursa:** between the skin and the lower part of the tibial tuberosity (fig. 240).

9- A bursa between the tendons of insertions of the sartorius, gracilis and semitendinosus and the tibial collateral (medial) ligament.

10- The bursae separating the insertions of the sartorius, gracilis and semitendinosus.

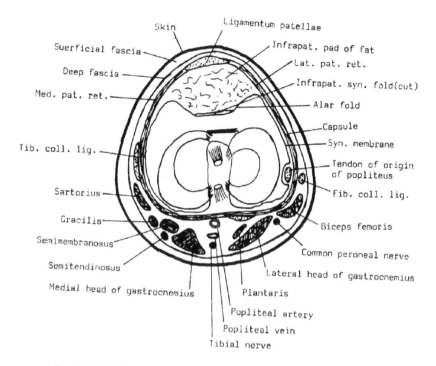

Fig. 246: Relations of the knee joint - Transverse section.

Arterial supply: by several arteries which form several anastomoses around the knee joint (fig. 247). These arteries are 10 in number and were previously described:

1- Descending genicular artery.

2- Descending branch of lateral circumflex femoral artery.

3- Superior lateral genicular artery.

4- Superior medial genicular artery.

5- Middle genicular artery.

6- Inferior lateral genicular artery.

7- Inferior medial genicular artery.

8- Anterior tibial recurrent artery.

9- Posterior tibial recurrent artery.

10- Circumflex fibular artery.

Nerve supply: The knee joint also receives articular branches from ten nerves. They were also previously described:

A- Articular twigs from the femoral nerve through the nerves supplying the three vasti muscles.

B- Genicular branch of obturator nerve which is a filament from the posterior branch of obturator nerve.

C- Three genicular branches of the tibial (medial popliteal) nerve.

D- Three genicular branches of the common peroneal (lateral popliteal) nerve.

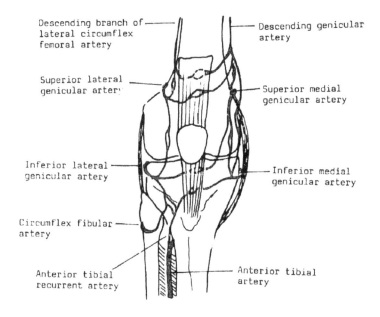

Fig. 247: Anastomoses around the knee joint.

Movements

1- *Flexion:* which is mainly done by the biceps femoris, semimembranosus and semitendinosus helped by the popliteus, sartorius and gracilis. When the sole of the foot is fixed on the ground, the gastrocnemius and plantaris help in flexion of the knee.

2- *Extension:* which is done by the quadriceps helped by the tensor fasciae latae.

3- *Medial rotation:* which is done by the popliteus helped by the semimembranosus, semitendosus, sartorius and gracilis.

4- *Lateral rotation:* which is done by the biceps femoris.

Flexion of the knee is accompanied by a small amount of medial rotation of the leg while extension is accompanied by a small amount of lateral rotation of the leg.

During flexion and extension, the menisci glide with the tibial condyles on the femoral condyles. But during rotation in the standing position, the menisci move with the femoral condyles on the tibial condyles.

A limited degree of abduction and adduction of the knee can occur in the standing position with the knee slightly flexed.

Locking and unlocking of the knee: At the end of extension of the knee in the standing position, there is an amount of lateral rotation of the knee or an amount of medial rotation of the femur on the tibia. This is known as *locking of the knee* and is done by the biceps femoris. It is so called because this movement turns the lower limb into a continuous uninterrupted rigid column carrying the body weight into the ground.

At the beginning of flexion of the knee, there is a slight amount of medial rotation of the leg or an amount of lateral rotation of the femur on the tibia. This is known as *unlocking of the knee* and is done by the popliteus muscle.

Stability: Although large, the knee is not a secure joint from the skeletal point of view due to the following factors:

1- The relatively long bones (femur and tibia) sharing in the joint and accordingly the wide range of leverage actions produced by the thigh and leg.

2- Maladaptation of the articular surfaces.

However, the strength and stability of the knee depend on the following factors:

A- The strong ligaments of the joint.

B- The strong muscles surrounding the joint.

Superior (Proximal) Tibiofibular Joint

This is a plane synovial joint between the articular surface of the head of the fibula and the fibular facet on the posterolateral aspect of the lateral condyle of the tibia.

The two bones are connected together by a *fibrous capsule* which is

attached to the margins of the articular surfaces. The capsule is lined by *synovial membrane* and is strengthened on the outside by *anterior* and *posterior tibiofibular ligaments.*

Relations

Superolaterally: fibular collateral ligament of the knee joint and tendon of biceps femoris.

Posteromedially: tendon of popliteus and its synovial sheath. The sheath may communicate with the cavity of the superior tibiofibular joint.

Arterial supply: twigs from the anterior and posterior tibial recurrent arteries (branches of the anterior tibial artery).

Nerve supply: twigs from the common peroneal, recurrent genicular and nerve to popliteus.

Middle Tibiofibular Joint
(Interosseous Membrane of the Leg)

This is a fibrous membrane connecting the interosseous borders of the tibia and fibula (fig. 248). Its fibers are directed obliquely downwards and laterally from the tibia to the fibula.

At its upper end it presents a gap for the anterior tibial vessels close to the medial side of the neck of the fibula. Two inches above the ankle, it presents a small opening for the perforating branch of peroneal artery and accompanying veins. The lower end of the membrane is continuous with the interosseous tibiofibular ligament.

Both surfaces of the membrane give partial origin to muscles of the anterior and posterior compartments as previously described.

The membrane receives twigs from the nerve to popliteus.

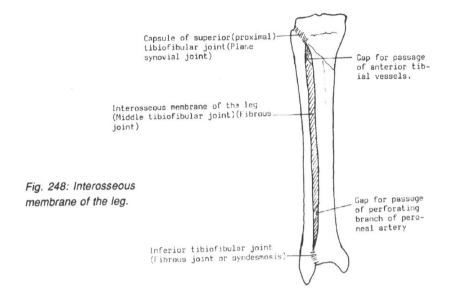

Capsule of superior(proximal) tibiofibular joint(Plane synovial joint)

Gap for passage of anterior tibial vessels.

Interosseous membrane of the leg (Middle tibiofibular joint)(Fibrous joint)

Fig. 248: Interosseous membrane of the leg.

Gap for passage of perforating branch of peroneal artery

Inferior tibiofibular joint (Fibrous joint or syndesmosis)

Inferior (Distal) Tibiofibular Joint

This is a fibrous joint (syndesmosis) where the rough impression on the medial side of the lower part of the shaft of the fibula is received into the fibular notch of the tibia; both bones being firmly interconnected by a strong *interosseous tibiofibular ligament* (fig. 248). This ligament prevents separation of the lower ends of the two bones under the effect of body weight.

Anteriorly, the interosseous ligament is covered by a thin *anterior tibiofibular ligament*. Posteriorly, it is also covered by a thin *posterior tibiofibular ligament*.

Transverse tibiofibular ligament: is a stong ligament which connects the posterior border of the inferior articular surface of the tibia with the malleolar fossa of the fibula (fig. 254). This ligament shares in the ankle joint.

Arterial supply: twigs from the perforating branch of peroneal artery and the medial malleolar branches of the anterior and posterior tibial arteries.

Nerve supply: twigs from the deep peroneal, tibial (posterior tibial) and saphenous nerves.

Movements: very slight gliding movements during dorsiflexion of the ankle joint.

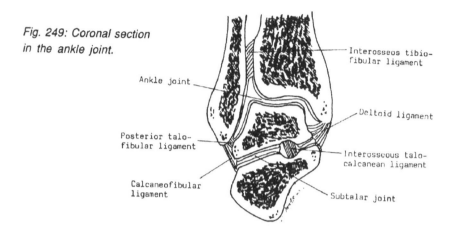

Fig. 249: Coronal section in the ankle joint.

Ankle joint

Posterior talo-fibular ligament

Calcaneofibular ligament

Interosseos tibio-fibular ligament

Deltoid ligament

Interosseous talo-calcanean ligament

Subtalar joint

Ankle Joint

This is a hinge synovial joint.

Articular surfaces

Superior articular surface: is a hollowed articular surface which is formed by the articular surface of the lower end of the tibia including the medial malleolus and the articular facet on the medial surface of the lateral malleolus (figs. 249, 250).

The lower ends of both tibia and fibula are strongly interconnected by the interosseous tibiofibular ligament, forming together a socket for the body of the talus. The socket is deepened posteriorly by the transverse tibiofibular ligament. The socket is wider anteriorly than posteriorly.

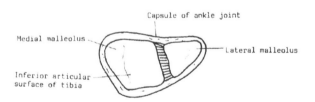

Fig. 250: Superior articular surface of ankle joint.

Medial malleolus

Inferior articular surface of tibia

Capsule of ankle joint

Lateral malleolus

Inferior articular surface: is formed by the trochlear surface of the talus which covers the superior surface of the body of the talus, extending onto the medial and lateral surfaces of the body (fig. 251). Conforming with the superior articular surface, the trochlear surface is wider anteriorly than posteriorly.

Capsule: is thin anteriorly and posteriorly, but is thickened medially by the medial (deltoid) ligament and laterally by the lateral ligament.

Synovial membrane: lines the capsule and forms a short upward recess between the lower ends of the tibia and fibula known as the *recessus sacciformis.* The synovial membrane also covers the inner surface of the transverse tibiofibular ligament.

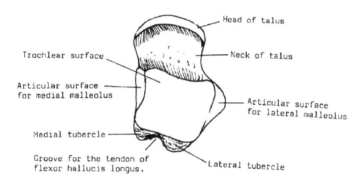

Fig. 251: Inferior articular surface of ankle joint (Trochlear surface of talus).

Ligaments of the joint

1- *Anterior ligament:* is the thin anterior part of the capsule. It connects the anterior border of the inferior articular surface of the tibia with the neck of the talus.

2- *Posterior ligament:* is the thin posterior part of the capsule. It extends from the posterior border of the inferior articular surface of the tibia and the lower border of the transverse tibiofibular ligament to the posterior surface of the talus (fig. 254).

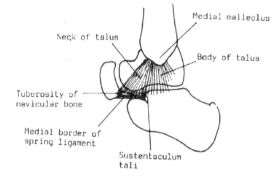

Fig. 252: Medial view of ankle joint showing the attachment of the deltoid ligament.

3- **Medial ligament:** is called the *deltoid ligament* as it is triangular in shape (fig. 252). It is a very strong ligament which is attached by its apex to the notch on the lower border of the medial malleolus. Its base is attached to five structures; arranged anteroposteriorly they are: tuberosity of navicular bone, medial border of spring ligament, neck of talus, sustentaculum tali and body of talus. By this attachment, the deltoid ligament pulls up the spring (plantar calcaneonavicular) ligament, thus supporting the head of the talus and keeping the longitudinal arch of the foot.

4- **Lateral ligament:** is formed of three bands (fig. 253):

    a- *Anterior talofibular ligament:* which connects the anterior border of the lateral malleolus with the neck of the talus.

    b- *Calcaneofibular ligament:* which connects the tip of the lateral malleolus with a tubercle on the lateral surface of the calcaneus (fig. 60).

    c- *Posterior talofibular ligament:* which connects the malleolar fossa of the fibula with the lateral tubercle of the talus.

Fig. 253: Lateral view of the ankle joint showing the three bands of the lateral ligament of the ankle joint.

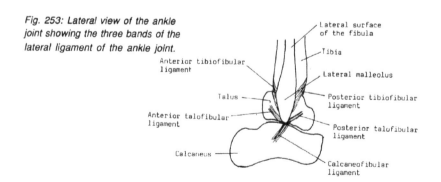

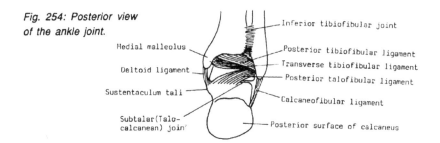

Fig. 254: Posterior view
of the ankle joint.

Medial malleolus

Deltoid ligament

Sustentaculum tali

Subtalar(Talo-
calcanean) join'

Inferior tibiofibular joint

Posterior tibiofibular ligament

Transverse tibiofibular ligament

Posterior talofibular ligament

Calcaneofibular ligament

Posterior surface of calcaneus

Relations (fig. 255)

Anteriorly: The ankle joint is related to the following structures arranged mediolaterally: tibialis anterior, extensor hallucis longus, anterior tibial vessels, deep peroneal (anterior tibial) nerve, extensor digitorum longus and peroneus tertius.

Posteriorly: The ankle is related to the following structures arranged mediolaterally: flexor digitorum longus, posterior tibial vesels, tibial (posterior tibial) nerve, flexor hallucis longus and tendo calcaneus.

Medially: tibialis posterior above and flexor digitorum longus below.

Laterally: peronei longus and brevis.

Arterial supply: twigs from several arteries which form a number of anastomoses around the ankle joint (fig. 256). These arteries were previously described:

    A- Anterior lateral and anterior medial malleolar arteries: branches of the anterior tibial artery.

    B- Lateral and medial tarsal arteries: branches of dorsalis pedis artery.

    C- Perforating branch and calcanean branches of peroneal artery.

    D- Malleolar branch and calcanean branches of posterior tibial artery.

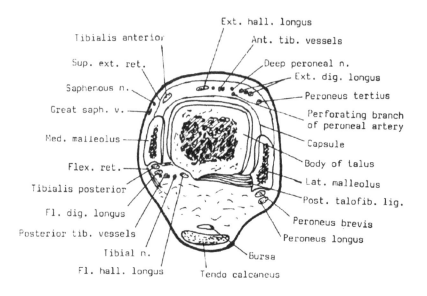

Fig. 255: Relations of the ankle joint.

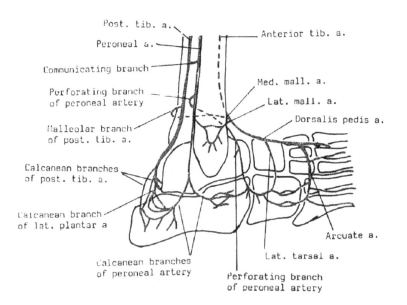

Fig. 256: Anastomoses around the ankle.

Lateral malleolar network: is formed by anastomoses between the anterior lateral malleolar artery (branch of anterior tibial artery), lateral tarsal artery (branch of dorsalis pedis artery), perforating and calcanean branches of the peroneal artery and branches from the lateral plantar artery.

Nerve supply: from the deep peroneal (anterior tibial) and tibial (posterior tibial) nerves.

Movements

1- *Dorsi flexion:* which is done by the muscles of the anterior compartment of the leg: tibialis anterior, extensor hallucis longus, extensor digitorum longus and peroneus tertius.

2- *Plantar flexion:* which is done by the muscles of the posterior and lateral compartments of the leg: gastrocnemius, plantaris, soleus, tibialis posterior, flexor digitorum longus, flexor hallucis longus, peroneus longus and peroneus brevis.

3- *Side to side movement:* A slight side to side movement of the talus can be produced when the ankle joint is in a position of plantar flexion as decribed below.

Locking and unlocking of the ankle joint: During dorsiflexion, the wide anterior part of the trochlear surface of the talus is lodged into the narrow posterior part of the superior articular surface (socket). In this position, the ankle joint is *locked* as the foot cannot be moved from side to side.

During plantar flexion, the narrow posterior part of the trochlear surface is lodged in the wide anterior part of the socket. In this position, the ankle joint is *unlocked* as the foot can be moved slightly from side to side.

Accordingly, the ankle joint is locked during dorsiflexion and unlocked during plantar flexion.

Joints And Ligaments Of The Foot

Subtalar (Talocalcanean) joint: is a gliding multiaxial synovial joint between the concave facet on the plantar surface of the body of the talus and the convex facet on the middle third of the dorsal surface of the calcaneus (posterior articular surface) (figs. 257, 258).

The shape of the articular surfaces renders this joint to be multiaxial where gliding movements are allowed in several directions with movements of other intertarsal joints specially the talocalcaneonavicular joint.

Talocalcaneonavicular joint: is a ball and socket synovial joint (figs. 257), 258). The ball is formed by the head of the talus. The socket is formed by the posterior (proximal) articular surface of the navicular bone, upper surface of the spring ligament (plantar calcaneonavicular ligament), sustentaculum tali and the facet on the anterior third of the superior surface of the calcaneus (fig. 259). This joint is a very important joint as it allows inversion and eversion of the foot.

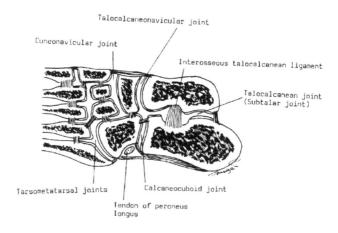

Fig. 257: Oblique section in the foot showing the intertarsal and tarsometatarsal joints.

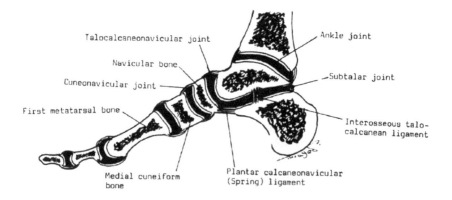

Fig. 258: Longitudinal section in the medial part of the foot.

Inversion is mainly done by the two tibialis: anterior and posterior. Eversion is done by the three peronei: longus, brevis and tertius (See page 141). Inversion is limited by tension of the peronei muscles and the interosseous talocalcanean ligament. Eversion is limited by tension of the tibialis anterior and the deltoid ligament.

The capsule of the talocalcaneonavicular joint is formed by four ligaments which fuse together at their edges to close the joint. These ligaments are:

1- Lower part of the deltoid ligament medially.

2- Interosseous talocalcanean ligament posteriorly and inferiorly.

3- Lateral calcaneonavicular ligament laterally.

4- Talonavicular ligament superiorly.

Plantar calcaneonavicular (Spring) ligament: is a very strong triangular ligament extending from the sustentaculum tali to the plantar surface of the navicular bone (figs. 259, 261). Its upper surface is coated with cartilage to share in the talocalcaneonavicular joint where it articulates with and supports the head of the halus. Its lower surface is closely related to the tendon of tibialis posterior which supports the ligament. Its medial border gives attachment to the deltoid ligament which braces up the ligament. All these supports show the importance of the spring ligament in supporting the head of the talus, thus maintaining the longitudinal arch of the foot. Although it is called spring ligament, it is a strong nonstretchible ligament.

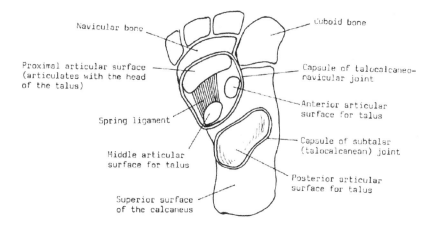

Fig. 259: Socket of the talocalcaneonavicular joint seen from its dorsal aspect after dislocation of the head of the talus.

Interosseous talocalcanean ligament: is a short ligament which fills the sinus tarsi thus connecting the sulcus tali with the sulcus calcanei (fig. 257). This ligament intervenes between the talocalcanean and talocalcaneonavicular joints.

Lateral calcaneonavicular ligament: connects the anterior part of the superior surface of the calcaneus with the lateral surface of the navicular bone, forming the medial limb of the *bifurcate ligament* (fig. 260).

Talonavicular ligament: connects the dorsal surface of the neck of the talus with the dorsal surface of the navicular bone (fig. 260).

Calcaneocuboid joint: is a plane synovial joint between the anterior surface of the calcaneus and the posterior surface of the cuboid (fig. 257). The capsule of the joint is formed by four ligaments which fuse together at their edges to close the joint. These ligaments are:

1- Dorsal calcaneocuboid ligament dorsally and laterally.

2- Medial calcaneocuboid ligament medially.

3- Plantar calcaneocuboid (short plantar) ligament ventrally.

4- Long plantar ligament ventrally.

The calcaneocuboid joint allows some gliding movements which accompany inversion and eversion of the foot.

The calcaneocuboid and talonavicular joint lie in the same transverse plane, forming together the ***transverse tarsal joint.***

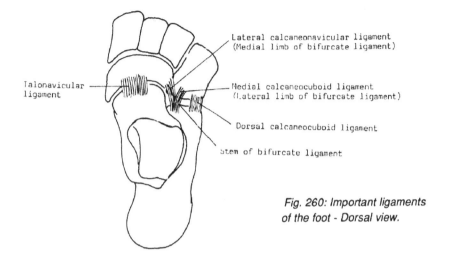

Fig. 260: Important ligaments
of the foot - Dorsal view.

Dorsal calcaneocuboid ligament: a thin ligament which connects the dorsal aspects of the calcaneus and cuboid bones (fig. 260).

Medial calcaneocuboid ligament: connects the superior surface of the calcaneus with the medial surface of the cuboid, forming the lateral limb of the *bifurcate ligament.*

Bifurcate ligament: is a strong Y- or V-shaped ligament which is attached by its stem to the anterior part of the superior surface of the calcaneus (fig. 260). The stem divides into medial and lateral limbs:

    A- **Medial limb:** is formed by the lateral calcaneonavicular ligament.

    B- **Lateral limb:** is formed by the medial calcaneocuboid ligament.

Plantar calcaeocuboid (Short plantar) ligament: a strong ligament which connects the anterior part of the plantar surface of the calcaneus with the plantar surface of the cuboid (fig. 261). This ligament is largely covered by the long plantar ligament except medially where its medial edge can be seen on the medial side of the long plantar ligament (fig. 261).

Long plantar ligament: is a strong ligament which has a wide attachment to the plantar surface of the calcaneus in front of the calcanean tuberosity (fig. 261), The ligament extends forwards where its fibers are differentiated into deep and superficial parts.

The *deep part* is attached to the margins of the groove on the plantar surface of the cuboid bone, forming a fibrous sheath for the tendon of peroneus longus and converting the groove into an ossefibrous tunnel for the tendon and its synovial sheath.

The *superficial part* of the ligament divides into slips which are attached to the bases of the seconds, third and fourth metatarsal bones.

The long plantar ligament plays an important role in supporting the longitudinal arch of the foot.

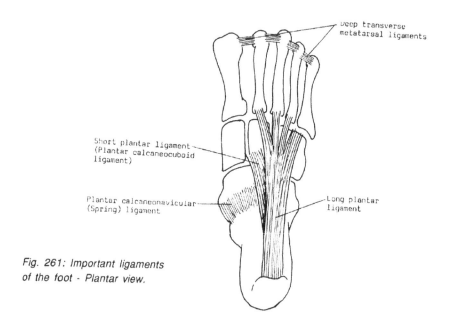

Fig. 261: Important ligaments of the foot - Plantar view.

Cuneonavicular joint: is a plane synovial joint between the three facets on the anterior (distal) surface of the navicular bone and the three cuneiform bones.

Intercuneiform joints: are the plane synovial joints between the three cuneiform bones.

Cuneocuboid joint: is a plane synovial joint between the lateral cuneiform and the medial surface of the cuboid bone.

Cubonavicular joint: is a fibrous joint (syndesmosis) between the cuboid and navicular bones where the two bones are interconnected by dorsal, interosseous and plantar ligaments. However, the interosseous ligament is frequently replaced by a small plane synovial joint between the adjacent surfaces of the two bones. This joint when present is frequently continuous with the cuneonavicular joint.

Movements of the intertarsal joints: Apart from inversion and eversion which occur in the talocalcaneonavicular joint, the intertarsal joints allow slight gliding movements which occur under the effect of body weight when the foot is put to the ground and reversed gliding movements when the foot is raised up from the ground.

Tarsometatarsal joints: are plane synovial joints between the distal row of tarsal bones and the bases of the metatarsal bones (fig. 257). The three cuneiform bones articulate with the first three metatarsal bones while the cuboid articulates with the fourth and fifth metatarsal bones.

Intermetatarsal joints: are plane synovial joints between the adjacent surfaces of the bases of the metatarsal bones.

Metatarsophalangeal joints: are ellipsoid synovial joints between the heads of the metatarsal bones and the bases of the proximal phalanges. The capsule of each joint is strengthened by an *alar ligament* on each side.

The plantar surfaces of the metatarsal heads are interconnected by four fibrous bands called the *deep transverse ligaments of the sole* which prevent separation of the heads under the effect of body weight. The plantar digital vessels and nerves and lumbrical muscles cross the plantar surfaces of these ligaments while the interossei cross their dorsal surfaces.

The plantar ligament of the metatarsophalangeal joint of the big toe is replaced by two *sesamoid bones* which lie in the two parts of the flexor hallucis brevis (See page 179). The two sesamoid bones articulate with the plantar surface of the head of the first metatarsal bone in the first metatarsophalangeal joint.

The metatarsophalangeal joints allow flexion, extension, abduction and adduction movements. Abduction and adduction movements are done in relation to the axis of the second toe.

Interphalangeal joints: are hinge synovial joints between the heads of the phalanges and the bases of the phalanges distal to them. The joint capsule are strengthened on each side by *collateral ligaments.* Being hinge (uniaxial) joints, the interphalangeal joints only allow flexion and extension movements.

Arches of the Foot

The skeleton of the foot is built up in a segmental pattern describing an arch form in order to carry its functions as a weight bearing and locomotive part of the body.

The foot describes an arch form both in the longitudianl and transverse directions (figs. 262, 263 and 264). Accordingly, the arches of the foot are classified into longitudinal and transverse arches.

A- **Longitudinal arch:** is subdivided into a *medial* (fig. 262) and a *lateral* (fig. 263) longitudinal arch. Both arches have a common *key stone* which is the talus and a common *posterior pillar* which is the calcaneus (fig. 262). But, the *anterior pillar* differs in both medial and lateral longitudinal arches.

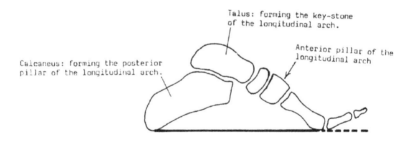

Fig. 262: Medial longitudinal arch of the foot.

Fig. 263: Transverse arch of the foot.

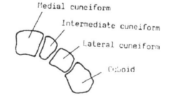

1- *Medial longitudinal arch:* The talus forms the key stone of the arch while the calcaneus forms the posterior pillar (fig. 262). The anterior pillar is formed by the navicular, three cuneiform bones and the first three metatarsal bones.

2- *Lateral longitudinal arch:* is less high than the medial arch. Its key stone is also formed by the talus. The posterior pillar is formed by the calcaneus. The anterior pillar is formed by the cuboid and the fourth and fifth metatarsal bones.

The lateral longitudinal arch is lower and less mobile than the medial longitudinal arch. Under the effect of body weight it flattens much more than the medial arch and gets into contact with the ground, transmitting a part of the body weight directly to the ground.

B - **Transverse arch:** is most marked at the distal row of the tarsus and at the bases of the metatarsal bones (fig. 264). This arch is not complete; reaching the ground laterally but is high medially. When both feet are put close together, both transverse arches constitute a complete transverse arch from the lateral border of one foot to the lateral border of the other foot.

Factors maintaining the arches of the foot

1- *Shape of the bones:* which are so constructed to keep an arch form when they are articulating together (fig. 262).

2- *Ligamentousattachments:* which play a great role in supporting the longitudinal arch. These are the spring (plantar calcaneonavicular) ligament, deltoid ligament which pulls up the spring ligament and the short and long plantar ligaments (figs. 264).

3- *Longtendons:* The long tendons reaching the foot play an important role in supporting the arches of the foot. The tendon of tibialis posterior is highly important in supporting the longitudinal arch helped by the tendons of flexor hallucis longus, flexor digitorum longus and tibialis anterior. The tendon of peroneus longus is highly important in supporting the transverse arch.

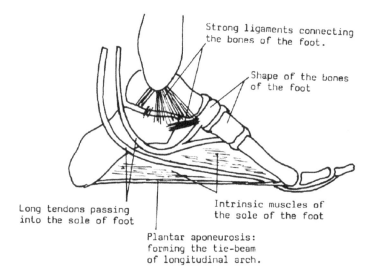

Strong ligaments connecting
the bones of the foot.

Shape of the bones
of the foot

Long tendons passing
into the sole of foot

Intrinsic muscles of
the sole of the foot

Plantar aponeurosis:
forming the tie-beam
of longitudinal arch.

Fig. 264: Factors maintining the arches of the foot.

4- **Short muscles of the sole of the foot:** The tone of the intrinsic muscles of the sole of the foot is very important in maintaining the arches of the foot. The flexor digitorum brevis (first layer) helps in supporting the longitudinal arch. The transverse head of adductor hallucis (third layer) helps in supporting the transverse arch.

5- **Plantar aponeurosis:** forms the *tie-beam* of the longitudinal arch and plays an important role in maintaining it.

NB.: The arches of the foot show great variations in their degree of development. During infancy, the arches are almost absent or poorly developed with the foot almost flat. Then, the arches gradually develop during childhood.

Applied anatomy: *Flat foot* is a common condition where the arches of the foot are lost. During standing, the sole of the foot forms a flat surface applied to the ground (fig. 267). It is the most frequent affection of the foot.

Flat foot is mostly an acquired condition. Many factors lead to flat foot, the most important of which are:

1- Prolonged standing without movement.

2- Rapid increase in body weight.

3- Repeated carrying of heavy weights.

4- Improper shoes.

5- Debilitating diseases.

6- Weakness of the ligaments.

7- Paralysis or loss of tone or weakness of the muscles of the leg which are inserted into the foot and the instrinsic muscles of the sole of the foot.

N.B.: The arches of the foot may be abnormally high. This condition is known as *"Pes cavus"* (Fig. 266).

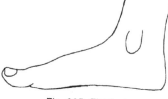

Fig. 265: Flat foot.

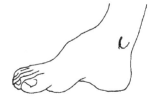

Fig. 266: Pes cavus.

HISTOLOGY

*   **Skin** – stratified squamous keratinized *layers of epidermis* (**deep to superficial**)

Stratum basale
Stratum spinosum
Stratum granulosum
Stratum corneum

*   Epidermis is devoid of blood vessels Stratum lucidum

*   **RS** – pseudostratified
*   *Nasopharynx* – respiratory epithelium
*   *Oropharynx* – striated squamous nonkeratinized
Alveolar sac – simple squamous
   Alveoli →Type –1 pneumocytes – simple squamous (thin)
                →Type –2 pneumocytes – cuboidal like

*   **GIT** – Esophagus – upper 2/3   - pseudostratified
                             lower 1/3   - squamous nonkeratinized

1. (SI) Small intestine – columnar absorptive (villi present)
2. Large intestine – villi absent (Paneth cells unique to SI secrete bactericidal enzymes)
3. Duodenum – Brunner's gland
4. Ileum - Payer's patches
5. Liver - sinusoids – lined by fenestrated endothelial cells and scattered kupffer cells
6. *Bile canaliculi* – (lined by hepatocytes)

$\downarrow$

Hering's canal

$\downarrow$

Hepatic duct (right and left)

$\downarrow$

Common hepatic duct

* **Kidney** – PCT, DCT - cuboidal
- PCT is the **only** site in kidney that has "***brush border***" (like small intestine, brush border helps in reabsorption of substances like glucose, etc.)

* **Bladder and ureter** – transitional epithelium
* **Urethra** – prostatic – transitional epithelium penile – stratified epithelium
* **Epididymis** – pseudostratified epithelium **with stereo cilia**
* **Vagina** – stratified squamous
* **Uterus** – simple columnar

Simple Squamous Epithelium (Single layer of flattened cells with disk-shaped central nuclei and sparse cytoplasm; the simplest of epithelia)

Function: allows passage of materials by diffusion and filtration in sites where protection is not important, secretes lubricating substances in serosae

Location: kidney glomeruli; air sacs of lungs; lining of heart, blood vessels, and lymphatic vessels; lining of ventral body cavity (serosae)

Simple Cuboidal Epithelium (Single layer of cubelike cells with large, spherical central nuclei.)

Function: secretion and absorption

Location: kidney tubules, ducts and secretory portions of small glands, ovary surface

Simple Columnar *Nonciliated* Epithelium

Function: absorption; secretion of mucus, enzymes, and other substances

Location: nonciliated type lines most of the digestive tract (stomach to anal canal), gallbladder, and excretory ducts of some glands

Simple Columnar *Ciliated* Epithelium (Single layer of tall cells with round to oval nuclei; some cells bear **cilia**; layer may contain mucus-secreting unicellular glands [**goblet cells**].)

Function: ciliated type propels mucus (or reproductive cells) by ciliated action

Location: ciliated variety lines small bronchi, uterine tubes, and some regions of the uterus

Stratified Squamous Epithelium (Thick membrane composed of several cell layers. Basal cells are cuboidal or columnar and metabolically active. Surface cells are flattened [squamous]. In the keratinized type, the surface cells are full of deratin and dead. Basal cells are active in mitosis and produce the cells of the more superficial layers.)

Function: protects underlying tissues in areas subject to abrasion

Location: nonkeratinized type forms the moist lining of the esophagus, mouth, and vagina; keratinized type forms the epidermis of the skin, a dry membrane

Areolar (Loose) Tissue (Gel-like matrix; three fiber types; contains fibroblasts, macrophages, mast cells, and white blood cells.)

Function: Hold *organs* in place and attach *epithelial tissue* to other underlying tissues. It also serves as a reservoir of water and salts for surrounding tissues.

Location: It surrounds blood vessels and nerves and penetrates with them even into the small spaces of muscles, tendons, and other tissues. It may be found in tissue sections from almost every part of the body.

Adipose Tissue (Gel-like matrix; cells closely packed, with nuclei pushed to the side.)

Function: provides reserve fuel, insulates against heat loss, supports and protects organs

Location: under skin, around kidneys and eyeballs, within abdomen, in breasts

---

Reticular Tissue (Network of reticular fibers and sparsely scattered cells.)

Function: Fibers form a soft internal skeleton that supports other cell types, including white blood cells, mast cells, and macrophages.

Location: lymphoid organs (lymph nodes, bone marrow, spleen)

Dense Regular Connective Tissue (Closely packed bundles of collagen fibers running in same direction, parallel to direction of pull.)

Function: attaches muscles to bones or to muscles, attaches bones to bones, withstands great tensile stress when pulling force is applied in one direction

Location: tendons, most ligaments, aponeuroses

Dense Irregular Connective Tissue (Bundles of collagen fibers are much thicker and arranged irregularly.)

Function: able to withstand tension exerted in many directions, provides structural strength

Location: fibrous capsules of organs and joints, dermis of the skin, submucosa of digestive tract

Elastic Tissue (Predominantly composed of elastic fibers; fibroblasts occupy some spaces between fibers.)

Function: allows recoil of tissue following stretching, maintains pulsatile flow of blood through arteries, aids passive recoil of lungs following inspiration

Location: walls of large arteries, within certain ligaments associated with vertebral column, within the walls of the bronchial tubes

Hylaine Cartilage (Chondrocytes are round, one cell per lacunae, and surrounded by the matrix they produce. Matrix is type-2 collagen, proteoglycans [chondotin sulfate].)

Function: supports and reinforces, has resilient cushioning properties, resists compressive stress

Location: forms most of the embryonic skeleton, covers the ends of long bones in joint cavities, forms the costal cartilages of the ribs, cartilages of the nose, trachea, and larynx.

Fibrocartilage (Composed of chondrocytes residing in lacunae and a hydrous extracellular matrix.)

Function: tensile strength with the ability to absorb compressive shock

Location: inververtebral discs

Elastic Cartilage (Covers ends of bones made of chondrocytes and elastic fibers.)

Function: maintains the shape of a structure while allowing great flexibility

Location: supports external ear

Compact Bone (Contains few spaces. The strongest form of bone tissue. It is found beneath the periosteum of all bones and makes up the bulk of the diaphyses of long bones.)

Function: bone supports and protects

Location: bones

Blood (Contains matrix called plasma and various types of cells: red [carry nutrients and wastes], white [fight infection and include neutrophils, lymphocytes, monocytes, eosinphils, basophils].)

Function: transport of respiratory gases, nutrients, wastes, and other substances

Location: contained within blood vessels

Skeletal Muscle (Striated, multiple nuclei per cell, very long cylindrical shape.)

Function: move bones/body

Location: attached to bones

Cardiac Muscle (Striated, one nucleus per cell, branched ends.)

Function: movement/contraction of the heart

Location: heart

Smooth Muscle (No striations. Cells are tapered at each end, one nucleus per cell.)

Function: movement in hollow organs

Location: hollow organs

Neuron - Nerve Cell (Long extension from the main body of the cell, one nucleus per cell, dendrites.)

Function: transmit impulses

Location: central nervous system and peripheral nervous system

Mitosis (Interphase. Most of the cell life spent in this phase.)

Three phases of the cell cycle that occur between cell divisions. Made up of the G1 (gap), S (synthesis), G2 (gap 2), and M (mitosis) phases (G1 phase-S phase-G2 phase-M phase)

Mitosis (Prophase)

First and longest phase of mitosis, in which centrioles appear and move to opposite ends of the cell, forming a mitotic spindle.

Mitosis (Metaphase)

Second phase of mitosis, in which the chromatids line up at the center of the nucleus and attach to the spindle fibers.

Mitosis (Anaphase)

Third phase of mitosis, in which the chromatids are pulled away from each other by the spindle fibers.

Mitosis (Telophase)

Final stage of mitosis, in which a nuclear membrane forms around each set of chromosomes. They appear as chromatin threads rather than rods.

BIOCHEMISTRY

Basic Concepts

In most of the biochemical reactions, usually the end product of the reaction is the main stimulator / inhibitor of the rate limiting enzyme of that reaction. If end product goes up, it inhibits the rate-limiting enzyme and thus inhibits the reaction. If the end product level goes down, it stimulates the rate-limiting enzyme, and thus the reaction. *Action of hormones is important too.*

Example: The purpose of the TCA cycle is to produce ATP. Main end products of the TCA cycle are NADH and FADH2, which enter in ETC and give ATP. The rate-limiting enzyme of the TCA cycle is isocitrate dehydrogenase. When NADH level goes up (when ETC doesn't use NADH in conditions causing hypoxia), it inhibits isocitrate dehydrogenase and thus inhibits the TCA cycle. When more ATP is used, that means an increase in ADP (because ATP produces energy by giving its phosphate), and it stimulates isocitrate dehydrogenase to meet the need of ATP.

First, remember all rate-limiting enzymes of all important reaction. In the exam, most of the time, they ask factors that stimulate / inhibit those reactions by correlating reactions with clinical conditions. Know how our body uses those end products of all important reactions so you can correlate them better with clinical conditions they present in the exam.

Y *RATE-LIMITING ENZYMES OF IMPORTANT REACTIONS*:

* Glycolysis – PFK-1
* Glycogenesis – glycogen synthase
* Glycogenolysis – glycogen phosphorylase
* Gluconeogenesis – fructose-1, 6-biphosphate (F-1, 6-BP)

* HMP shunt – G6PD
* TCA cycle – isocitrate dehydrogenase
* FA synthesis – acetyl co-A carboxylase
* Beta-oxidation – carnitine acyltransferase-1
* Heme synthesis – δ ALA synthase (ALA - aminolavulinate)
* Purine synthesis – PRPP amidotransferase
* Cholesterol synthesis – HMG co-A reductase

-	ENZYMES	Stimulated By	Inhibited By
1	hexokinase (low Km, in most tissue) glucose → glucose-6-P		glucose-6-P
2	glucokinase (high Km, in liver) glucose → glucose-6-P (irreversible)	insulin high glucose	fasting
3	PFK-1 (phosphofructokinase-1) fructose-6-P → F-1, 6 BP (irreversible) (insulin [+] PFK-2 F6P F-2, 6 BP)	AMP F-2, 6 BP insulin	ATP citrate glucagon
4	glycogen synthase (form α-1, 4 glycosidic bond)	insulin glucose	epinephrine (epi) glucagon
5	glycogen phosphorylase (break α-1, 4 glycosidic bond and release glucose-1-P)	epi, glucagon AMP Ca+2	insulin ATP
6	F-1, 6 BP (opposite to PFK-1)	ATP	AMP
7	pyruvate carboxylase (in mitochondria) pyruvate → oxaloacetate	acetyl co-A	
8	pyruvate dehydrogenase pyruvate → acetyl co-A (irreversible)	insulin, PEP, AMP	acetyl co-A, ATP, NADH
9	PEPCK (cytoplasm, requires GTP) (oxaloacetate → PEP) (PEP = phosphoenolepyruvate)	glucagon cortisol	
10	G6PD (G6P → 6-phosphogluconate → ribulose-5-P → ribose-5-P) (form 2 NADPH)	insulin NADP	NADPH
11	isocitrate dehydrogenase (isocitrate → α-ketoglutarate)	ADP	NADH
12	acetyl co-A carboxylase (acetyl co-A → malonyl co-A)	insulin citrate	
13	carnitine acyltransferase-1	glucagon	malonyl co-A insulin

14	δ ALA synthase (glycine + succinyl co-A → δ ALA)	require vit-B6	heme
15	PRPP amidotransferase (↑ activity leads to hyperuricemia)		IMP AMP GMP allopurinol 6-MP
16	HMG co-A reductase (cholesterol synthesis)	insulin	glucagon

- Our body needs energy in the form of ATP, and we get ATP from glucose. Period! Substrates to produce glucose are carbohydrate, fat and protein (from food and from our body storage).

- *Carbohydrate from food*: Glycolysis (to produce ATP), glycogenesis (to store in body as a glycogen). Disaccharides like lactose and sucrose are broken to glucose + galactose (by lactase) and glucose + fructose (by sucrase) respectively. These monosaccharide forms are then absorbed into blood and transported to liver and other tissues for glycogenesis and glycolysis. Once the body's need of glucose has fulfilled, the remaining glucose is then converted into glycogen in the liver and some used in HMP shunt and some in AA synthesis. After glycogen storage, if glucose still remains, it is then converted into triglycerides (TGs) in adipose tissues.

- *Fat from food*: The lipase (activated by acid) breaks down the fat (TGs) into monoglycerides (glycerol) and fatty acids. The bile emulsifies the fatty acids so they may be easily absorbed. Short- and some medium-chain fatty acids are absorbed directly into the blood via intestine capillaries and travel through the portal vein just as other absorbed nutrients do. However, long-chain fatty acids and some medium-chain fatty acids are absorbed into the fatty walls of the intestine villi and reassembled again into triglycerides. Chylomicrons carry dietary TGs. Within the villi, the chylomicron enters a lymphatic capillary called a lacteal, which merges into larger lymphatic vessels. It is transported via the lymphatic system and the thoracic duct, which empties the chylomicrons into the bloodstream via the left subclavian vein. At this point, the chylomicrons can transport the triglycerides to where they are needed (liver).

- *Proteins from food*: Pancreatic enzymes clave peptide bonds and releases AA. Absorbed into intestinal epithelial cells by secondary active transport and from epithelial cells, AA diffuses directly into blood.

- *During fasting*: Glycogenolysis occurs until stored glycogen deprived. After that, gluconeogenesis begins to provide glucose to the brain.
- After prolonged fasting (>1 week), brain use ketone bodies (2/3) and glucose (1/3)
- In all conditions, RBCs use only glucose because they lack mitochondria.

- *Essential AA and Fatty Acid (FA)*: *Essential* means our body can't synthesize them so we have to ingest them in the form of food.

- *Essential AA*: PM AT TV HILL: phenylalanine, methionine, arginine, threonine, tryptophan, valine, histidine, isoleucine, leucine, lysine
- *Essential FA*: α-linolenic acid (ALA, 18:3, ω-3 fatty acids); linoleic acid (LA, 18:2, ω-6 fatty acids)

- *How do we get energy from food*? Glucose is oxidized and released energy. This energy is transferred to NAD+ by reduction to NADH as part of glycolysis and the TCA cycle. NADH is then enter in ETC to produce ATP.

- *Glycolysis*: Glucose → G-6-P → F-6-P → F-1, 6-BP → PEP → Pyruvate
- End product of glycolysis is pyruvate.
- When oxygen is available / less ATP is required, pyruvate is converted to acetyl co-A to enter the TCA cycle and produce ATP through ETC
- When less oxygen available / more ATP is required (*ex.*, during exercise), pyruvate is converted to lactate and produces ATP

$$PEP \xrightarrow[\text{ATP} \to \text{ADP}]{\text{pyruvate kinase}} \text{pyruvate (irreversible)}$$

$$\text{pyruvate} \xrightarrow[\text{NAD}^+ \to \text{NADH}]{\text{pyruvate dehydrogenase}} \text{acetyl co-A (irreversible)}$$

$$\text{pyruvate} \xrightarrow[\text{NADH} \to \text{NAD}^+]{\text{lactate dehydrogenase}} \text{lactate (produces 2 ATP)}$$

$$\text{pyruvate} \xrightarrow[\text{glutamate} \to \alpha\text{-ketoglutarate}]{\text{alanine transaminase}} \text{alanine (reversible)}$$

$$\text{pyruvate} \xrightarrow[\text{ATP} \to \text{ADP}]{\text{pyruvate carboxylase}} \text{oxaloacetate (gluconeogenesis)}$$

- Lactate produced from pyruvate in anaerobic reaction can be used to synthesis glucose (gluconeogenesis in liver through Cori cycle). Pyruvate to Lactate produce only 2 ATP to use by our body whereas lactate to glucose conversion consumes 6 ATP of our body so there is a loss of 4 ATP, which explains why this cycle can't continue without external energy (food) and we can't survive without eating! This process also produces NAD+, which is required to continue glycolysis.
- *Glycolysis*: It produces 2 ATP (substrate level phosphorylation), 2 NADH, and 2 pyruvate molecules (aerobic).
  2 ATP per glucose molecule (anaerobic)
  6 or 8 ATP (depends upon which shuttle is used to carry NADH, aerobic)
  NADH – carried by *malate shuttle* (3ATP) *or glycerol-3-P shuttle* (converts in FADH2 and gives 2 ATP)
- *TCA cycle*: *Three* important shuttles
  citrate ⟶ FA synthesis
  succinyl co-Aheme ⟶ (to activate ketone bodies)

malate $\longrightarrow$ gluconeogenesis

fumarate $\longleftarrow$ urea cycle

acetyl co A is the entry point in TCA cycle

- As already mentioned above, end products of TCA cycle are NADH and FADH2, which enter in ETC and produce ATP.
- NADH – carried by *malate shuttle* (give 3ATP) *or glycerol-3-P shuttle* (converts in FADH2 and gives 2 ATP)
- FADH2 (produced by glycerol-3-P shuttle and succinate dehydrogenase [complex-2]) directly transfer electron to coenzyme-Q in ETC.

Important Concept

- In pyruvate dehydrogenase deficiency, pyruvate doesn't convert into acetyl co-A. Increased pyruvate will then convert into lactate and alanine, so in pyruvate dehydrogenase deficiency → ↑ lactate and alanine
- Pyruvate kinase deficiency → anaerobic glycolysis → ↑ 2, 3 BPG → O2 dissociation curve shift to the right

---

- *Electron in ETC pass in following order*: complex-1 (NADH dehydrogenase) coenzyme-Q

  complex-3 (cytochrome b/c1) cytochrome C (inhibited by cyanide)

  complex-4 (cytochrome a/a3) $\longrightarrow$ transfer electron to O2

- *Uncouplers:*↓ proton gradient in ETC leads to ↓ ATP synthesis, ↑ O2 consumption, ↑ oxidation of NADH, and therefore, energy is released as heat. *Ex.,* 2, 4 dinitrophenol (2, 4-DNP), Aspirin, brown adipose tissue in newborns

- *Gluconeogenesis*: Synthesis of *glucose* from other substrates during *fasting*; occurs in liver (major) and in the cortex of kidney (small part)

- Substrate: pyruvate, lactate, oxaloacetate, glycerol, and glucogenic AA (*except* lysine and leucine)

- FA *cannot* be converted *directly* into glucose in animals, the *exception* being odd- chain FA that yields propionyl CoA, a precursor for succinyl CoA.

- Before glycerol can enter the pathway of gluconeogenesis, it must be converted to their intermediate glyceraldehyde 3-phosphate.
- Alanine is converted in pyruvate, which is then used to synthesize glucose.

- *Gluconeogenesis*: lactate → pyruvate → oxaloacetate → malate (in mitochondria) → oxaloacetate (in cytoplasm) → PEP → F-1, 6-BP → F-6-P → G-6-P → glucose
- *Gluconeogenesis*: glyceraldehyde-3-P → F-1, 6-P → F-6-P → G-6-P → glucose

- Our body use this glucose to generate energy (ATP) during fasting
- *Glycolysis*: glucose → G-6-P → F-6-P → F-1, 6-BP → PEP → pyruvate

- *Important reaction of glycolysis intermediate when excess of glucose is available*: F-1, 6-BP ↔ glyceraldehyde-3-P + dihydroxyacetone phosphate (DHAP) [fructose bisphosphate aldolase] (↔ means reversible process, enzyme has been written in brackets, [], with each end product)

- In liver (after eating), glycerol (came from food) ↔ glycerol-3-P [glycerol kinase] (used for TGs synthesis in adipose tissue for storage)
- In adipose tissue, DHAP (produced during glycolysis from F-1, 6-BP in liver) ↔
- glycerol-3-P [glycerol-3-P dehydrogenase] (used in synthesis of TGs for storage)

- During fasting, *in adipose tissue*, TGs ↔ free FA + glycerol [glucagon stimulate hormone-sensitive lipase]. Glycerol from adipose tissue now goes to liver.
- In liver, glycerol (came from adipose tissue) ↔ glycerol-3-P (glycerol kinase) ↔ DHAP (glycerol-3-P dehydrogenase) ↔ glyceraldehyde-3-P (triosephosphate isomerase) → F-1, 6-P → F-6-P → G-6-P → *glucose*
- Glucose-6-P and glycerol kinase enzymes—present only in liver, that's why gluconeogenesis (major) occurs in liver. Glucokinase (glycolysis) is also present in liver only.

- Beta oxidation: When glycogen store depleted, TGs from adipose tissue break into free FA and glycerol via hormone-sensitive lipase. Free FA is then converted into acetyl co-A, which is used in TCA cycle to produce ATP, but when acetyl co-A is exceeded and TCA cycle can't handle the load (low TCA intermediate, especially oxaloacetate, which is also used for gluconeogenesis), acetyl co-A is then used to form ketone bodies.
- Acetoacetate is the first ketone body to form.
- Acetone and β-hydroxybutyrate are formed from acetoacetate.
- Acetone is 3-carbon ketone bodies that are *not* used as energy fuel. Acetone is excreted as a waste product, and that's why we get a specific fruity smell in patients with diabetic ketoacidosis, which is due to acetone.
- Free FA is needed to be activated first before they are carried to mitochondria for beta oxidation. It is done by the enzyme fatty acyl co-A synthetase.
- Fatty acid + CoA + ATP ↔ Acyl co-A + AMP + PP_i (by fatty acyl co-A synthase)
- *Carnitine shuttle*: Fatty acyl co-A then transfers fatty acyl group to carnitine via carnitine acyltransferase-1. Fatty acyl carnitine is a shuttle across the inner membrane. Carnitine acyltransferase-2 transfer fatty acyl group back to a co-A to formed fatty acyl co-A in the mitochondria.
- Fatty acyl co-A is *then* degraded to acetyl co-A + acyl co-A. This process continues until it gives acetyl co-A + acyl co-A for FA with even number of carbons. For FA with odd number of carbons, it continues until it gives acetyl co-A + propionyl co-A.
- During each step, it gives one FADH2, one NADH. Acetyl co-A enters the TCA cycle and gives ATP. That's how beta oxidation provides energy.

- *Propionyl co-A*: Propionyl co-A is a product of odd-chain fatty-acid oxidation, a product of metabolism of isoleucine and valine and a product of alpha- ketobutyric acid (which is a product of threonine and methionine), propionyl co- A → methylmalonyl co-A → succinyl co-A. (First reaction is conducted by propionyl co-A carboxylase, which requires biotin as a cofactor. Second reaction is catalyzed by methylmalonyl co-A mutase, which requires vit-B12 as a cofactor.) Succinyl co-A then enters the TCA cycle.

- *FA synthesis, from glucose,* which is still there after body's demand is over, *through glycolysis:* oxaloacetate + acetyl co-A ↔ citrate (citrate synthase)
- Citrate is transported to the cytoplasm where it again converts to acetyl co-A. Acetyl co-A is converted into malonyl co-A by acetyl co-A carboxylase enzyme.
- Fatty acids are formed by the action of fatty acid synthase from acetyl co-A and malonyl co-A precursors.

- *Glycogen synthesis, from glucose,* which is still there after body's demand has over, *through glycolysis:* glucose → glucose-6-P → glucose-1-P → UDP glucose → UDP and (1, 4-α-D-glucosyl)n+1 → Branches are made by branching enzyme
- *Only* those glucose molecules *that are bound to UDP nucleotide* used in glycogen synthesis.
- Enzymes responsible for above reactions respectively are glucokinase/hexokinase → phosphoglucomutase → uridyl transferase (also called UDP-glucose pyrophosphorylase) → glycogen synthase → Branching enzyme (amylo-α[1:4]-α[1:6] transglycosylase)
- Glycogen synthase: catalyses the reaction of UDP-glucose and (1, 4-α-D- glucosyl)n to yield UDP and (1, 4-α-D-glucosyl)n+1. In other words, *this enzyme converts excess glucose residues one by one into a polymeric chain for storage as glycogen.*

- *Glycogenolysis:* glycogen → glycogen n-1 + glucose-1-P by glycogen phosphorylase. It breaks down glucose polymer at α-1–4 linkages until 5 linked glucoses are left on the branch. Now debranching enzymes involve that moves the remaining glucose units to another nonreducing end. This results in less glucose units available to glycogen phosphorylase. The final action of the debranching enzyme leads to the original glucose-1-P connected 1, 4 to another branch being released. Glucose-1-P → glucose-6-P by phosphoglucomutase. *Glucose-6-P then enters glycolysis to provide ATP.*

- *HMP shunt (pentose phosphate pathway)*: *Glucose-6-phosphate* does HMP shunt. *Fructose-6-phosphate* produced in HMP shunt is a reentry to glycolysis.
- Important of HMP shunt: to generate NADPH (for reductive biosynthesis reactions within cells) and ribose-5-phosphate (for the synthesis of the nucleic acids and nucleotides)
- Importance of NADPH: To maintain the reduced state of glutathione (GSH). Reduced glutathione converts reactive H_2O_2 into H_2O by oxidizing itself (GSSH). In G6PD deficiency, there is very low NADPH, so glutathione remains in its oxidizing phase so RBC can't handle oxidative stress leads to hemolysis.

- Pyruvate dehydrogenase, alpha-ketoglutarate dehydrogenase, branched-chain ketoacid dehydrogenase → require thiamin (vit-B1), co-A, NAD, FAD, lipoic acid.
- ↑ transketolase in RBCs in thiamin (vit-B1) deficiency.

- *Amino acid synthesis*: There are twenty main amino acids. Out of twenty, eight are essential AA. Our body synthesizes remaining twelve AA.
- Amino acids are synthesized from TCA cycle intermediate (glutamate).
- Alpha-ketoglutarate + NH_4^+ ↔ glutamate
- Afterward, alanine and aspartate are formed by transamination of glutamate. All of the remaining amino acids are then constructed from glutamate or aspartate, by transamination of these two amino acids with one α-keto acid.

- $NH4^+$ is the source of nitrogen for all the amino acids
- Alanine and aspartate are synthesized by the transamination of pyruvate and oxaloacetate, respectively. Glutamine is synthesized from NH4+ and glutamate, and asparagine is synthesized similarly. Proline and arginine are derived from glutamate. Serine, formed from 3-phosphoglycerate, is the precursor of glycine and cysteine. Tyrosine is synthesized by the hydroxylation of phenylalanine (an essential amino acid).
- *Importance of AA*: Nitric oxide, a short-lived messenger, is formed from arginine. Porphyrins are synthesized from glycine and

succinyl co-A, which condense to give δ-aminolevulinate, which is a part of heme synthesis.

- Aminotransferases (AST and ALT) – both require vit-B6 (pyridoxine). In muscle – transfer amino group to glutamate. In liver – alanine to aspartate.
- Glutamate dehydrogenase convert glutamate to α-ketoglutarate (TCA cycle intermediate)
- AST and CPS-1 (carbamoyl phosphate synthetase-1) are direct donors of nitrogen in the urea cycle

- *Urea cycle (Ornithine cycle)*: It produces urea from ammonia. Ammonia is toxic to the brain. Urea cycle takes place only in liver. Both mitochondria and cytosol.
- It consumes 4 ATP and releases 5 ATP so we get 1 ATP from urea cycle
- *Reactions*: NH_4^+ + 2ATP + HCO_3^- → carbamoyl phosphate (CPS-1) + 2ADP + P (mitochondria) CPS-1 + ornithine → citrulline + P [ornithine transcarbamoylase] (mitochondria) citrulline + aspartate + ATP → argininosuccinate + AMP + PP (argininosuccinate synthase) [cytosol] argininosuccinate → arginine + fumarate (argininosuccinate lyase) [cytosol] arginine + H_2O → ornithine + urea (arginase) [cytosol]
- Fumarate → malate [fumarase] → oxaloacetate [malate dehydrogenase]
- Oxaloacetate → aspartate [transaminase] / oxaloacetate → PEP (*gluconeogenesis*)

- *Importance of essential FA*: Used to make eicosanoids (prostaglandins, prostacyclins, thromboxane, and leukotrines)
- Eicosanoid biosynthesis begins when cell is activated by mechanical trauma, cytokines, growth factors or other stimuli. Phospholipids from cell membrane → arachidonic acid [phospholipase A_2] → prostaglandins (PG) [cyclooxygenase (COX)] / arachidonic acid → HPETE [lipoxygenase] (leukotrines synthesis) arachidonic acid → PGH [cyclooxygenase] → thromboxane A_2 [thromboxane synthase] arachidonic acid → PGH [cyclooxygenase] → Prostacyclins [prostacyclin synthase] arachidonic acid → PGH [cyclooxygenase] → PGE_2 [PGE synthase] → PGF_2
- *Clinical Importance*: *Steroids* inhibit phospholipase (inhibit synthesis of both prostaglandins and leukotrines). *NSAIDs*

inhibit COX (inhibit synthesis of prostaglandins). *Ziluton* inhibits lipoxygenase (inhibit synthesis of leukotrines) *Low-dose Aspirin* inhibits thromboxane synthase (inhibits platelate aggregation)

- *Glucose Transport*
  GLUT-1 – brain, RBCs (do not need insulin for uptake)
  GLUT-3 – most tissue (do not need insulin for uptake)
  GLUT-2 – Liver
  GLUT-4 – Adipose tissue and skeletal M. (insulin-stimulated glucose uptake)

- *Citrate shuttle* – transport acetyl co-A group from mitochondria to cytoplasm for FA synthesis.

- *Carnitine shuttle*: After FA is activated to fatty acetyl co-A, fatty acyl co-A, then transfer fatty acyl group to carnitine via carnitine acyltransferase-1. Fatty acyl carnitine is a shuttle across the inner membrane. Carnitine acyltransferase-2 transfer fatty acyl group back to a co-A to formed fatty acyl co-A in the mitochondria.

- *Farnesyl phosphate*: an intermediate in cholesterol synthesis pathway, used for the following:
  - Synthesis of co-Q
  - Synthesis of dolichol phosphate (required cofactor in N-linked glycosylation in RER)
  - Prenylation of proteins that need to be held in the cell membrane by the lipid tail

- Enzymes in Inner Mitochondrial Membrane succinate dehydrogenase (complex-2)
  F0-F1-ATP synthetase carnitine acyltransferase-2

- Enzymes in Outer Mitochondrial Membrane fatty acyl co-A synthetase carnitine acyltransferase-1

- Carbamoyl Phosphate Synthase (CPS) cytoplasm – pyrimidine synthesis mitochondria – urea cycle
  (Both are different enzymes with different locations but similar name.)

- *Fatty acyl synthase*: activate FA by attaching co-A (first step in both FA synthesis and beta-oxidation)
- *Fatty acid synthase*: FA synthesis
- (Both are different enzymes, so don't confuse.)

Y *PROCESSES IN MITOCHONDRIA*
- Ketone body synthesis
- FA oxidation
- Production of acetyl co-A
- TCA cycle
- ETC (electron transport chain)

Y *PROCESSES IN CYTOPLASM*
- Glycolysis
- FA synthesis
- Cholesterol synthesis
- HMP shunt

Y *PROCESSES IN BOTH MITOCHONDREA and CYTOPLASM*
- Gluconeogenesis
- Urea cycle
- Heme synthesis

- *Lipoproteins*: lipid + protein
- Chylomicrons - carry triacylglycerol (fat) from the intestines to the liver, skeletal muscle, and to adipose tissue
- VLDL - carry (newly synthesized) triacylglycerol from the liver to adipose tissue
- IDL - intermediate between VLDL and LDL, not usually detectable in the blood
- LDL - carry cholesterol from the liver to cells of the body (bad cholesterol)
- HDL - carry cholesterol from the body's tissues to the liver (good cholesterol)

- *Chylomicron Metabolism*
- After lipids are absorbed from small intestine, these lipids (triglycerides, phospholipids, and cholesterol) are assembled with apolipoprotein B-48 into chylomicrons. These nascent

chylomicrons are secreted into the lymphatic circulation, bypass the liver circulation, and are drained via the thoracic duct into the bloodstream.

- In the circulation, HDL particles donate apolipoprotein C-II and apolipoprotein E to the nascent chylomicron; the chylomicron is now considered mature. Apolipoprotein C-II activates lipoprotein lipase (LPL), an enzyme on endothelial cells lining the blood vessels. LPL catalyzes a hydrolysis reaction that ultimately releases glycerol and fatty acids from the chylomicrons. Glycerol and fatty acids can be absorbed in peripheral tissues, especially adipose and muscle, for energy and storage.
- The hydrolyzed chylomicrons are now considered chylomicron remnants. The chylomicron remnants absorb into liver via interaction with apolipoprotein E. This interaction causes the endocytosis of the chylomicron remnants, which are subsequently hydrolyzed within lysosomes. Lysosomal hydrolysis releases glycerol and fatty acids into the cell, which can be used for energy or stored for later use.

- *VLDL Metabolism*
- The liver is another important source of lipoproteins, principally VLDL. Triacylglycerol and cholesterol are assembled with apolipoprotein B-100 to form VLDL particles (nascent VLDL).
- In the circulation, HDL donates its apolipoprotein C-II and apolipoprotein E to VLDL particles (mature VLDL).

- Now apolipoprotein C-II activates LPL, causing hydrolysis of the VLDL particle and the release of glycerol and fatty acids. These products can be absorbed from the blood by peripheral tissues, principally adipose and muscle. The hydrolyzed VLDL particles are now called VLDL remnants *or* intermediate density lipoproteins (IDL). The VLDL remnants absorb into liver via interaction with apolipoprotein E. They can be further hydrolyzed by hepatic lipase.
- Hydrolysis by hepatic lipase releases glycerol and fatty acids, leaving behind IDL remnants, called low-density lipoproteins (LDL), which contain relatively high cholesterol content. LDL circulates and is absorbed by the liver and peripheral cells. Binding of LDL to its target tissue occurs through an interaction between LDL receptor and apolipoprotein B-100 or E on the LDL particle.

Absorption occurs through endocytosis, and the internalized LDL particles are hydrolyzed within lysosomes, releasing lipids, chiefly cholesterol.

- LPL (lipoprotein lipase) → induced by insulin
- HSL (hormone stimulated lipase) → induced by epinephrine

Y *COLLAGEN SYNTHESIS*
- Hydroxyproline is an amino acid unique to collagen
- Glycine (gly) is found at almost every third residue (Gly – x-y-Gly-x-y- etc.)
- Proline (pro) makes up about 9% of collagen
- Proline and lysine – hydroxylated in RER by prolyl and lysyl hydroxylase (require vit-C)
- Procollagen (triple helical structure) glycosylated in golgi and secreted from cell
- Cross-linking involves lysyl oxidase (require O2, Cu+2)

- Tetrahydrofolate (THF): THF is a carrier of activated one-carbon unit and plays an important role in the metabolism of amino acids and nucleotides. This coenzyme carries one-carbon units *at three oxidation states*, which are interconvertible: *most reduced*—methyl; *intermediate*—methylene; and *most oxidized*—formyl, formimino, and methenyl. Methionine → S-adenosylmethionine [methionine adenosyltransferase] → adenosylhomocystine [methyltransferase] → homocystine → methionine [homocystine methyltransferase transfer methyl group from N5-methyl-THF] (This enzyme requires vit-B12 as a cofactor; therefore in vit-B12 deficiency, stored folate (N5-methyl-THF) can not be used, and so secondary folate deficiency is created, which produces megaloblastic anemia) / homocystine → cystathione [cystathione synthase] (requires vit-B6).
- Cystathione → cystine + α-ketobutyrate [cystathione γ lyase]
- α-Ketobutyrate → propionyl co-A [α-ketobutyrate dehydrogenase]

- Vit-B12: It is used as a cofactor in propionyl co-A metabolism, which is a product of odd-chain FA, valine, isoleucine, methionine, and threonine.

- Methylmalonic aciduria (seen in vit-B12 deficiency) – distinguished megaloblastic anemia from folate deficiency

Y *Heme Transport and Storage*
- Feroxidase (also known as ceruloplasmin, copper protein) oxidize Fe^{+2} to Fe^{+3} for transport and storage.
- Transferrin carries Fe^{+3} in blood
- Ferritin stores normal amount of Fe^{+3} in tissue
- Hemosiderin binds excess Fe^{+3} to prevent escape of free Fe+3 into blood where it is toxic.

•

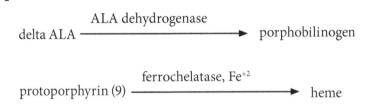

- Lead inhibits both ALA dehydrogenase and ferrochelatase.

- Vit-B$_6$ deficiency: ↓ protoporphyrin and ↓δ ALA
- Iron deficiency: ↑protoporphyrin and N δ ALA
- Lead poisoning: ↑protoporphyrin and ↑δ ALA

Y *Purine and Pyrimidine Metabolism*
- Purines are synthesized as nucleotides (bases attached to ribose 5-phosphate).
- Pyrimidines are assembled before being attached to 5-phosphoribosyl-1- pyrophosphate (PRPP)
- *Purine synthesis*: ribose-5-Phosphate (HMP shunt) → PRPP (by ribose-phosphate diphosphokinase) → 5-phosphoribosylamine [amidophosphoribosyltransferase] → IMP (*It is a precursor of both adenine and guanine.* Amino acids involved in synthesis of IMP are glycine, glutamine, and aspartic acid. Also used THF as a cofactor) IMP → XMP → GMP / IMP → adenylosuccinate → AMP
- *Pyrimidine Synthesis*: glutamine → carbamoyl phosphate [carbamoyl phosphatase II] → carbamoyl aspartic acid → dihydroorotate → orotate → OMP (used PRPP) → UDP → UTP → CTP (Glutamine and ATP. *Uracil is a precursor of both C and T*)

- *Purine degradation*: Final common product is uric acid. When a cell dies (apoptosis), the nuclease frees nucleotides. *Guanine*: nucleotide → guanosine [nucleotidase] → guanine [purine nucleoside phosphorylase] → xanthine [guanase] → uric acid [xanthine oxidoreductase]. *Adenine*: nucleotide → adenosine → inosine [adenosine deaminase, deficiency of which causes severe combined immunodeficiency {SCID}] / nucleotide → IMP [AMP deaminase] → inosine [nucleotidase]. Now from inosine → hypoxanthine [purine nucleoside phosphorylase] → xanthine [xanthine oxidoreductase] → uric acid [xanthine oxidoreductase]
- *Purine salvage*: Salvage pathways are used to recover bases and nucleosides that are formed during degradation of RNA and DNA. hypoxanthine → IMP [HGPRT] Guanine → GMP [HGPRT] adenine → AMP [adenine phosphoribosyltransferase]\

- *Clinical Biochemistry*

Y *GLYCOGEN STORAGE DISEASES*

- *Von Gierke's Disease*: glucose-6-phosphatase deficiency
  Severe fasting hypoglycemia, lactic acidosis, hyperuricemia, hepatomegaly, ketosis, hyperlipidemia

- *Medium-chain acyl co-A dehydrogenase (MCAD) deficiency*: severe fasting hypoglycemia, *no* ketosis, dicarboxylic acidosis

- Pompe's disease (Pump–heart): lysosomal alpha-1, 4 glucosidase deficiency cardiomegaly (*usually death occurs by age of two years*) glycogen-like material in inclusion bodies

- McArdle's disease (Muscle): muscle glycogen phosphorylase deficiency muscle cramps and weakness on exercise glycogen present in muscle biopsy

- *Myopathic carnitine deficiency*: carnitine deficiency in muscle muscle cramps and weakness on exercise triglycerides (TGs) present in muscle biopsy

- *Hers* disease: *H*epatic glycogen phosphorylase deficient mild fasting hypoglycemia, hepatomegaly

- Cori's disease: debarnching enzyme deficiency short outer branches, single glucose residue at outer branch

- Anderson's (amylopectinosis): branching enzyme deficiency Very few branch toward periphery.
  Infantile hypotonia, cirrhosis, usually death occur by age of 2 years

- *Lesch-Nyhan Syndrome*
- Defective purine metabolism
- Deficient HPRT (HGPRT)
- Child has tendency to compulsively bite his finger (*self-mutilation*)
- Mental retardation
- Hyperuricemia is due to ↓ IMP (hypoxanthine $\xrightarrow{\text{HPRT}}$ IMP)

- *Tay-Sachs Disease*
- Hexosaminidase A deficient
- Ganglioside accumulate in cells
- Charry red macula, *no* hepatomegaly, and cervical lymphadenopathy

- *Niemann-Pick*
- Sphingomyelinase deficiency
- Sphingomyelin accumulate in cells
- Characteristic foamy macrophage, *cherry-red macula*, hepatomegaly, and cervical lymphadenopathy (*Hepatomegaly is absent in Tay-Sachs.*)

- *Gaucher's Disease*
- gluocerebrosidase deficiency
- glucocerebroside accumulate in cells
- characteristic macrophage (crumpled paper inclusion)

- *Ashkenazi Jews* (Eastern European) → two diseases → Tay-Sachs and Gaucher's disease (type – I)
- *Ceremide* is common substance from all sphingolipid derived. Serine is AA joined with fatty acyl co–A to form ceremide.

- *Phenylketonuria*
- Phenylalanine hydroxylase deficiency (phenylalanine → tyrosine)
- *Musty odor* from child, mental retardation
- *Aspartame* (artificial sweeteners) must be strictly avoided by phenyketonurics
- ↑Phenylalanine level in pregnant woman → mental retardation in infants

- *Homogentisate Oxidase Deficiency*
- Accumulation of homogentisic acid in blood and excretion in urine
- Ochronosis (accumulation of black/brown pigments in cartilages)

- *Maple Syrup Urine Disease*
- Branched chain ketoacid dehydrogenase deficiency
- Impaired metabolism of valine, leucine, isoleucine
- Maple syrup odor in urine
- Ketosis, coma, and death if not treated

- *Acute Intermittent Porphyria*
- Uroporphyrinogen-1 synthase deficient
- Episodic variable expression
- Acute abdomen ("*belly full of scars*"), brief psychosis
- *No* photosensitivity (↑δ ALA, PBG)
- Never give *barbiturates*, pyrazinamide, gresiofulvin

- *Porphyria Cutanea Tarda*
- Uroporphyrinogen decarboxylase deficient
- *Photosensitivity* (↑uroporphyrin 1, urinary uroporphyrin - *diagnostic test*)
- Chronic inflammation to overt blistering and shearing in exposed area of skin.
  Tx., stop alcohol and estrogen use.

- *Homocystinuria*: arthrosclerosis in childhood, recurrent DVT

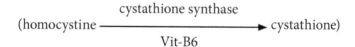

$$\text{homocystine} \xrightarrow[\text{Vit-B6}]{\text{cystathione synthase}} \text{cystathione}$$

- *Causes*: cystathione synthase deficiency, vit- B_6 deficiency, homocystine methyltransferase deficiency, folic acid, and vit- B_{12} deficiency
- Methionine is degraded via the homocystine-cystathione pathway, so methionine is elevated in patient with cystathione synthase deficiency via activation of homocystine methyltransferase by excess substrate homocystine.

- *Genetic Deficiency of the Urea Cycle* (Both mitochondrial enzymes)
- Carbamoyl-P-synthase and ornithine transcarbamoylase deficiency
- Both have same signs and symptoms but increase in uracil and orotic acid seen in ornithine transcarbamoylase deficiency differentiate both.
- Increase in NH_4^+, which is toxic to the brain
- *Tx.*, low protein diet (Urea is produced from AA degradation.)

- *Hartnup disease*: defect in epithelial transport of neutral AA, including tryptophan
- Signs and symptoms are *similar to pellagra*
- Niacin – helpful in controlling symptoms
- Defective transport leads to dietary AA in stool and excess *free AA in urine*

- *Cystinuria*: Most common aminoaciduria characterized by defect in reabsorption of *COAL—c*ystine, *o*rnithine, *a*rginine, *l*ysine
- Associated with *Staghorn calculi in kidney*

Galactosemia/Galactosuria	Fructosemia/Fructosuria
25. Galactokinase deficiency	*8. Fructokinase deficiency*
- ↑ Galactose in blood	- ↑Fructose in blood
- *Cataract* (aldose reductase)	- *No* Cataract
- Galactokinase traps galactose in cell by phosphorylation as galactose-1-phosphate	- Fructokinase traps fructose in cell by phosphorylation as fructose-1-phosphate
- *Gal-1-uridyltransferase deficiency*	- *Aldolase B deficiency*

- Converts galatose-1-phosphate into glucose-1-phosphate	- Converts fructose-1-phosphate into DHAP and glyceraldehydes
- If deficient, galactose-1-phosphate accumulates in cells and produces symptoms	- If deficient, fructose-1-phosphate accumulates in cells and produces symptoms.
- Liver, *brain,* and other tissue.	- Liver, *kidney*
- Symptoms evident while on breast milk, so *early onset* of symptoms after birth	- Symptoms are *not* evident while on breast milk, *so late onset* of symptoms after birth
- *Cataract*	- *No* cataract
- Hypoglycemia, lactic acidosis, jaundice, *mental retardation*	- Hypoglycemia, lactic acidosis, jaundice, *proximal renal tubular disorder* resembling Fanconi's syndrome
- Avoid milk and milk products	- Avoid honey and table sugar, which contain sucrose

■ *Menkes Disease*: X-linked recessive
Mutation in the gene encoding a Cu+2 efflux protein. Cu+2 accumulates in the cell and creates Cu+2 deficiency.

Y *HYPERLIPIDEMIAS*

■ Type-1 (familial hyperchylomicronemia)- ↑ chylomicrons (↑ TGs) – lipoprotein lipase deficiency – xanthomas present but *no* ↑ risk for atherosclerosis

■ *Type-2a* (familial hypercholesterolemia) - ↑ LDL only (LDL receptors deficiency) - ↑ cholesterol

■ Type-2b (combined hyperlipidemia) - decreased LDL receptor and increased apo B - ↑ LDL and VLDL (↑ cholesterol and TGs)

■ Type-3 (familial dysbetalipoproteinemia) - defect in apo E synthesis - ↑ chylomicrons remnants and IDL (↑ cholesterol and TGs)

■ Type-4 (familial hyperlipemia) - increased VLDL production and decreased elimination - ↑ VLDL (↑ cholesterol and TGs)

- Type-5 (endogenous hypertriglyceridemia) – carbohydrate induced (DM, alcohol) - ↑ VLDL (↑ TGs) but normal cholesterol

- *Fragile X-Syndrome*
- CGG repeat sequence
- Mental retardation, *enlarged testis*, prominent jaw, large ears

- *Ehlers-Danlos Syndrome*
- defect in type-I and type-III collagen synthesis and structure
- Hypermobile joints, *Aortic dissection* (MCC of death), poor wound healing

- *Osteogenesis Imperfecta*
- Blue sclera, brittle bones
- Defective synthesis of type-I collagen

- *Albinism*: deficiencies of tyrosine hydroxylase (copper dependent tyrosinase), *blocking production of melanin from aromatic AA tyrosine*—white hair, pinkirises, very pale skin, and a history of burning easily when exposed to the sun. Patients are at increased risk of squamous cell CA and melanoma.

- *Miscellaneous*

- Histidine is the only AA with good buffering capacity at physiologic pH.

- Fat-free diet – decrease prostaglandins (essential FA products)

- Km = (S) concentration at which half Vmax produced S = substrate
  Km – measure affinity of the enzyme
  Low Km (high affinity) – less substrate require
  High Km (low affinity) – more substrate require Competitive inhibitors – Km-↑, Vmax – no effect
  Noncompetitive inhibitors – Km – no effect, Vmax - ↓

CELL BIOLOGY

* *Replication*: DNA synthesis
* *Transcription*: RNA synthesis
* *Translation*: Protein synthesis

* *DNA*: deoxyribonucleic acid
* *RNA*: ribonucleic acid

<table>
<tr><td colspan="2" align="center">Basic Concepts
Nucleic acid = chain of nucleotides
Nucleotides = nitrogenous base + sugar + phosphate
Nucleosides = nitrogenous base + sugar</td></tr>
<tr><td align="center">DNA</td><td align="center">RNA</td></tr>
<tr><td>▪ Two strands of chain of nucleotides</td><td>▪ Single strand of chain of nucleotides</td></tr>
<tr><td>▪ Deoxyribose sugar (doesn't contain –OH group at 2nd position)</td><td>▪ Ribose sugar</td></tr>
<tr><td>▪ Complementary base to A is T</td><td>▪ Complementary base to A is U</td></tr>
</table>

Nitrogenous bases: A, C, G, T, U
Purines: two rings (A, G; *short name, two rings*)
Pyrimidines: one ring (C, T, U; *long name, one ring*)
Base pairing: A-T (DNA), A-U (RNA), G-C (Both DNA and RNA)

A-T / A-U – double bond, G-C – triple bond

A is identified by NH3 group

A = Adenine
C = Cytosine
G = Guanosine
T = Thymine

Uracil (U) is a precursor of both C and T (C contains NH2 and T contains CH3)
Amination of U → C (deamination of C gives U)
Methylation of U → T (demethylation of T gives U)

Deamination of A and G gives hypoxanthine and xanthine respectively.

Because of base pairing, *amount* of purines and pyrimidines are *same* in both DNA and RNA; therefore, amount of A = amount of T (DNA), amount of A = amount of U (RNA), and amount of G = amount of C.

Ribose sugar contains OH group at 2nd position
deoxyribose Sugar *doesn't contain* OH group at 2nd position

RNA is *antiparallel and complementary* to DNA *template strand*; RNA is *identical* to DNA *coding strand* (except U substitutes for T in RNA)

Sequences are always specified as 5'→ 3'

- Denaturation occurs by heat, and renaturation occurs by cooling.
- Supercoiling – more twisting
  - DNA gyrase (topoisomerase-2) – negative supercoiling (remove positive)
  - topoisomerase-1 – positive supercoiling (remove negative)
- In nature, DNA remains in a slight negative supercoiling
- Histone proteins (lysine and arginine) – +ve charged, help condensing DNA
- Core histones – H2A, H2B, H3, and H4
- Linker histones – H1 and H5
- Without H1 – (10 nm fibers) sensitive to endonucleases (Ten nm fibers are the first fibers to be destroyed in apoptosis.)

- Basic PH – decrease histone activity – fibers susceptible to endonucleases

- *DNA synthesis*: DNA is a double-stranded structure. First, we need something to start the process, and then we need something to separate it, then need something to maintain the process. At the end, we need something to end the process. During this process, we need something that makes sure the process is going smoothly without mutations.
- DNA synthesis always occurs in 5'→ 3' direction, and the newly synthesized strand is antiparallel and complementary to the template strand, so the template strand would be 3'→ 5' direction.
- To start the process – protein binds to DnaA box in prokaryote (pro)
- Separation of DNA double strands – helicase (DnaB protein)
- To continue process – need SSB protein (single-strand binding protein), which prevents reannealing (rejoining of strands). DNA gyrase is needed to relieve the stress by creating negative supercoiling. Need primase and RNA polymerase to prime each DNA template to begin synthesis.
- Maintaining the process – DNA is synthesized in two forms. Continuous (leading strand) and short fragment forms (lagging strand). Both forms require DNA polymerase 3. Short fragments are called Okazaki fragments. After beginning of synthesis, RNA primers are removed by DNA polymerase 1 (exonuclease). Short fragments are joined by ligase.
- Checking mutations: in bacteria, all three DNA polymerases (I, II, and III) have the ability to proofread, using 3' → 5' exonuclease activity.
- Termination: because bacteria have circular chromosomes, termination of replication occurs when the two replication forks meet each other on the opposite end of the parental chromosome.

- *DNA synthesis in eukaryotes*: process occurs same way as above with following differences:
- DNA replication in eukaryotes occurs only in the S phase of the cell cycle. However, pre-initiation occurs in the G1 phase.
- The G1/S checkpoint (or restriction checkpoint) regulates whether eukaryotic cells enter the process of DNA replication and subsequent

division. Cells that do not proceed through this checkpoint are quiescent in the G0 stage and do not replicate their DNA.

- Synthesis of the leading strand occurs by DNA polymerase δ.
- Synthesis of the lagging strand occurs by DNA polymerase α.

- In eukaryotes, only the polymerases that deal with the elongation (γ, δ and ε) have proofreading ability (3'→ 5' exonuclease activity).
- Termination: because eukaryotes have linear chromosomes, DNA replication often fails to synthesize to the very end of the chromosomes (telomeres), resulting in telomere shortening.
- Within the germ cell line, which passes DNA to the next generation, the enzyme telomerase extends the repetitive sequences of the telomere region to prevent degradation. Telomerase can become mistakenly active in *somatic cells*, sometimes *leading to cancer formation.*
- Telomerase is a reverse transcriptase enzyme that carries its own RNA molecule, which is used as a template when it elongates telomeres.

- *Ribosomes*: 70s (30s and 50s) in pro; 80s (40s and 60s) in eu
- *tRNA*: Acceptor arms carry AA (amino acids); anticodon arm— anticodons complementary and antiparallel to the codon in mRNA.
- *mRNA*: carry coded information for protein synthesis
- *rRNA*: central component of the ribosome, provide a mechanism for decoding mRNA into amino acids and to interact with the tRNA during translation by providing peptidyl transferase activity.
- *snRNA (small nuclear RNA)*: participate in splicing mRNA (remove introns)
- *RNA*: tRNA – smallest species; mRNA and hnRNA – largest species. On electrophoresis – smallest species migrate farthest

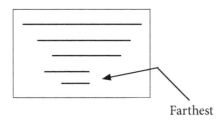

Farthest

- *RNA synthesis*: RNA synthesis always occurs in a 5'→ 3' direction, and newly synthesize strands are antiparallel and complementary to template strand so template strand would be 3'→ 5' direction.
- Only one DNA strand acts as template. (Both strands are used in DNA synthesis.)
- RNA synthesis doesn't require primers.
- It occurs in cytoplasm in prokaryotes and in nucleus in eukaryotes.
- mRNA is not modified in prokaryotes, but mRNA is modified through RNA splicing, 5' end capping, and the addition of a polyA tail in eukaryotes.
- Transcription is divided into 5 stages: pre-initiation, initiation, promoter clearance, elongation, and termination.
- *Pre-initiation*: RNA polymerase with other cofactors simply binds to DNA to initiate process. Proximal (core) promoters (TATA promoters) are found around -30 bp to the start site of transcription.

- *Initiation*: In prokaryotes, *a sigma factor* (number 70) that helps in finding the appropriate thirty-five- and ten-base pairs downstream of promoter sequences to initiate transcription. In eukaryotes, *transcription factors* mediate the binding of RNA polymerase and the initiation of transcription.
- *RNA polymerase in prokaryotes*: a core enzyme consisting of 5 subunits (2 α subunits, 1 β subunit, 1 β' subunit, and 1 ω subunit)
- *RNA polymerase in eukaryotes*: RNA polymerase I synthesizes a pre-rRNA 45S, which matures into 28S, 18S and 5.8S rRNA that will form the major RNA sections of the ribosome. RNA polymerase II synthesizes precursors of mRNA and most snRNA. RNA polymerase III synthesizes tRNA, rRNA 5S found in the nucleus and cytosol.
- *Promoter clearance*: RNA polymerase clears promoter. It is an ATP dependent process.
- *Elongation*: RNA polymerase traverses the template strand to create an RNA copy. It produces an exact copy of the coding strand (except that thymine is replaced with uracil, and the nucleotides are composed of a ribose sugar).
- *Termination in prokaryotes*: Rho-independent transcription termination. RNA transcription stops when the newly synthesized RNA molecule forms a G-C rich hairpin loop, followed by a run of *Us*, which makes it detach from the DNA template. In the

rho-dependent type of termination, a protein factor called rho destabilizes the interaction between the template and the mRNA, thus releasing the newly synthesized mRNA from the elongation complex. *In eukaryote*: It is less well understood. It involves cleavage of the new transcript, followed by template-independent addition of polyA at its new 3' end, in a process called polyadenylation.

■ *Modification in eukaryotes*: *RNA splicing* (in which introns are removed and exons are joined; splicing is done in a series of reactions that are catalyzed by the spliceosome, a complex of small nuclear ribonucleoproteins [snRNP]), *5' cap* (7-methyguanine), *3' cap* (poly-A sequence)

■ *Synthesis of protein*: occurs in cytoplasm where ribosomes are located
■ Same as replication and transcription, translation proceeds in four phases: activation, initiation, elongation, and termination

---

Basic Concepts

1. The ribosome consists of three sites: the *A site*, the *P site*, and the *E site*. The *A site* is the point of entry for the aminoacyl tRNA (*except* for the first aminoacyl tRNA, fMet-tRNA$_f^{Met}$, which enters at the P site). The *P site* is where the peptidyl tRNA is formed in the ribosome. *The E site* is the exit site for the tRNA after it gives its amino acid to the growing peptide chain.

2. Prokaryotic initiation factors (IF): *IF1* blocks the A site to insure that the fMet-tRNA can bind only to the P site and that no other aminoacyl-tRNA can bind in the A site during initiation, while *IF3* blocks the E site and prevents the two subunits from associating. *IF2* is binds fmet-tRNA$_f^{Met}$ and helps its binding with the small ribosomal subunit.

9. Eukaryotic initiation factors (eIF): There are many different eIF, but eIF2 is the most important one. The eIF2 is a GTP-binding protein responsible for bringing the initiator tRNA to the P-site of the pre-initiation complex. It has specificity for the methionine-charged initiator tRNA, which is distinct from other methionine-charged tRNAs specific for elongation of the polypeptide chain. Once it has placed the initiator tRNA on the AUG start codon in the P-site, it hydrolyzes GTP into GDP and dissociates. This signals the beginning of elongation.

10. Start codon: AUG (methionine)

11. Stop codon: UAG, UGA, UAA

12. Shine-Dalgarno sequence (AGGAGG): It exists in prokaryotic only. It is a ribosomal binding site generally located 6–7 nucleotides upstream of the start codon AUG on mRNA. The complementary sequence (CCUCCU) is called the anti-Shine-Dalgarno sequence and is located at the 3' end of the 16S rRNA of small 30s ribosomal subunit. When the Shine-Dalgarno sequence and the anti-Shine-Dalgarno sequence pair, initiation begins.

13. In eukaryotic, when 40s subunit of ribosome binds to 5' cap on mRNA through initiation factors, initiation begins.

14. Elongation in both prokaryote and eukaryote (eEF2): Once initiator tRNA with methionine (formyl-methionine in prokaryote) is inserted at P-site and large ribosomal subunits join the complex, the A-site opens and elongation begins. So when new amino acid (AA) attached with tRNA is inserted to A-site, tRNA attached to AA in the P-site released tRNA and form peptide bonds with newly added AA in A-site. This process is catalyzed by peptidyl trasferase enzyme, an activity intrinsic to the 23S ribosomal RNA in the 50S ribosomal subunit. A-site AA still has its tRNA and new peptide bond. When new AA is come to join A-site amino acid, tRNA of A-site amino acid release and peptide bond form between A-site AA and newly came AA. This process is going on until it reaches to stop codon. Translocation is the process in which tRNA is moved to E-site for exit. This requires GTP.

15. Termination in both: Once stop codon comes in way of elongation process, termination of translation occurs and releasing factors release newly formed peptide chain.

16. Post-translational modification: It occurs only in eukaryotes. This may include the formation of disulfide bridges or attachment of any of a number of biochemical functional groups, such as acetate, phosphate, various lipids (dolichol phosphate), and carbohydrates (phosphorylation of mannose in Golgi apparatus).

17. When when tRNA is attached with AA, it is called "charged" tRNA. It consumes 2 ATP. When AA is inserted to A or P sites, it consumes 2 GTP. So it requires 4 high energy phosphate bonds to insert one AA.

18. Puromycin (similar to the tyrosinyl aminoacyl-tRNA) binds to the ribosomal A site and participates in peptide bond formation, producing peptidyl-puromycin. However, it does not engage in translocation and quickly dissociates from the ribosome, causing a premature termination of polypeptide synthesis.

19. Streptomycin causes misreading of the genetic code in bacteria and inhibits initiation by binding to the 30s ribosomal subunit.

20. Tetracyclines block the A site on the ribosome, preventing the binding of aminoacyl tRNA.

21. Chloramphenicol blocks the peptidyl transfer step of elongation on the 50s ribosomal subunit

22. Macrolides and lincosamides bind to the 50s ribosomal subunits inhibiting the Peptidyl trasferase reaction or translocation or both

23. *Important concepts from translation can be asked in exam*: When do initiations occur in both? How many phosphate bonds are required in the process of inserting one AA? Mechanism of action of different antibiotics on translation? Which factor is inhibited by pseudomonas and diphtheria? (Ans: eEF2)

- **DNA repair:**
  - Thymine dimers: *Due to UV radiation*; excision endonucleases recognize and excise it. (This enzyme is deficient in xeroderma pigmentosa.) DNA polymerase and ligase are repair enzymes.
  - Mismatched bases: deficiency in the ability to repair mismatched base pairs in DNA leads to hereditary nonpolyposis colorectal cancer (HNPCC)

- **Regulation of Gene Expression**

- **Prokaryote:** lactose operon; attenuation

- **Lactose Operon**
  - *Lactose* induces gene expression for lactose metabolism by preventing the repressor protein binding to operator sequence.
  - *Glucose* represses gene expression for lactose metabolism by decreasing cAMP in the cell and thus preventing cAMP dependent activator binding to CAP site (cAMP dependent activator protein site).
  - *In the absence of lactose*, repression protein binds to operator protein and prevents gene expression.

- **Attenuation:** Premature termination of transcription. (Not possible in eukaryotes because in eukaryotes, transcription and translation do not occur simultaneously.. Both transcription and translation are independent events in eu.)
  - *High histidine*: rho-independent terminator to form; RNAP stops transcription
  - *Low-histidine*: prevent terminator formation; RNAP continues transcription and transcription of message produce all enzymes required for histidine biosynthesis

- **Eukaryote** (Regulation of Gene Expression)
- *Upstream Promoter Elements*
  - TATA box – (-25) General transcription factor (TFIID) binds here.
  - GC rich – SP-1 binds here.
  - CCAAT box – (-75) NF-1 binds here.
- *Enhancers*: (response elements) activator proteins bind here.

- *Silencers*: repressor proteins bind here.
- *Transcription factors*
  - *DNA binding domain*
    Zinc fingers (steroid hormone receptors)
    Leucine zippers (cAMP dependent transcription factors)
    Helix-turn-helix (homeodomain protein)
- *Activation Domain*
  - Binds to other transcription factors
  - Recruit chromatin modifying proteins such as histone acetylase (favor gene expression) *or* deacetylase (favor inactivate chromatin)
- ■ *Homeodomain proteins*: control embryonic gene expression and are regulated by homeobox (HOX) / homeotic gene and paired box (PAX) gene.

- ■ *Waardenburg-Klein Syndrome*
  - Mutation in PAX3 gene
  - Dystonia canthorum (lat displacement of inner corner of eye)
  - Pigmentary abnormality
  - Congenital deafness, defects in structures arising from the neural crest

- ■ *Neucleolus*: rRNA synthesis and then transport them to ribosome in cytoplasm

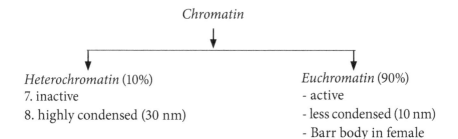

Chromatin

Heterochromatin (10%)
7. inactive
8. highly condensed (30 nm)

Euchromatin (90%)
- active
- less condensed (10 nm)
- Barr body in female

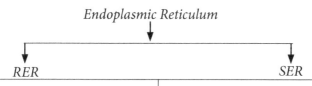

Endoplasmic Reticulum

RER	SER
• Lack ribosomes • *Function of SER:* 　▢ Lipid and steroid synthesis 　▢ Gluconeogenesis via G-6-phosphatase 　▢ Detoxification 　▢ Regulation of calcium concentration	• Ribosomes present • *RER is key in multiple functions:* 　▢ Lysosomal enzymes with a mannose-6- phosphate marker added in the *cis-*Golgi network 　▢ Secreted proteins 　▢ Integral membrane proteins 　▢ N-linked glycosylation • Abundant RER in neuron cell body stains intensely with basic dyes is referred to as Nissl substance

- *Golgi Apparatus*
  - Cis face – RER
  - Trans face – plasma membrane
  - Posttranslational modification

- *Peroxisome*: contains enzymes that produce H_2O_2 which is degraded by enzyme catalase—detoxification and long chain FA (fatty acid) metabolism—degradation of ethanol to acetaldehyde occurs in peroxisome and SER

- *Mitochondria*
  ▢ Outer membrane – highly permeable
  ▢ Inner membrane – impermeable
  　▢ Inner membrane compartmentalized into numerous cristae, which expand the surface area of the inner mitochondrial membrane and enhance its ability to produce ATP
  　▢ Matrix, the space enclosed by inner membrane, contains a highly concentrated mixture of hundreds of enzymes.

- Cytoskeleton: Microtubule, Intermediate Filaments, and Microfilaments
- *Microtubule*: polymers of α- and β-tubulin dimers
  - Involved in many cellular processes including mitosis, cytokinesis, and vesicular transport (anterograde and retrograde)
- *Intermediate Filaments*
  - Vimentins – being the common structural support of many cells (endothelial cells, Vascular smooth muscle, fibroblast, chondroblast)
  - Keratin – found in skin cells, hair, and nails
  - Neurofilaments of neural cells
  - Lamin – giving structural support to the nuclear envelope
- *Microfilaments*
  - Composed of actin filaments (thinnest filaments of the cytoskeleton)
  - Responsible for resisting tension and maintaining cellular shape
  - Participation in some cell-to-cell or cell-to-matrix junctions
  - Essential to transduction
  - Along with myosin in muscle contraction

- Gap junction: area of communication between adjacent cells
  - Directly connects the cytoplasm of two cells, which allows various molecules and ions to pass freely between cells.
  - One-gap junction is composed of two connexons (or hemichannels) that connect across the intercellular space,

- Cilia: two types of cilia: motile cilia (constantly beat in a single direction) and nonmotile or primary cilia, which typically serve as sensory organelles
  - Two central microtubules surrounded by nine microtubules
  - Nine microtubules connect each other with nexin link
  - *Dynein arm* is attached to each A subtubule
  - Dynein arm binds to ATP

- Hemidesmosomes anchor epithelial cells to basement membranes.
- Hydrophobic interactions are responsible for retaining integral membrane proteins within cell membranes (lipid bilayer)

- Receptors in cAMP and PIP2 pathways all have characteristic 7-helix membrane spanning domains.
- Trimeric G protein include Gi, Gs, Gq, and Gt. All have 7-helix membrane spanning structure.
- Zinc finger receptors – steroids, thyroxine, vit-A, vit-D.

■ *I-cell disease (mucoliposis)*: A deficiency in N- acetylglucosamine phosphotransferase results in I-cell disease in which the whole family of enzymes is sent to the wrong destination.
- Lysosomes missing the *hydrolase enzyme* that normally degrade glycoconjugates
- This enzyme is *present in other body fluid and plasma in I-cell disease.*
- The absence of the mannose-6-phosphate on the hydrolase results in their secretion into other body fluids rather than their incorporation in lysosomes.
- Phosphorylation of mannose done by N- acetylglucosamine phosphotransferase.
- I-cell disease is characterized by huge inclusion bodies in cells
- *Symptoms of I-cell disease*: skeletal abnormality, coarse features, mental retardation, restricted joint movement

- Fabry's Disease: Sphingolipidosis, in which ceremidetrihexoside accumulate in cells leading to renal failure, Telangiectasia and skin rashes. Alpha-galactoside A (lysosomal enzyme) is deficient. X-linked.

- Hunter's disease (mucopolysaccharidosis type-2): Iduronate sulfate sulfatase deficiency. Dermatan and heparin sulfate accumulate in cells. X-linked.

- Hurler Disease, Scheie Disease, Hurler-Scheie Disease (mucopolysaccharidosis type-1) – alpha-L-iduronidase deficiency
  Severe symptoms – *Hurler's disease*
  Normal intelligence and who live into adult life – *Scheie Disease*
  Normal intelligence but severe symptoms – *Hurler/Scheie Disease*
  Characterized by accumulation of dermatan and heparin sulfate in cells Autosomal Recessive

- *Chediak-Higashi syndrome*: Defect in microtubule polymerization. Delayed fusion of phagosomes with lysosomes in leucocytes, thus preventing phagocytosis of bacteria

- *Cilium diseases*: A defect of the primary cilium in the renal tube cells can lead to polycystic kidney disease (PKD). Lack of functional cilia in Fallopian tubes can cause ectopic pregnancy. Kartagener's syndrome (primary ciliary dyskinesia, immotile cilia syndrome): genetic defect in dynein arm—situs inversus, recurrent sinusitis

Cardiovascular System

* $CO = HR \times SV$ (CO = cardiac output)
  $$CO = \frac{MAP}{TPR}$$

* $SV = EDV - ESV$
* $\text{Ejection Fraction} = \frac{SV}{EDV} = \frac{EDV - ESV}{EDV}$

- *Cross-sectional area*: single vessel with large diameter has small cross-sectional area than more vessels with small diameter.
  | Velocity is *inversely* proportional to cross-sectional area.
  | Aorta has small cross-sectional area; therefore, velocity in aorta is high
  | In respiratory system, velocity decreases as air moves from trachea to alveoli because cross-sectional area increases due to severe branching of trachea

- *Vascular resistance* **is the resistance to flow that must be overcome to push blood through the circulatory system. Total peripheral resistance (TPR) is the sum of the resistance of all peripheral vasculature in the systemic circulation.**

- **Resistance is inversely proportional to radius^4 (r4) that means a decreased radius will greatly increase the resistance—e.g., vasoconstriction**
- It also depends on the capacitance of the blood vessel

- The amount of pressure lost in a particular segment is proportional to the resistance of that segment. E.g. In a capillary bed, resistance is high (*small diameter*), so pressure loss is high. Therefore, pressure loss from 120/80 in aorta to 30–50 in capillary bed. *Highest pressure loss occurs in arterioles* (capillary bed is made by joining of arterioles and venules).

- *Effect of GRAVITY:*
  Gravity reduces the rate of blood return from the body veins *below* the heart back to the heart and thus reduces stroke volume and cardiac output. *Compensation:* **the veins below the heart quickly constrict (increase TPR) and the heart rate increases.**

- *Characteristics of Auto-Regulating Tissues (No involvement of nervous system)*
- **Keep blood flow constant when blood pressure varies**
- Seen in the kidney, the heart, and the brain; skeletal muscles during exercise
- Blood flow α tissue metabolism (increase metabolism → increase blood flow)
- **In the kidneys: maintain renal blood flow and glomerular filtration rate,** *Myogenic mechanism*: **as blood flow increases, the afferent arterioles are stretched, they contract,** and subsequently reduce blood flow. – *Tubuloglomerular feedback*: the macula densa senses the low blood pressure and causes vasoconstriction to maintain GFR.
- In the heart: state of high metabolic activity (increased metabolism, increase blood flow) mediated by the equilibrium of ATP, ADP, AMP, and adenosine in the myocardial cell—lack of oxygen, the equilibrium is shifted toward adenosine. Adenosine causes vasodilation and, therefore, increases the supply of oxygen. (Adenosine is formed in the myocardial cells during hypoxia, ischemia, or vigorous work due to the breakdown of high-energy phosphate compounds. It causes vasodilation in the small- and medium-sized resistance arterioles—it can cause a coronary steal phenomenon, where the vessels in healthy tissue dilate as much as the ischemic tissue and more blood is shunted away from the ischemic tissue that needs it most. This is the principle behind adenosine stress testing.)

- In the brain: flow α arterial PCO_2 (CO_2 = vasodilator) ($\uparrow$ arterial PCO2 [hypoventilation) → $\uparrow$ cerebral blood flow; $\downarrow$ arterial PCO2 (hyperventilation) → $\downarrow$ cerebral blood flow) – large $\downarrow$ in PO_2 → $\uparrow$ cerebral blood flow (In these conditions low art PO_2 determine cerebral blood flow, *not* PCO_2.)

* As already mentioned above, the heart has high metabolic activity. The tissue extracts almost all the O_2 they can from the blood, even under basal conditions. Therefore, the lowest venous Po$_2$ in a resting individual is in coronary sinus – highest venous Po$_2$ is in Renal veins

Left coronary artery	Right coronary artery
- Very little if any blood flow can occur during systole (due to mechanical compression, which is more prominent in subendocardium)	- Significant flow can occur during systole due to less mechanical compression
- Most blood flow occur during diastole (phase-1)	

* *Pulmonary Circuit*
  High flow, low resistance ($R = \Delta P / Q$), low pressure Very compliant circuit – both arteries and veins
  ./ Hypoxic vasoconstriction (exception)
  ($\downarrow O_2$ → $\uparrow CO_2$, normally CO_2 acts as a vasodilator, but in a lung, it acts as vasoconstrictor)
  ./ $\uparrow$ Cardiac Output α $\uparrow$ pressure and flow in pulmonary circuit means $\downarrow$ resistance
  $\downarrow$ CO α $\downarrow$ pressure and flow in pulmonary circuit means $\uparrow$ resistance
  $\downarrow$ CO α $\uparrow$ pulmonary vascular resistance

- Carotid sinus (dilatation of the wall of internal carotid artery) → baroreceptors (medulla, provides a negative feedback loop to increase blood pressure) → sensory (CN – 9, 10) and motor (CN – 10 [vagus nerve]) → medulla only interprets afferent (aff.) activity as an index of BP ($\uparrow$ BP → $\uparrow$ aff. activity; $\downarrow$ BP → *no* aff. activity) →

($\uparrow$ aff. activity → $\uparrow$ efferent activity [CN-10] → $\downarrow$ CO and $\downarrow$ TPR; CO = cardiac out put, TPR = total peripheral resistance)

- Carotid body (at the origin of external and internal carotid arteries) – chemoreceptor (see in "Respiratory System")

- *Cardiac action potential*: **Automaticity is the ability of the cardiac muscles to depolarize spontaneously, i.e., without external electrical stimulation from the nervous system. It is most often demonstrated in the sinoatrial (SA) node ("pacemaker of the heart"). Abnormalities automaticity result in rhythm changes. During a cardiac cycle, once an action potential is initiated, there is a period of time that a new action potential cannot be initiated. This is called the effective refractory period (ERP) of the tissue. ERP acts as a protective mechanism and keeps the heart rate in check and prevents arrhythmias and coordinates muscle contraction. Conduction system of heart: SA node—AV node—bundle of His—Purkinje fibers—ventricular wall. The AV node delays impulses by approximately 0.12 seconds before allowing the impulses through to the His-Purkinje conduction system. This delay in the cardiac pulse is extremely important: it ensures that the atria have ejected their blood into the ventricles first before the ventricles contract.**

21. AP of Ventricles

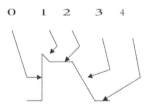

24. Phase-0: $\uparrow$ Na$^+$ influx causes depolarization
25. Phase-1: slight repolarization due to K$^+$ current and closing of Na$^+$
26. Phase-2: Ca++ channel open ($\uparrow$ influx of Ca++), voltage gated K+ closed (plateau depend on this), K+ efflux continue through unvoltage gated channel
27. Phase-3: Ca^{++} channel closed and voltage gated K$^+$ channel open

28. Under resting condition voltage gated K$^+$ channel is open. Depolarization is a signal for closing them.

27. *AP of SA node*:

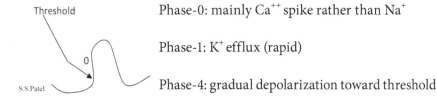

Phase-0: mainly Ca^{++} spike rather than Na$^+$

Phase-1: K$^+$ efflux (rapid)

Phase-4: gradual depolarization toward threshold

mainly due to ↓ K$^+$ conductance once threshold reach, AP generate

* *Sympathetic*: Beta-1 receptors are present here, which work through Gs protein so when it stimulates, it increases heart rate by increasing Ca^{++} conductance → threshold reached sooner.
* *Parasympathetic*: M2 receptors are present here, which work through Gi protein, so when it stimulates, it decreases heart rate by increasing K$^+$ conductance → takes a long time to reach threshold

* **Preload: the Pressure Stretching the Ventricle of the Heart**
* Heart muscle at the end of diastole is below Lo; therefore, ↑ in preload in *normal* heart – ↑ force of contraction
* **Afterload: The tension produced by a left ventricle in order to contract. Increased afterload is seen in aortic stenosis, hypertension.**
* Frank-Starling law of the heart: Under *normal physiologic state*, the greater the volume of blood entering the heart during diastole (end-diastolic volume), the greater the volume of blood ejected during systolic contraction (stroke volume). The law is true for normal physiologic condition because, for example, in CHF, end-diastolic volume is increase but SV is not increased.

* ↑ Contractility → ↓ systolic interval
  ↑ Heart rate → ↓ diastolic interval
* Isovolumatric → both valves closed
- *Pathophysiology of Main Valvular Heart Diseases*

- Aortic Stenosis (AS)
  | Increase ventricular systolic pressure-systolic murmur
  | Stenosis means small opening, so pressure gradient between LV and aorta during ejection
  | Concentric hypertrophy due to increased afterload

- Mitral Insufficiency (MI)
  | Systolic murmur
  | No pressure gradient between atrium and ventricle
  | Left atrium and ventricle, both enlarge
  | Increase atrial pressure in systole in MI

- Aortic Insufficiency (AI)
  | ↑ Preload (↑ in force of contraction → slight ↑ in ventricular systolic pressure)
  | ↑ PP (↑ SP and ↓ DP)
  | Eccentric hypertrophy due to increase volume load in LV
  | Diastolic murmur

- Mitral Stenosis (MS)
  | Stenosis means small opening, so pressure gradient between atrium and ventricle
  | Only left atrium is enlarged
  | Diastolic murmur
  | Increased atrial pressure in diastole is seen in MS

* *Pressure-volume loop*:

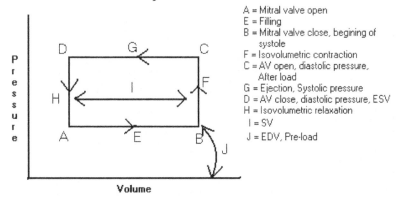

A = Mitral valve open
E = Filling
B = Mitral valve close, begining of systole
F = Isovolumetric contraction
C = AV open, diastolic pressure, After load
G = Ejection, Systolic pressure
D = AV close, diastolic pressure, ESV
H = Isovolumetric relaxation
I = SV
J = EDV, Pre-load

Think of two parameters
(1) Preload   If ↑ ⟶ loop shift to right
       If ↓ ⟶ loop shift to left
(2) Ventricular systolic pressure (peak pressure)

* J = preload
* G = systolic pressure
* B = beginning of systole
* D = beginning of diastole
* C = diastolic pressure

(Remember and understand landmarks in figure very well, most likely to get on exam)

* It is always a pressure difference that causes the valves to open and close.
  E.g., What causes MV to open? (Open in ventricular diastole.)
  → MV opens because pressure in left ventricle goes below than pressure in left atrium.
* Opening of AV → terminates isovolumatric contraction and begins ejection phase

CELL AND MUSCLE PHYSIOLOGY

* *Diffusion*: Transport of molecules from a region of higher concentration (conc.) to one of lower concentration. It is proportional to concentration gradient across the membrane, surface area, and solubility of substance in the medium. It inversely depends on thickness of membrane.

* *Osmosis*: Water diffuses from *high concentration to low concentration*
   1. Higher water conc. means low solute conc. means low osmolarity
   2. High water conc. = low solute conc. = low osm
   3. Low water conc. = high solute conc. = high osm
   4. Therefore water diffuse from *low osm to high osm*
   5. Isotonic solution = 300 mOsm = 150 mM NaCl = 300 mM glucose

* *Protein (Carrier) Mediated Transport*
   1. First transportation increases as conc. increases, but once saturation occurs, it becomes steady, even though conc. increases and shows plateau.
   2. Plateau is a characteristic of all protein-mediated transport.

* In *simple diffusion* graph, show a straight line relationship, i.e., as concentration increases rate of diffusion is increased (i.e., *no* carrier in simple diffusion).

* *Facilitated Transport*: *passive* process, carrier-mediated transport
   1. Requires *no* ATP

2. Always down a concentration gradient like simple diffusion but requires carrier

*   *Active Transport*: requires ATP
    1. Against concentration gradient.
    2. Primary active transport: directly use ATP.
    3. Secondary active transport: indirectly depends on ATP, two main forms.
    4. Counter-transport: In counter-transport, two species of ion or other solutes are pumped in opposite directions across a membrane. One of these species is allowed to flow from high to low concentration, which yields the entropic energy to drive the transport of the other solute from a low-concentration region to a high one. An example is the sodium-calcium exchanger or antiporter, which allows three sodium ions into the cell to transport one calcium out.
    5. Cotransport: Uses the downhill movement of one solute species from high to low concentration to move another molecule uphill from low concentration to high concentration (against its electrochemical gradient). An example is the glucose symporter, which cotransports one glucose molecule into the cell for every two sodium ions it imports into the cell.
    6. Endocytosis is the proccess by which cells ingest materials. The cellular membrane folds around the desired materials outside the cell. The ingested particle is trapped within a pouch, vacuole, or inside the cytoplasm. Often enzymes from lysosomes are then used to digest the molecules absorbed by this process.
    7. Endocyctosis can be split up into two main types: pinocytosis and phagocytosis.
    8. In pinocytosis, cells engulf liquid particles.
    9. In phagocytosis, cells engulf solid particles.
    10. Exocytosis is the process by which cells excrete waste and other large molecules from the protoplasm.

* *Body Compartments:* ↗ 2/3 ICF
  Total body water ↘ 2/3
  interstitial (60% of body weight) ↗ 1/3 ECF
  ↘ 1/3 vascular

■ Concentration of NA^+ determines the effective osm between ICF and ECF
■ Concentration of plasma protein determines the effective osm between interstitial and vascular fluid.
■ If you give fluid by any route, i.e., infusion *or* orally, ECF volume enlarges.
■ If you lose fluid by any route, ECF volume decrease.

Therefore in any question, first determine osm of ECF (i.e. increase *or* decrease) then think of water movement accordingly. (Remember, water always move from low osm to high osm).

* Movement of sodium between blood and interstitial fluid is via diffusion through channel between endothelial cells.

* *Vol^m measurement:* $V \times C = A$
  V - Volume of the compartment
  C - Concentration of tracer in that compartment
  A - Amount of tracer
* *Blood vol^m vs Plasma vol^m :*
  Blood vol^m = *Plasma vol^m*
  (HCT = hematocrit)
  1 – HCT
* *CHANGES IN RBC VOLUME*
  1. In isotonic saline (300 mOsm = 150 mM NaCl) – *no* change in volume.
  2. In hypotonic saline, RBC swells.
  3. In hypertonic saline, RBC shrinks.
  4. The presence of a substance such as *UREA* that penetrates the cell membrane quickly does *not* affect osmotic movement of water.
  5. Osmotic movement of water depends on presence of any salt like NaCl that affect osmolarity.

6. There is *no* osmotic effect at equilibrium.
7. When there is NaCl *or* any salt + slowly penetrating substance (like glycerol) present in a solution then consider both of its osm as total osm so initially there is increase in osm of solution but as slowly penetrating substance penetrate membrane slowly and reach at equilibrium there is decrease in osm.

■ Sweating ⟶ loss of hypotonic fluid → increase ECF osm
■ Drinking tape water (very few solute, same as infusing hypotonic fluid) → dilute ECF → decrease ECF osm
■ Infusing isotonic saline → *no* change in ECF osm but increase ECF volume therefore *no* osmotic movement between ECF and ICF therefore ICF volume *not* change

* *Concentration force*: determined by conc. difference across the membrane
  1. Nernst equation convent conc. force into mV.(Ex)
  2. If there are tenfold conc. differences across the membrane, then the conc. force has a magnitude of *60 mV.*

* *Electrical force*: electrical difference across the membrane.
  1. In vivo magnitude is determine by membrane potential (Em).
  2. The direction of force is based on the fact that *like charges repel and opposite charges attract.*
     E.g., If Em -70mv; then a force of 70mv attracts all positive ions and repels all negative ions.

* If Em and Ex both are in same direction then net force is Em + Ex.
* If Em and Ex are in opposite directions, then net force is the difference between Em and Ex and directed along the axis of the larger force.
* If Em and Ex both are equal and opposite directions, then net force is zero and ion is in the state of equilibrium. So an equilibrium = Em=Ex.

* All cells have ungated K^+ channels.

■ *Action potential*: a self-regenerating wave of electrochemical activity that allows nerve cells to carry a signal over a distance

*   A typical action potential is initiated at the axon hillock when the membrane is depolarized sufficiently (i.e., when its voltage is increased sufficiently). As the membrane potential is increased, both the sodium and potassium ion channels begin to open up. This increases both the inward sodium current and the balancing outward potassium current. For small voltage increases, the potassium current triumphs over the sodium current, and the voltage returns to its normal resting value, typically –70 mV. However, if the voltage increases past a critical threshold, typically 15 mV higher than the resting value, the sodium current dominates. This results in a runaway condition whereby the positive feedback from the sodium current activates even more sodium channels. Thus, the cell fires, producing an action potential.

*   Action potentials that do reach the ends of the axon generally cause the release of a neurotransmitter (ACh) into the synaptic cleft. This may combine with other inputs to provoke a new action potential in the postsynaptic neuron or muscle cell.

*   The principal ions involved in an action potential are sodium and potassium cations; sodium ions enter the cell, and potassium ions leave, restoring equilibrium.

*   *Hyperpolarization*: Sometimes more potassium channels open than usual, which leads to membrane potential reach close to the potassium equilibrium voltage. This is called a hyperpolarization, which persists until the membrane potassium permeability returns to its usual value.

*   *Refractory period*: the opening and closing of the sodium and potassium channels during an action potential may leave some of them in a refractory state, in which they are unable to open again until they have recovered.

*   *Absolute refractory period*: So many ion channels are refractory that no new action potential can be fired. Significant recovery requires that the membrane potential remain hyperpolarized for a certain length of time.

*   *Relative refractory period*: enough channels have recovered that an action potential can be provoked, but only with a stimulus much stronger than usual.

*   Refractory period ensure that the action potential travels in only one direction along the axon.

* A cell's resting membrane potential is very sensitive to changes in the extracellular potassium.
  (K^+) ion conc. *not* to Na+ conc.
  Hypokalamia $\longrightarrow$ ↑ efflux of k^+ → hyperpolarize the cell
  Hyperkalemia $\longrightarrow$ ↓ efflux of k^+ → depolarization of the cell

  ./ Preventing the opening of voltage-gated Na+ channel in response to depolarization will prevent the depolarization of AP.

  ./ Preventing the opening of voltage-gated K^+ channel slows repolarization as k+ efflux continues *via ungated K+ channel.*

* *Conduction Velocity of AP*
- *Cell diameter*: increase diameter – increase conduction velocity
- *Myelin*: increase myelin – increase conduction velocity
- Large myelinated fibers = fast conduction
- Small unmyelinated fibers = slow conduction

* *Synaptic transmission*: As mentioned above, AP travels down the axon and releases ACh in the presynaptic cleft, which opens sodium-potassium channels in the postsynaptic neurons or muscle cells. Their opening causes the initiation of AP that spreads across the surface of the skeletal muscles.

* *ACh*: enzymatic degradation by AChE (acetylcholine esterase) is the major factor in terminating Ach action
* NE → E by PNMT (Phenylethanolamine N-methyltransferase)
* Reuptake of NE is a major factor in terminating NE action.
* Some of NE is converted to deaminated derivatives by MAO.

9. *Skeletal Muscles Contraction*
* A band – *no* change during contraction
* H band – shortens

• I band – shortens
• *A band* contains most of *myosin filaments* and some actin filaments (H band is inside A band)
• Actin – troponin (binding site for Ca+2) and tropomysin (covers the attachment site of the crossbridge in *resting* muscle)

- Overlap of actin and myosin is required for maximum achievable force during contraction, but *if both actin filaments overlap in resting stage*, then it decreases maximum achievable force during contraction. *If muscles are overstretched in resting stage*, then also very few actin-myosin coupling occur and decrease force during contraction.
- Preload align actin-myosin overlap in resting condition.
- As already mentioned above, AP spread across the surface of the skeletal muscles, it then travels through T-tubular membranes (an extension of the surface membrane) and activate dihydropyridine receptors in T-tubular membrane that pull the junctional foot process away from the calcium-releasing channels in sarcoplasmic reticulum and release calcium into intracellular environment
- As long as calcium is attached to troponin, crossbridge cycles continue. Contraction is terminated as calcium is sequestered by the sarcoplasmic reticulum. (Contraction is the continuous cycling of crossbridges. Intracellular release of calcium attached to troponin, which leads to bonds formation between actin and myosin. However bonds are *NOT* maintained; rather, there is continuous cycling of those crossbridges.)
- ATP is used to power the mechanical aspect of contraction in the form of active tension and/or active shortening of muscles

- *Red muscles (type-I, slow oxidative, slow twitch)*: utilized for long term

  - Small muscle mass (less powerful)
  - Low ATPase activity
  - Maintain aerobic glycolysis (mitochondria)
  - Has myoglobin (red color; myoglobin stores O2 and speeds up delivery of O2 to mitochondria)

- *White Muscles (type-II, fast twitch)*: utilized for short term
- Large mass per motor unit (more powerful)
- High ATPase activity
- High capacity of anaerobic glycolysis
- *No* myoglobin
- Ex., ocular muscles of eye (not large, but fast)

Skeletal	Cardiac	Smooth
No gap junction, so AP doesn't move from cell to cell, so each fibers are innervated	Gap junction present, so AP can move from cell to cell electrical syncytium	Gap junction present, so AP can move from cell to cell electrical syncytium
Troponin, to bind calcium	Troponin, to bind calcium	*Calmodulin*, to bind calcium
High ATPase activity	Intermediate ATPase activity	Low ATPase activity

ENDOCRINOLOGY

* Important concepts: hormone synthesis; positive and negative feedback system to regulate hormone levels; other factors that regulate hormones; M/A of hormones; effect of hormones in our body; primary, secondary and tertiary hyper- and hypostatus of the gland
* Hypothalamus: secretes releasing hormones that stimulate the pituitary gland to secrete stimulating hormones; GnRH (LHRH, FSHRH), TRH, CRH, GHRH, PIH, somatostatin (GHIH)
* Pituitary gland: secretes all stimulating hormones that stimulate secretion of hormones from different glands; LH, FSH, TSH, ACTH, GH, prolactin (anterior), oxytocin, and ADH (posterior)
* Positive and negative feedback: When the level of free hormone is decreased in the bloodstream, the hypothalamus stimulates the pituitary gland to secrete stimulating hormones to increase the free level of decreased hormone. This is called positive feedback. When the free level of hormone is increased in the bloodstream, the hormone itself inhibits release of the releasing hormone from the hypothalamus or inhibits release of stimulating hormones from the pituitary gland. This is called negative feedback. Most of the hormones in our body remain attached to the plasma protein or remain stored in the gland and are released into bloodstream when the need arises.
* Hormones that are not regulated by the pituitary gland: aldosterone, epinephrine, insulin, glucagon
* *Concepts*: It is a free hormone level that plays important role in positive and negative feedback. Example, estrogen can *increase the circulating level of binding proteins*. Therefore, transient decrease in the level of free hormones occurs, which stimulates a positive feedback loop that leads to an increase in the free hormone level back to normal. Therefore in pregnancy, *total* plasma hormone

increases, but *free* plasma hormone remains constant. Same thing happens when person is on OCP.

* *Concept*: Damage to the pituitary stalk (connection between the hypothalamus and the pituitary gland) leads to a decrease in all anterior pituitary hormones *except* prolactin, the level of which is increased because of the decreased level of PIF (prolactin inhibiting factor).

* Mechanism of action of hormones (see pharmacology notes for details)
* *Lipid-soluble hormones* (steroids, thyroid hormones):
  t1/2 is proportional to affinity of hormone to plasma protein carrier. Receptors are inside the cell and stimulate the synthesis of specific proteins to exert their action. (t1/2 – long [hours, day]).
* *Water-soluble hormones* (peptides, proteins):
  Receptors are on the outer surface of the cell membrane; production of second messenger, which modifies action of intracellular proteins (t1/2 – short [minutes]).
* All hormones in the hypothalamic-anterior pituitary system are water soluble.
* Chronic high circulating levels of a hormone can cause the number of receptors on a hormone target cells to decrease.
* *Permissive action*: one type of hormone must be present before another hormone can act

* In the hypothalamic pituitary system, hormonal release is pulsatile *except* the thyroid system.

Metabolism	Insulin	Glucagon	Epinephrine	Cortisol	GH
glycogen synthesis	increase by stimulating glucokinase and glycogen synthase	decrease by inhibiting glucokinase and glycogen synthase	decrease	decrease	decrease
glycogen degradation in liver for gluconeogenesis	decrease by inhibiting phosphorylase and glucose-6-phosphatase	increase by stimulating phosphorylase and glucose-6-phosphatase	increase by stimulating phosphorylase and glucose-6-phosphatase	increase gluconeogenesis by providing more substrate in form of AA, free FA and glycerol	increase gluconeogenesis by providing more substrate in free FA and glycerol
fat synthesis by adipose tissue	increase by stimulating lipoprotein lipase (endothelium of capillary)	decrease by inhibiting lipoprotein lipase	decrease	decrease	decrease
fat degradation for gluconeogenesis	decrease by inhibiting hormone sensitive lipase	increase by stimulating hormone sensitive lipase (it does *not* increase lipolysis in adipose tissues)	increase lipolysis in adipose tissue leads to increase delivery of free FA and glycerol to liver	increase lipolysis in adipose tissue leads to increase delivery of free FA and glycerol to liver	increase lipolysis in adipose tissue leads to increase delivery of free FA and glycerol to liver
protein synthesis	increase by increasing AA uptake by muscles	decrease	decrease	decrease	increase (anabolic hormone)
protein degradation for gluconeogenesis	decrease	increase	increase	increase delivery of AA to liver	

Hormone secretion	Stimulated by	Inhibited by	Other comments
epinephrine (80% of adrenal medulla)	exercise, emergency, exposure to cold		
norepinephrine (20% of adrenal medulla)	when one goes from a lying to a standing position		most circulating norepinephrine arises from post-ganglionic sympathetic neurons
cortisol	ACTH	negative feedback	peak cortisol secretion occurs in the early morning
adrenal androgens	ACTH	negative feedback	
insulin	glucose (increase ATP in B-cells), GIP (gastric inhibitory peptide), CCK, secretin, gastrin, glucagon, AA (arginine)	somatostatin, alpha-2 agonist	
glucagon	hypoglycemia, AA (arginine)	somatostatin, insulin	
aldosterone	angiotensin-II, elevated plasma K+	weightlessness	see renin-angiotensin system below
ADH (vasopressin)	increased serum osmolarity	weightlessness	
ANP (atrial natriuretic peptide)	in response to right atrium stretching, increase salt intake, weightlessness		
thyroid hormone	TSH	negative feedback (regulated by free T4)	

GH	deep sleep, exercise, AA (arginine), hypoglycemia	somatostatin, IGF-1 (somatomedin-C), elevated glucose	secreted in pulses and mainly at night; requires the presence of normal plasma levels of thyroid hormones
PTH	hypocalcemia	negative feedback (regulated by free Ca+2)	
LH	LHRH	testosterone (male), increased estrogen in follicular phase, increased progesterone in luteal phase (female), suckling of the baby (inhibits GnRH)	

23. *Adrenal Hormones*

 * *Zona glomerulosa*: aldosterone; controlled by *angiotensin-II, K⁺*
 * *Zona fesciculata*: cortisol; controlled by ACTH
 * *Zona reticularis*: androgen; controlled by ACTH
 * *Medulla*: epinephrine; *controlled by ANS*

 * If problems develop with anterior pituitary secretion, glucocorticoids secretion may be affected, but the mineralocorticoid system remains intact, which is controlled by angiotensin-II, K^+.

 * Urinary 17-OH steroids are usually an index of cortisol secretion.
 * Urinary 17-ketosteriods are an index of all androgens, adrenal and testicular.

 * Desmolase is a rate-limiting enzyme in all steroid hormone synthesis that converts cholesterol into pregnenolone.

 * Congenital defects in any of the enzymes leads to *deficient cortisol secretion* and *congenital adrenal hyperplasia*
 * Enzymes ⟶ 17 alpha-OH, 21 beta-OH, 11 beta-OH

    17 alpha-OH deficiency:
    Decreased cortisol, decreased androgen
    Increased 11 deoxycorticosterone (weak mineralocorticoid, responsible for HTN)

    21 beta-OH deficiency:
    Decrease cortisol, decrease mineralocorticoid
    Increase adrenal androgens (responsible for ambiguous genitalia)

    11 beta-OH deficiency: Decrease cortisol
    Increase 11 deoxycorticosterone Increase adrenal androgens

 * *Other Important Actions of Cortisol*

* It increases blood pressure by increasing the sensitivity of the vasculature to epinephrine and norepinephrine. In the absence of cortisol, widespread vasodilatation occurs.
* Stimulates gastric acid secretion, thus promoting gastric ulcer formation.
* It lowers bone formation, thus favoring development of osteoporosis in the long term.
* Glucagon increases liver glycogenolysis, but without cortisol, fasting hypoglycemia rapidly develops.
* Anti-inflammatory effects by reducing histamine secretion and stabilizing lysosomal membranes. The stabilization of lysosomal membranes prevents their rupture, thereby preventing damage to healthy tissues.
* It causes hyperkalemia.

* *Actions of Aldosterone*
  * Increases Na^+ absorption by increasing the number of Na^+ channel in luminal membrane
  * Promotes activity of Na^+/K^+ ATPase pump
  * Increases excretion of K^+ and H^+
  * For one H^+ secreted, one HCO_3 moves into the ECF
* *Renin-Angiotensin System*
  * Decreases BP in afferent arteriole—JG cells present in afferent arteriole.
  * Decreases Na^+ delivery to macula densa cells—tall columnar cells lined DT near afferent arteriole.
  * Increase B1-noradrenergic input to JG cells.
  * Above three factors lead to release of renin from JG cells that convert angiotensinogen into angiotensin-1, which is converted into angiotensin-II by ACE (angiotensin converting enzyme) in the lung.
  * Angiotensin-II (vasoconstriction and increase aldosterone secretion).
  * Alveolar capillary contains ACE, *not* pneumocytes.

* Elevated plasma K^+ (hyperkalemia) directly stimulates zona glomerulosa to secrete aldosterone.

* *Weightlessness* (*example*, standing on the ground, sitting on a chair on the ground, flying in a plane, during an orbital maneuver in a spacecraft, etc.): because blood no longer pools in the extremities, a large portion of the redistributed blood ends up in the atria and large veins of the chest and abdomen, which stimulate baroreceptors → decrease aldosterone and decrease ADH and lose Na^+ and ECF vol^m.

■ 1^0 Hyperaldosteronism (Conn's syndrome) – HTN + hypokalamia
■ 1^0 Adrenal insufficiency (Addison's disease) – increase ACTH, hyperpigmentation

■ *ADH (Vasopressin)*
Maintain osmolarity (increased osmolarity → increased secretion of ADH from post pituitary)
MA: increased permeability of renal collecting duct for water by placing water channels in the membrane

■ *Atrial Natriuretic Peptide (ANP)*:
  • Increased GFR by dilation of afferent arterioles and constriction of efferent arterioles
  • Increased Na+ loss and water loss by inhibition of reabsorption of sodium and water in CD (collecting duct)
  • Increased secretion in weightlessness

* *The Endocrine Pancreas*
  ■ *α cells*: (20% of islet cells) at the periphery, secrete *glucagon*
  ■ *β-cells*: (60–75% of islet cells) near the center, secrete *insulin + C peptide*
  ■ *Delta cells*: (5% of islet cells) between α and B cells, secrete *somatostatin*

■ Tissues that require insulin for effective glucose uptake are: adipose tissues, *resting* skeletal muscles. Glucose uptake occurs by insertion of glucose transporters in the membrane of above tissues (see biochemistry notes).
■ Tissues in which glucose uptake is *not* affected by insulin are nervous tissue, RBCs, kidney tubules, intestinal mucosa, and beta-cells of pancreas.

■   Insulin decreases formation of ketone bodies by the liver.

*   Insulin pumps K^+ into cells. Therefore it is used to treat life-threatening hyperkalemia (e.g hyperkalemia of renal failure). Simultaneous administration of glucose is required to prevent severe hypoglycemia.

*   *Actions of glucagon*: mediated by increase
cAMP 1^0 Target tissue ⟶ liver hepatocytes
Skeletal muscles are *not* target tissue for glucagon

*   All hormones that increase degradation of AA increases ureagenesis.

*   *Growth Hormone*

    Acts on   Acts on
_   GH ⟶ liver and skeletal muscles ⟶   Somatomedins
                                and release of (especially IGF-1)

\-   IGF-1 is also called Somatomedin-C

*   *IGF-1*: $t_{1/2}$ - very long (20 hrs)
1.   Plasma IGF-1 serves as a reflection of 24 hrs GH secretion.
2.   GH secreted in pulses and mainly at night.
3.   Increases synthesis of cartilage (chondrogenesis) in the epiphyseal plates of long bones.
Increases bone length.
4.   At puberty, increases in GH secretion is facilitated by the pubertal increase in androgen secretion.
5.   Secretion of GH requires the presence of normal plasma levels of thyroid hormones.

*   *GH deficiency*: prepuberty ⟶ dwarfism
*   *Hypersecretion of GH*: prepuberty ⟶ gigantism
                     postpuberty ⟶ acromegaly

*   *Adrenal Medulla*
•   80% epinephrine and 20% nonepinephrine

- Plasma norepinephrine ($t_{1/2}$ -2 mins only) levels double when one goes from a lying to a standing position.
- Secretion of epinephrine by adrenal medulla increase by exercise, emergency, exposure to cold

* *Actions of Epinephrine*:
  Increases metabolic rate (needs presence of thyroid and adrenal cortex hormones), increases glycogenolysis in *both* liver and skeletal muscle (glucagon – only liver), increase lactate output by skeletal muscle;
  lactate ⟶ glucose (Cori cycle in liver)

* *Calcium*:
  - 99% of total calcium – bone (hydroxyapatites)
  - 0.1% of calcium – interstitial fluid (mostly ca^{+2})
  - 0.5% of – plasma (50% Ca^{+2} and 50% protein bound)
  - 1% of – ICF (Ca^{+2} and protein bound calcium)
  - Whether calcium and phosphate are laid down in bone *or* are resorbed from bone depends on the product of their concentration.
  - Increase interstitial fluid concentration of either Ca^{+2} or phosphate increase bone mineralization
  - Decrease interstitial fluid concentration of either Ca^{+2} or phosphate promotes bone resorption.
  - Free Ca^{+2} precisely regulated, *not* phosphate

* *Action of PTH* stimulates osteoclast and 1-α-hydroxylase (increase production of active form of vit-D [1–25-$(OH)_2$-D]), increases Ca^{+2} level by bone resorption (osteoclast) and by absorption of Ca^{+2} from gut and kidney (vit-D).
* *Action of vit-D*: increases absorption of both Ca^{+2} and phosphorus (PO4) from intestine and increases absorption of Ca^{+2} and decreases absorption of PO4 from kidney
* Bone resorption leads to increased concentration of both phosphate and Ca^{+2}

* *Calcitonin*: (parafollicular cells [c cell] of thyroid gland) decreases plasma Ca^{+2} by decreasing activity of osteoclast

* *Osteoblast*: deposits bone matrix (collagen), located on surface of bone
* *Osteocyte*: Osteoblast when surrounded by mineralized bone. It differentiates into osteocytes.
* *Osteoclast*: Resorbed bone, arises from monocytes migrating to bone. Several monocytes fused to form the multinucleated osteoclast.
* *Paget's disease of bone*: increase alkaline phosphatase, myelophthisic anemia
* *Osteomalacia (rickets in children)*: increase in osteoid but poor mineralization due to dietary deficiency of Ca^{+2}, vit-D *or* sunlight (also increase *osteoblast*)
* *Osteoporosis*: sparse trabaculae
* *Osteoarthritis*: "wear and tear" – enzymatic degradation of *type-2* collagen in *cartilage*

  1. Increase alkaline phosphatase ⟶ osteoblastic activity.
  2. Increase urinary excretion of hydroxyproline ⟶ breakdown product of collagen

* Abnormally high vit-D promotes bone resorption.
* Receptors for both PTH and vit-D are on osteoblast. Osteoblast has communication with osteoclast, which carries out bone resorption.

* *Thyroid hormones*:
  * Thyroid epithelial cells (follicle cells, form follicles) synthesize and secrete T4 and T3.
  * Thyroid epithelial cells form thyroglobulin (Tg, protein; Tg is referred to as colloid).
  * Iodine is stored as an iodination of tyrosine residue of thyroglobulin in follicle lumen.
  * Iodide (I⁻) actively transport in follicle cell.
  * *Thyroperoxidase* is an important enzyme that carries out iodination of tyrosine and coupling of MIT and DIT to form T4 and T3.
  * When iodine is abundant → mainly T4 is formed.
  * When iodine is scare → mainly T3 is formed.
  * T4 - 3, 5, 3', 5'

T3 - 3, 5, 3' (5' deiodinase) in peripheral tissue; reverse T3 - 3, 5, 5' (inactive)

- T4 converts into T3 to exert its effect in our body (T3 is an active form of thyroid hormone), but only free T4 regulates TSH. (Free T4 converts into T3 in hypothalamus, which inhibits TRH and thus TSH)
- T4 and T3 are carried into blood by thyroid-binding globulin, transthyretin, and albumin. TBG has higher affinity to thyroid hormones, but its concentration is lower than other two.
- Microsomal deiodenase removes iodine from free DIT and MIT (released by proteolysis of thyroglobulin during secretion of T4 and T3) but *not* from T4 and T3.

* *Actions of Thyroid Hormone*
  - Permissive *or* acts synergistically with growth hormone. (A stippled epiphysis is a sign of hypothyroidism in children.)
  - Increases metabolic rate by increase Na^+/K^+ - ATPase activity in most tissue.
  - Required for maturing of nervous tissue. (Mental retardation if low level in infancy.)
  - Required for conversion of carotene to vit-A (night blindness and yellow skin in hypothyroid).
  - Accelerates cholesterol clearance from plasma.
  - Increase number and affinity of beta-adrenergic receptors in heart (causes arrhythmia when in access).
  - Goiter is an enlarged thyroid gland and can occur in hypo-, hyper-, and euthyroid.

* *Male Reproductive System*
  LH, FSH, TSH, and hCG—all glycoproteins. Alpha subunit is same in all four. Only beta subunit is different in all four
  - *LH* → Leydig cells → testosterone
    It acts through cAMP / protein kinase
  - Testosterone provides negative feedback to regulate LH
  - Androgen binding protein (ABP) synthesized by Sertoli cells and secreted into the lumen of the seminiferous tubules helps maintain a high local concentration.
  - FSH + testosterone → increase synthesis of ABP

- Testosterone receptors are located on the nuclear chromatin of the Sertoli cell.

- FSH receptors are located on plasma membrane of Sertoli cells; FSH acts through cAMP / protein kinase.
- *Both* FSH and Leydig cell testosterone are required for normal spermatogenesis.
- *Inhibin* provides negative feedback to regulate FSH.
- GnRH secreted in pulsatile fashion.
- *Methyl testosterone* – synthetic androgen – used by athletes.
- At puberty, if T4 is normal, increase androgen ⟶ increase GH ⟶ increase IGF-I
- Near the end of puberty, androgens promote the mineralization (closure) of the epiphysis of long bones. After closure, lengthening can *no* longer occur.
- Androgens stimulate protein synthesis – increase muscle mass.

* PANS does *not* innervate arterioles in systemic tissue (penis is an exception).
* Erection is caused by dilation of the blood vessels in the erectile tissue of the penis via parasympathetic response.
* Emission is mediated by sympathetic transmitters.
* Ejaculation → contraction of bulbospongious and ischiocavernosus → (somatic innervation). Therefore complete ejaculation requires intact SANS and somatic innervation.

* *The Menstrual Cycle*
  Follicular phase → increase estrogen
  Ovulation → LH surge
  Luteal phase → increase progesterone with estrogen
  Menses → withdrawal of hormones

* *Follicular Phase (Proliferative Phase)*
  - FSH secretion is slightly elevated, which causes proliferation of granulosa cells—increase estrogen (E).
  - E acts locally to increase granulosa cells' sensitivity to FSH, the follicle with best blood supply, secrete more estradiol than others, and become dominant follicle.

- LH (stimulates) → theca cells → increase androgen (goes to) → granulosa cells → aromatase converts androgen → estrogen.
- Increased E – stimulates female sex accessory organ and secondary sex characteristics Endometrial cell proliferation
  Thinning of cervical mucus
  Inhibits FSH and LH

* *Ovulation*: When E rises above certain level, it *no* longer inhibits FSH and LH. Instead, it stimulates FSH and LH ([-] feedback to [+] feedback loop)
  - Only LH surge is essential for induction of ovulation and formation of corpus lutem; therefore, if estrogen (E) is still rising, ovulation has *not* occurred.
  - Follicular rupture occur 24–36 hrs after LH surge.
  - LH removes restraint upon meiosis and first meiotic division is completed and 1st polar body extruded

* *Luteal phase*: LH surge causes granulosa cells and theca cells to be transformed into luteal cells.
  ./ E + FSH → granulosa cells produce LH receptors
  ./ Luteal cells form progesterone and some E
  ./ Progesterone ⟶ Inhibits LH release
  ⟶ Endometrium become Secretory
  ⟶ Mucus → thick
  ⟶ Increase basal temp. (0.5^0 - 1^0 F)

* *Menses*: Progesterone inhibits LH, which is required for corpus lutem. Decrease LH → demise of the corpus lutem.
  - Decreased progesterone due to decreased LH and decreased sensitivity of luteal cells to LH 1 week after ovulation
  - Lower level of progesterone no longer support the endometrium, necrosis of tissue occurs, spiral arterioles break, and menses ensues.

* Decreased P metabolites and rapidly increased E metabolites → follicular phase
* Increased P metabolites ⟶ luteal phase/pregnancy

* Length of luteal phase (last 14 days) doesn't vary

* *Placental Hormones*
   Human chorionic somatomammotropin (hCS), also called human
      placental lactogen (hPL)
   - *hPL* → growth stimulating activity, anti-insulin activity
   - *hCG* requires to maintain pregnancy from *implantation to 3rd*
      month.
   - *Placenta* secrete enough progesterone and estrogen, which
      maintain pregnancy from 3rd *month to term*
   - Plasma oxytocin is *not* elevated until the baby enters the birth
      canal
   - Oxytocin → stimulate uterine synthesis of PGs
   - Progesterone and E → stimulate growth of mammary tissue
   - E → stimulate prolactin secretion
   - E → inhibits milk synthesis

* At parturition, plasma E drops, withdrawing block on milk
   synthesis. As a result, the number of prolactin receptors in
   mammary tissue increase several fold, and milk synthesis begins.
* Oxytocin contract myoepithelial cells → milk ejection
* Suckling of the baby → stimulate oxytocin and prolactin release
   (sucking inhibits PIF in hypothalamus)
* Suckling of the baby → inhibits GnRH (FSH and LH), therefore
   inhibits ovulation, and menstruation cease.
* Aromatase: convert testosterone to estrogen
   Male – Sertoli cells, adipose tissue
   Female – granulosa cells, adipose tissue
* Estradiol (ovarian follicle) > estrone (peripheral tissues) > estriol
   (placenta)

GI PHYSIOLOGY

* *Digestion of Food*

* *Phases of Gastric Secretion*
* *Cephalic phase.* This occurs before food enters the stomach. Taste and smell send signals to the cerebral cortex that sends signal through the vagus nerve and releases acetylcholine. ACh stimulates gastric secretion. Acidity in the stomach is *not* buffered by food at this point, and thus acts to inhibit parietal (secretes acid) and G cells (secretes gastrin).
* *Gastric phase.* This phase takes three to four hours. It is stimulated by distention of the stomach, presence of food in stomach, and increase in pH. Distention activates long and myentric reflexes that release Ach, which releases more acid into the stomach. As protein enters the stomach, it binds to hydrogen ion, which raises the pH of the stomach around 6. This leads to increased release of gastrin, which in turn releases more HCl.
* *Intestinal phase.* This phase has two parts, the excitatory and the inhibitory. When partially digested food enters the duodenum, it triggers intestinal gastrin to be released. Enterogastric reflex inhibits vagal nuclei, activating sympathetic fibers and causing the pyloric sphincter to tighten to prevent more food from entering and inhibits local reflexes.
* *Oral Cavity*: Digestion begins in the oral cavity. Saliva is secreted in large amounts (1–1.5 liters/day) by three pairs of exocrine salivary glands (parotid, submandibular, and sublingual) in the oral cavity, and is mixed with the chewed food by the tongue. There are two types of saliva. One is a thin, watery secretion, and its purpose is to wet the food. The other is a thick, mucous secretion, and it acts as a lubricant and causes food particles to stick together and form a bolus. It contains digestive enzymes such as salivary amylase (breaks polysaccharides

such as starch into disachharides such as maltose). It also contains mucin, a glycoprotein that helps soften the food into a bolus.

* Swallowing transports the chewed food into the esophagus, passing through the oropharynx and hypopharynx. The mechanism for swallowing is coordinated by the swallowing center in the medulla and pons. The reflex is initiated in the pharynx as the bolus of food is pushed to the back of the mouth.

* *Esophagus*: The wall of the esophagus is made up of two layers of smooth muscles, which contract slowly over long periods of time. The inner layer of muscles is arranged circularly, while the outer layer is arranged longitudinally. The epiglottis, a flap of tissue at the top of the esophagus, closes during swallowing to prevent food from entering the trachea. The chewed food is pushed down the esophagus to the stomach through peristaltic contraction of these muscles. It takes only about seven seconds for food to pass through the esophagus, and no digestion takes place in the esophagus.

* *Stomach*: Food enters the stomach through the cardiac orifice where it is further broken apart and thoroughly mixed with gastric acid, pepsin, and other digestive enzymes to break down proteins. The acid itself doesn't break down food molecules; rather, it provides an optimum pH for the reaction of the enzyme pepsin and kills many microorganisms that are ingested with the food. The parietal cells of the stomach also secrete intrinsic factor (IF), which is required for an absorption of vit-B12. Food in the stomach is in semiliquid form, which upon completion is known as chyme. It secretes mucous, which protects stomach mucosa from acid exposure. Pepsinogen is also secreted from the stomach, and it requires H^+ to convert into pepsin (active form).

* *Small intestine*: After being processed in the stomach, food is passed to the small intestine via the pyloric sphincter. The majority of digestion and absorption occurs here after the milky chyme enters the duodenum. Here it is further mixed with three different liquids:

• Bile, which emulsifies fat to allow absorption, neutralizes the chyme and is used to excrete waste products such as bilin and bile acids.
• Pancreatic juice made by the pancreas.
• Intestinal enzymes of the alkaline mucosal membranes. The enzymes include maltase, lactase, and sucrase (all three of which process only sugars), trypsin and chymotrypsin.

- The pH becomes more basic in small intestine, which activates pancreatic and small intestinal enzymes that break down various nutrients into smaller molecules to allow absorption into the circulatory or lymphatic systems. Blood containing the absorbed nutrients is carried away from the small intestine via the hepatic portal vein and goes to the liver for filtering, removal of toxins, and nutrient processing.

- The small intestine and remainder of the digestive tract undergoes peristalsis to transport food from the stomach to the rectum and allow food to be mixed with the digestive juices and absorbed.

- *Peristalsis*: The circular muscles and longitudinal muscles are antagonistic muscles, with one contracting as the other relaxes. When the circular muscles contract, the lumen becomes narrower and longer and the food is squeezed and pushed forward. When the longitudinal muscles contract, the circular muscles relax, and the gut dilates to become wider and shorter to allow food to enter.

- Large intestine: After the food has been passed through the small intestine, the food enters the large intestine. The large intestine absorbs water from the bolus and stores feces until it can be egested. Food products that cannot go through the villi, such as cellulose (dietary fiber), are mixed with other waste products from the body and become hard and concentrated feces. The feces are stored in the rectum for a certain period, and then the stored feces are egested due to the contraction and relaxation through the anus. The exit of this waste material is regulated by the anal sphincter.

- Fat digestion: It requires lipase and bile. The lipase (activated by acid) breaks down the fat into monoglycerides and fatty acids (FA). The bile emulsifies the fatty acids so they may be easily absorbed. Short- and some medium-chain FA are absorbed directly into the blood via intestine capillaries and travel through the portal vein just as other absorbed nutrients do. However, long-chain FA and some medium chain fatty acids are too large to be directly released into the intestinal capillaries. They are absorbed into the walls of the intestine villi and reassembled again into triglycerides (TGs). The triglycerides are coated with cholesterol and protein (protein coat) into a compound called a chylomicron. Within the villi, the chylomicron enters a lymphatic capillary called a lacteal, which merges into larger lymphatic vessels. It is transported via the lymphatic system and the thoracic duct. The thoracic duct empties the chylomicrons into the bloodstream via the left subclavian vein. At this point the chylomicrons can transport the triglycerides to liver.

■ Digestive hormones:

- *Gastrin*: Secreted from G cells of the stomach. Stimulates the gastric glands to secrete pepsinogen (an inactive form of the enzyme pepsin) and HCl. It stimulates stomach motility and secretion. Secretion of gastrin is stimulated by distension, ACh (parasympathetic stimulation). The secretion is inhibited by low pH (acidity).

- *Secretin*: Secreted from the duodenum. Stimulates sodium bicarbonate secretion from the pancreas and bile secretion from the liver and gallbladder. It inhibits stomach motility and secretion. The hormone secreted in response to the acidic chyme.

- *Cholecystokinin (CCK)*: Secreted from the duodenum. Stimulates the release of pancreatic enzymes and emptying of bile from the gall bladder. It inhibits stomach motility and secretion. The hormone is secreted in response to fat in chyme.

- *Gastric inhibitory peptide (GIP)*: Secreted from the duodenum. It inhibits stomach motility and secretion. Stimulate insulin secretion. Secreted in response to AA, fat, and carbohydrate.

- All four hormones describe above stimulate insulin release; therefore, oral glucose will increase insulin secretion more than IV glucose.

- Gastrin and CCK have same chemical structure.

* *Salivary Secretion*
    - Hypotonic (All secretions in GIT are isotonic. This is an exception.)
    - Low Na^+ and Cl^- because of the reabsorption of these ions
    - High K^+ and $HCO3^-$ because of the secretion of these ions

* *Gastric Secretions*
    - Gastric secretion contains high H^+, K^+, Cl^- but low Na^+

* *Pancreatic Secretion*

Enzymes Secreted in Active Form

- Pancreatic amylase
- Pancreatic lipase (needs colipase to be effective)
- Cholesterol esterase (sterol lipase)
- Phospholipase A2
- High HCO_3^- and low Cl^-

Enzymes Secreted in Inactive Form

- Proteases – Trypsinogen
  - Chymotrypsinogen
  - Procarboxypeptidase
- Trypsinogen enterokinase converts trypsinogen into trypsin, which then converts all proteases in their active form
- *Trypsin inhibitor* is also secreted by pancreas with proenzymes

■ *Bile Salts and Micelles*

1^0 bile acid (by liver) – Cholic acid
  Chenodeoxycholic acid
1^0 bile acid – *lipid soluble*

- Conjugate with glycine → *become water soluble* but still contain lipid-soluble segment
- Because they are ionized at neutral P^H, conjugated bile acids exist as salts of (Na^+) cations and therefore called bile salts.

2^0 bile acid (by intestinal bacteria) – deoxycholic acid (cholic acid) and lithocholic acid (chenodeoxycholic acid). Lithocholic acid is hepatotoxic → excreted.

29. *Micelle formation*: When bile salts become concentrated, they form micelles. These are water-soluble spheres with a lipid-soluble interior

- In the distal ileum and only in the distal ileum, bile salts are *actively* reabsorbed.

■ *Celiac disease*: sensitive to gluten – autoimmune disease – *flattening of villi* and generalized malabsorption – normal function returns if gluten is avoided by removal of wheat *or* rye flour from the diet – strong association with dermatitis herpetiformis

RENAL PHYSIOLOGY

- 7/8 of all nephrons are cortical nephrons
- 1/8 of all nephrons are juxtamedullary nephrons

- Juxtamedullary nephrons consist of the long loop of Henle and the terminal region of the collecting ducts.

- Individual nephrons that make up both kidneys are connected in parallel but flow through single nephron represents two arterioles and two capillary beds connected in series,

- Constrict efferent / dilate afferent → ↑ glomerular cap pressure → ↑ filtration
- FF = GFR/RPF (RPF = renal plasma flow, FF = filtration fraction)

- Filtered load = GFR × Px (Px = concentration in plasma) (amt/time) = (vol/time) × (amt/vol)

- Excretion = Ux × V
  (amt/time) = (vol/time) × (amt/vol)

- Reabsorption = filtration > excretion = filtration – excretion
- Secretion = excretion > filtration = excretion – filtration
- Net transport load = filtered load – excretion rate = (GFR × Px) – (Ux × V)

	Filtration	Reabsorption	Secretion
plasma protein	no	–	–
inulin, mannitol	yes	no	no
glucose, amino acid, urea, Na	yes	yes	no
PAH	yes	no	yes
creatinine	yes	no	small amount

- Clearance$_a$ = $U_a \times V / P_a$
- C_{INULIN} = GFR (b/c no reabsorption and secretion of inulin so it is equal to GFR)
- C_{PAH} = RPF (ERPF) (EPRF – effective renal plasma flow)
- Renal blood flow = ERPF / 1-Hct
- PAH clearance is only 90% as 10% flow perfuse renal capsule and is not cleared.
- PAH – carrier mediated secretion – increased PAH leads to increase in secretion initially, but later, as saturation of carriers occur, clearance decreases and becomes stable (see protein mediated diffusion).

30. *Proximal Tubule (PT)*
   - About 2/3 (66%) of filtered Na^+ is reabsorbed in PT
   - About 2/3 of filtered H_2O, K^+ and Cl^- follow Na
   - 80–90% of filtered HCO_3^- is reabsorbed and H^+ is secreted
   - Osmolarity at the end of PT is 300 mOsm (isotonic)
   - The most energy-demanding process of nephron
   - Normally all CHO, AA, proteins, peptides, and ketone bodies are reabsorbed in PT via secondary active transport

31. *The Loop of Henle*
   - Counter current multiplier
   - Descending limb is permeable to water
   - Ascending loop is permeable to NaCl
   - Anything that ↑ flow through the loop of Henle or vasa recta will ↓ the ability of the system to maintain a high medullary osmolarity and reduce the ability of the kidney to form a concentrated urine.
   - Normally, medullary interstitial fluid is hyperosmolar.

32. *Collecting Duct (CD):*

   ■ Without ADH, the CD is impermeable to water.

33. *Distal Tubule (DT) and CD*

   ■ ADH controls the final water and urea reabsorption.
   ■ Aldosterone controls the final NaCl reabsorption and K^+ secretion.
   ■ **Regulates pH by absorbing bicarbonate and secreting H^+ into the filtrate**
   ■ Arginine vasopressin receptor 2 is also expressed in the DCT.

   ■ In acidosis, H^+ moves inside the cell to buffer and K^+ moves out from the cell therefore hyperkalemia occurs in acidosis and hypokalemia occurs in alkalosis *except* diarrhea and carbonic anhydrase inhibitors (acetazolamide, etc.) in which acidosis and hypokalemia occur. (Remember, acidosis – hyperkalemia – hypercalcemia [$\uparrow$ free Ca^{+2}])
   ■ pH = 7.4, Pco_2 = 40 mmHg, HCO_3^- = 22–28 mmol/L (see pathology notes)
   ■ Anion gap – normal (5–11 mEq/L) = (Na – [Cl + HCO_3^-])

   ■ *Respiratory compensation*: occurs in metabolic disturbance
   ■ Metabolic acidosis – hyperventilation
   ■ Metabolic alkalosis – hypoventilation

   ■ *Renal compensation*: occurs in respiratory and/or metabolic disturbance
   ■ Acidosis (acidic urine) – $\uparrow$ loss of H+ in urine, $\uparrow$ production of HCO3- and reabsorption
   ■ Alkalosis (alkaline urine) - $\uparrow$ loss of HCO3- in urine

RESPIRATORY PHYSIOLOGY

- Total ventilation $V = V_T \times f$ (V_T = tidal volume, f = RR)
- Alveolar ventilation $V_A = (V_T - V_D) \times f$ (V_D = Dead space (150 ml))
- Dead space does *not* contain CO_2 at the end of inspiration
- Dead space does contain CO_2 at the end of expiration
- FRC is the volume of gas at the end of passive expiration (2700 ml). FRC is the neutral / equilibrium point for the RS (respiratory system)
- RV (residual volume, 1200 ml)
- VC (vital capacity, 5500 ml) = TLC – RV
- TLC (total lung capacity, 6700 ml)
- Positive end expiratory pressure (PEEP) – By not allowing intra-alveolar pressure to return to zero at the end of expiration, the lung will be kept at a larger volume. This will decrease the tendency to develop regional atelectasis.

- **Lung compliance (C) = $\Delta V / \Delta P$ (the ability of the lungs to stretch during a change in volume relative to an applied change in pressure). Fibrosis is associated with a *decrease* in pulmonary compliance. Emphysema/COPD is associated with an *increase* in pulmonary compliance due to the loss of alveolar and elastic tissue.**
- ↑ Recoil → ↓ compliance → more negative intrapleural pressure required to inflate the lung
- ↑ Negative intra-pleural pressure → ↑ capillary filtration → pulmonary edema
- Surfactant – ↑ compliance, ↓ recoil, ↓ capillary filtration
- **Pulmonary surfactant increases compliance by decreasing the surface tension of water. The main lipid component of surfactant, dipalmitoylphosphatidylcholine. The internal surface of the alveolus is covered with a thin coat of fluid. The water in this**

fluid has a high surface tension and provides a force that could collapse the alveolus. The presence of surfactant in this fluid breaks up the surface tension of water, making it less likely that the alveolus can collapse inward

- Airway resistance (R) α 1 / radius^4
- Increase lung volume $\alpha \downarrow$ R
- Increase negative intra-pleural pressure $\alpha \downarrow$ R

- Normal people can exhale only 80% of their VC in one second because during forced expiration, intrapleural pressure becomes more positive, and the airways are closed.

* *Obstructive Pulmonary Disease*
   - $\uparrow$ airway resistance
   - $\downarrow$ expiratory flow rate
   - $\uparrow$ TLC
* *Restrictive Pulmonary Disease*
   - $\uparrow$ in lung recoil
   - $\downarrow$ in all lung volume
   - FEV_1 / FVC - $\uparrow$ *or* N

- Medullary centers – The DRG (dorsal respiratory group) is involved in the generation of respiratory rhythm and is primarily responsible for the generation of inspiration. The VRG contains both inspiratory and expiratory neurons. The VRG (ventral respiratory group) is secondarily responsible for initiation of inspiratory activity, after the dorsal respiratory group. The VRG is responsible for motor control of inspiratory and expiratory muscles during exercise

- Apneustic center – Located in the lower pons, it promotes inspiration by stimulation of the inspiratory neurons in the medulla oblongata providing a constant stimulus (prolonged inspiration [apneustic breathing]). It controls the intensity of breathing. The apneustic center is inhibited by pulmonary stretch receptors

- Pneumotaxic center (pontine respiratory group [PRG]) – The PRG antagonizes the apneustic center (cyclically inhibits inspiration).

The PRG limits the burst of action potentials in the phrenic nerve, effectively decreasing the tidal volume and regulating the respiratory rate. Absence of the PRG results in an increase in depth of respiration and a decrease in respiratory rate.

■ *High Altitude*: Partial pressure of O_2 is decrease at high altitude so PAo_2 and Pao_2 decreased acutely and remain decrease in person who is living at high altitude for long time. Same way $PAco_2$ and $Paco_2$ remain decrease. Hb% saturation remains decrease because partial pressure is decreased at high altitude. P^H is increased (respiratory alkalosis) initially due to hyperventilation but it returns back to normal level in a person who is living at high altitudes for a long time. Erythropoietin secretion increase in response to hypoxia, which leads to increase RBC in blood after 3–4 wks in a person who is living at high altitude for long time. Increase in RBC brings systemic O2 content back to normal in a person who is living on high altitude for long time.

■ *Ventilation (V_A) and Perfusion (Q)*:
• Toward the apex – lower perfusing pressure and high resistance therefore less blood flow to the apex
• Toward the base – no loss in perfusing pressure and lower resistance therefore more blood flow to the base
• **The ventilation/perfusion ratio is higher in the apex of lung when a person is standing than it is in the base of lung**

* *Hypoxic vasoconstriction* – unique to pulmonary circuit – a physiological phenomenon in which pulmonary arteries constrict in the presence of hypoxia without hypercapnia (high carbon dioxide levels), redirecting blood flow to alveoli with higher oxygen tension

• Alveoli → pulmonary vein (pulmonary end capillary) → LV → systemic arteries
• $PAo_2 = 100$ mmHg (A = Alveolar)
• Pulmonary end capillary $PO_2 = 100$ mmHg
• $Pao_2 = 95$ mmHg (a = systemic arteries)

	PAo2	End capillary PO2	Pao2	
hypoventilation	↓	↓	↓	
diffusion impairment (structural problem)	↑	↓	↓	improve A-a gradient with supplemental oxygen
pulmonary shunt	↑	↑	↓	A-a gradient does *not* improve with supplemental oxygen

- Hypoxia *never* develops in left to right shunt

- *Atrial septal defect*: PO$_2$ increase first appears in the right atrium

- *Ventricular septal defect*: PO$_2$ increase first appears in the right ventricle

- *Patent ductus arteriosus*: PO$_2$ increase first appears in the pulmonary artery

IMMUNOLOGY

1. What happens when organisms enter to the body?

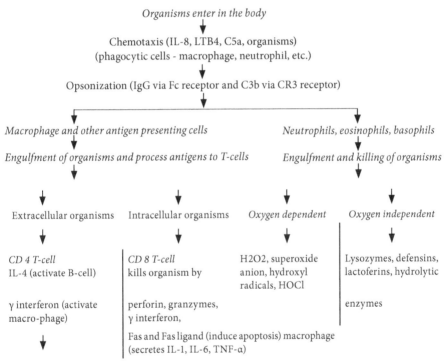

Organisms enter in the body
↓
Chemotaxis (IL-8, LTB4, C5a, organisms)
(phagocytic cells - macrophage, neutrophil, etc.)
↓
Opsonization (IgG via Fc receptor and C3b via CR3 receptor)

Macrophage and other antigen presenting cells

Engulfment of organisms and process antigens to T-cells

Neutrophils, eosinophils, basophils

Engulfment and killing of organisms

Extracellular organisms | Intracellular organisms | *Oxygen dependent* | *Oxygen independent*

CD 4 T-cell
IL-4 (activate B-cell)

CD 8 T-cell
kills organism by

H_2O_2, superoxide anion, hydroxyl radicals, HOCl

Lysozymes, defensins, lactoferins, hydrolytic

γ interferon (activate macro-phage)

perforin, granzymes, γ interferon,

enzymes

Fas and Fas ligand (induce apoptosis) macrophage (secretes IL-1, IL-6, TNF-α)

* cell (secrete immunoglobulins)

401

- When an organism enters in the body, IL-8, LTB4, C5a and the organism itself act as chemotactic agents to attract phagocytic cells (macrophage, neutrophil, etc.). Meanwhile IgG via Fc receptor and C3b via CR3 receptor attach to organism and mark them for engulfing by phagocytic cells. Now depending upon phagocytic cell, organisms are either presented to T-cells or killed directly. Macrophage and other antigen-presenting cells present organisms to T-cells whereas neutrophils and eosinophils kill them directly.

- *Macrophages* present *extracellular* organisms to *CD 4* cells while *intracellular* organisms to *CD 8.*

- *When organisms are presented to CD4 cells,* they secrete IL-4 (which activate B-cells) and gamma interferon (which activate macrophage, now to kill organisms). Macrophage secrete IL-1, IL-6, and TNF-α (acute phase reactants) and B-cells (transform into plasma cells) secrete immunoglobulins to kill organisms [*B-cell mediated immunity*: Naive mature B cells produce both IgM and IgD. After activation by antigen, these B cells proliferate and begin to produce high levels of IgM and IgD. If these activated B cells are also activated via their CD40 and IL-4 receptors (both modulated by T helper cells), they undergo antibody class switching to produce IgG, IgA, or IgE antibodies. During class switching, the constant region portion of the antibody heavy chain is changed, but the variable region of the heavy chain stays the same. Since the variable region does not change, class switching does not affect antigen specificity. Instead, the antibody retains affinity for the same antigens, but can interact with different effector molecules.]

- *Concept*: IgM is the only Ab where there is *NO* class switching required. So if *thymus (T-cells)* are *not* involved, there is *no* class switching and only IgM is produced.
- *When organisms are presented to CD8 cells*, they kill organisms directly by perforins, granzymes, gamma interferon, and Fas and Fas ligand (which induce apoptosis). (Cell-mediated immunity, T-cell mediated immunity)
- When *neutrophils* engulf organism, they kill them directly. Killing occurs through two pathways, oxygen dependent and oxygen independent.
- *Oxygen dependent*: Killing occurs by producing H_2O_2, superoxide anion, hydroxyl radicals, HOCl. This involves NADPH oxidase (produce superoxide anion) and myeloperoxidase enzymes (produce HOCl)
- *Oxygen independent*: Killing occurs by lysozymes, defensins, lactoferins, hydrolytic enzymes
- *Concept*: Oxygen-independent killing is still working in the patient with NADPH oxidase (chronic granulomatous disease) and myeloperoxidase disease
- *Concept*: In myeloperoxidase deficiency, H_2O_2 is still produce so organisms that lack catalase enzyme can be still killed by neutrophils. (*Example*: Streptococci are still killed, but *not* staphylococci, which produce catalase.)

- Important CD markers on different cells

CD Markers	Different Cells	Functions
▪ CD 3	▪ All T-cells	▪ TCR associated signal transduction molecule ▪ TCR = T-cell receptor
▪ CD 2	▪ All T-cells	29. Adherence to other cells, bind to LFA-3 30. LFA-3 = lymphocyte function associated antigen
29. CD 4	- Helper T-cells	- Interaction with MHC class 2 cells
▪ CD 28	10. Helper T-cells 11. Most CD 8 cells	- Costimulatory molecule needed for activation of T- cells - Binds on B-cells, macrophage, dendritic cells
• CD 40 ligand	• Activated helper T- cells	- Binds to CD 40 on B-cells - Essential for class switching (from IgM to IgG, IgA or IgE)
▯ CD 14	▯ Macrophage	
• CD 16, CD 56, CD 2	• NK cells • Lymphokine activated killer (LAK)	▪ *NO* CD 3, 4, 8, 19 on NK cells
• CD 19, CD 20, CD 21, CD 40	- B-cells	• *CD 40*: Require for class switching • *CD 21*: Serve as receptor for EBV (Ebstein-Bar Virus)
• CD 15, CD 30	• Reed-Sternberg cells	

- Important antigen receptors on different cells
  1. *TCR*: γδ (T-cells in skin and mucosal surface), αβ (T-cells at other sites)
  2. *BCR*: Ig M, Ig D
     - *MHC-1*: α 1, 2, 3 β_2
  3. *MHC-2*: αβ

- Receptors through which signal transduction occurs in B and T cells
- B-cells – α, β, CD 19, 20, 21
- T-cells – CD 3

5. Human Leukocyte Antigens and Different Classes

- The human leukocyte antigen system (HLA) is the name of the major histocompatibility complex (MHC) in humans. It is located on chromosome 6. Two different classes.
- *HLA class 1 (MHC-1)*: HLA-A, HLA-B, HLA-C
- *HLA class 2 (MHC-2)*: HLA-DP, HLA-DQ, HLA-DR

- Location of MHC-1 and MHC-2 Antigens
- *MHC-1*: all nucleated cells and platelets (*NO* MHC on RBC)
- *MHC-2*: antigen presenting cells (dendritic cells, langerhans cells, activated macrophage, B-cells, activated T-cells, and activated endothelial cells)

- Importance
- MHC-1 is necessary for antigen recognition by *CD8+ T-cells.*
- MHC-2 is necessary for antigen recognition by *CD4+ T-cells.*

- Difference
- *MHC-1*: Reacts with *ENDOGENOUSLY* produce peptides by virus, intracellular bacteria, intracellular parasites, and tumor cells
- *MHC-2*: Reacts with *EXOGENOUSLY PROCESSED* antigens

- Handling of organisms:
- *MHC-1*: It works with intracellular organisms *so after reacting with endogenously processed antigen*, β_2 microglobulin transports MHC class-1 molecules to the cell surface where it can be recognized by CD 8 T-cells and organisms are then killed by CD8 T-cells
- *MHC-2*: It works with extracellular organisms so once organisms engulfed, MHC class-2 molecule *fuse with vacuole containing exogenously processed antigen*, invariant chain is released and MHC-2-peptide complex is then transported to the cell surface where it can be recognized by CD 4 T-cells. Invariant chain prevents interaction between endogenously produced peptide and MHC-2 molecules intracellularly.

6. How does ADCC (antibody-dependent cellular cytotoxicity) and NK cells–mediated cytotoxicity differed?

- *ADCC*: IgG + NK cells → use CD 16 molecule (Fc receptor) to identify target cells
- *NK cells mediated cytotoxicity*: use CD 56 (*No* antibody involved. Ex., lysis of infected RBC)

7. Complement System

- *Classical pathway*: Activated by antigen-Ab reaction (IgG and IgM, IgM most efficient, *start point C1*, C1 - C4 - C2 - C3, C4bC2a is C3-convertase, C4bC2aC3b [C5-convertase] splits C5 into C5a and C5b, which then form C5b, 6, 7, 8, 9)
- *Alternative pathway*: C3 hydrolyze *spontaneously* in our body into C3a and C3b. If there is a pathogenic membrane surface nearby, C3b binds to it. If not, both C3a and C3b rejoin. Upon binding with a cellular membrane, C3b is bound by factor B to form C3bB. This complex in presence of factor D will be cleaved into Ba and Bb. Bb will remain covalently bonded to C3b to form C3bBb, which is the alternative pathway C3-convertase. Alternative pathway is also activated by simple presence of an organism in the body (LPS of cell wall of gram [-] bacteria), it *doesn't require antibodies*. (*Start point C3b*, C3b splits C5 into C5a and C5b, which then form C5b, 6, 7, 8, 9)

- Important Products of Complement Pathways: C3a, C4a, C5a; C3b and C5b6789

- Function of Complement System
- C3b – opsonization of pathogen
- C3a, C4a, C5a – play role in Chemotaxis
- C5b, 6, 7, 8, 9 – membrane attack complex – kill pathogen

- How to determine complements are working:
- ↓C2/C4 – classical pathway is working
- ↓Factor B – alternate pathway is working
- ↓C3 – both pathways are working

- C3-convertase can be inhibited by decay accelerating factor (DAF)
- C5a and C3a are known to trigger mast cell degranulation

- The inhibition of C1-complex is controlled by C1-inhibitor (C1 esterase). (C1-esterase also inhibits proteinases of the fibrinolytic, clotting, and kinin pathways. The kinin-kallikrein system makes bradykinin. Deficiency of C1-inhibitors leads to activation of plasma kallikrein, which produces bradykinin that is a potent vasodilator responsible for angioedema.)

- Important points to remember about different immunoglobulins:
- *IgG*: Main Ab in secondary immune response – highest concentration in the body – only Ab that can cross placenta – remain up to 4–6-months in the newborn – capable of opsonization.

- *IgM*: Main Ab in primary immune response – largest Ab in the body, has five Fc regions (circulates as a pentamer) – presence on IgM in newborn suggest recent infection – first Ab to appear in the serum after exposure to antigen – effective in complement fixation – isohemagglutinins, rheumatoid factors, and heterophile antibodies are all IgM

- *IgA*: present in secretions (Breast milk [colostrum], GI secretions, saliva, tears) – deficiency of IgA causes repetitive upper respiratory tract infections, *transfusion reaction*

- *IgD*: functions as a cell surface antigen receptor on undifferentiated B cells.

- *IgE*: involved in allergic response and immediate type of HS (type-1) – Fc region of IgE binds to basophils and mast cells – binding of antigen to two IgE molecules leads to mast cells degranulation and release of leukotrines, histamines, eosinophils, hemotactic factors, and heparin – IgE is also involved in killing of parasites (IgE + eosinophils mediated cytotoxic reaction – type-2 HS).

- What is the difference between papain and pepsin?
- *Papain*: If Ab reacts with papain and then Ag is added, Ag will be unaffected.
- *Pepsin*: If Ab reacts with pepsin and then Ag is added, Ag will agglutinate/precipitate.

- *Antigen specificity*: Variable region of both heavy and light chain. Class switching doesn't affect variable region of both heavy and light chain, therefore class switching doesn't affect specificity of antibody to that antigen.

- What are allotype and idiotype?
- *Allotype*: A genetically determined difference in molecules between two members of the *SAME SPECIES*.
- *Idiotype*: The *individual, unique* differences between antibodies of different *antigen-binding specificities*.

12. Important Interleukins, Other Immune System Cells, and Their Functions
    - IL-4 – class switch to *IgE*
    - IL-5 – class switch to IgA and ↑*eosinophils*
    - Macrophage – IL-1, IL-6, IL-8, TNF-α
    - IL-10 – downregulate CMI (cell mediated immunity), Th1 (helper T-cell 1)
    - γ interferon – downregulate Th2
    - Th1 – delayed-type hypersensitivity (DTH) (type-IV HS)
    - Th2 – Antibody mediated immunity
    - IL-1 – Pyrogenic (fever inducing)
    - IL-6 – Stimulate acute phase proteins
    - IL-3 – Stimulate bone marrow stem cells (granulocyte and monocytes)
    - IL-7 – Stimulate pre-B and pre-T cells (lymphoid cell development)
    - IL-2 – Stimulate B-cells to produce antibody and self-stimulation of T-cells. IL-2 is produced by Th1, NK, and Tc

13. Important Points to Remember about Hypersensitivities and Their Examples
    - *Type I hypersensitivity reaction (HS)*: Anaphylaxis (bee stung, severe allergic reaction due to peanut); mast cells and basophils degranulation (release of histamines) – bronchospasm, vasodilation, etc – *Tx*: epinephrine (SC, 1:1,000) (prevents mast cell degranulation by increasing cyclic AMP levels; relax smooth muscle of respiratory tract)

- *Type II HS*: Antibody to receptor (e.g., myasthenia gravis, Goodpasture's syndrome, Grave's disease) and cytotoxic reaction (*Ab binds to antigens, which activate complements causing cell destruction*, e.g., IgG + complement-mediated platelet destruction in ITP, IgE + eosinophils, and complement-mediated cytotoxic lysis of filaria, complement mediated lysis of RBCs, *rheumatic fever*, erythroblastosis fetalis)
- *Type III HS*: deposition of circulating immune complexes in different tissues and then activate complement system that produces damage (e.g., vasculitis, *rheumatoid arthritis*, SLE, arthus reaction; blockage of C3b by Ab helps in patient with disease due to type-3 HS)
- *Type IV HS*: CD4 cells mediated HS (e.g., tuberculosis, poison ivy, latex gloves)

- Which *HS reaction* is responsible for symptoms of nematodes infection and destruction of filaria?
- In nematode infection, the larva migrates to the lung and produce cough, wheezing, etc. These symptoms are due to *type-1 HS* reaction
- In filarial infection, destruction of microfilaria is IgE dependent cytotoxicity (*Type-2 HS*)
- How does destruction of toxoplasma occur?
- Usually IgE is involved in parasite destruction, but toxoplasma is an intracellular parasite and IgE is *not*
- involved in its destruction. *Th1, Tc, NK, ADCC involve in killing of Toxoplasma.*

---

14. Different types of graft:
    - Allograft – transplant between different genetic makeup within the same species
    - Isograft – transplant between genetically identical (monozygotic twins)
    - Autograft – transplant from one site to another on the same individual
    - Xenograft – transplant across species barriers (transplant a heart from baboon to human)

15. *Graft-versus-Host Disease*: when immunocompetent tissue (fresh whole blood, thymus, bone marrow) is transplanted into an immunocompromised host

- *Important point*: *T-cells from transplant tissue attack host tissues. (Type-4 Hypersensitivity(HS) reaction).*

- Different Types of Rejections
- Hyperacute rejection: mins. to hrs. – preformed antidonor antibody (*type-2 HS*)
- Acute rejection: days to weeks – primary activation of T-cells. (*Type-4 HS*)
- Chronic rejection: months to years – causes unclear. (*Type-4 HS*)
- Accelerated rejection: days (3–5) – reactivation of sensitized T-cells. Ex. If 1 kidney is rejected, then you transplant another kidney. If it is rejected a second time, then it rejects faster than first time.

- Important HLA association with different diseases:
- HLA-A3 – Hemochromatosis
- HLA-B27 – Ankylosing spondylitis
- HLA-DR2 – Multiple Sclerosis, goodpasture, narcolepsy, hay fever
- HLA-DR2, DR3 – SLE
- HLA-DR3 – Celiac sprue, dermatitis herpatiformis
- HLA-DR3, DR4 – Type-1 DM
- HLA-DR4 – Rheumatoid arthritis (RA), pemphigus vulgaris
- HLA-DR5 – Pernicious anemia, juvenile RA
- HLA-DR7 – Steroid-responsive nephrotic syndrome

- *Important Syndromes/Diseases due to Deficiency of Different Immune Components*

- Phagocyte dysfunction (CGD, Chediak-Higashi syndrome) – *extracellular bacteria (Staph. aureus)*
  + *fungi* (aspergillosis) (CGD – negative NBT [nitro-blue tetrazolium test])
- T-Cells deficiency (DiGeorge syndrome) – *intracellular organisms* (virus, candida, TB) but *NOT*
  Extracellular; 3rd and 4th pouch defect, *absent thymus*; Hypocalcaemia due to *absent parathyroid glands*

- B-cells deficiency (Bruton's agammaglobulinemia) – *extracellular pyogenic bacteria* but *NOT* intracellular
- SCID (severe combined immune deficiency) – *bacteria, virus, fungus (extracellular + intracellular)*; adenosine deaminase deficiency; neutrophils - ↑ or N, BandT cells - ↓↓↓

- Bruton's agammaglobulinemia – *tyrosine kinase deficiency* – arrest of B-cell maturation – virtually *absent B-cell* but pre-B cells present and low circulating immunoglobulins
- Wiskott-Aldrich syndrome – *deletion of* T and B cells – eczema, thrombocytopenia, and low IgM, association with *non-Hodgkin lymphoma.*
- Bruton's agammaglobulinemia and Wiskott-Aldrich syndrome are the only X-linked recessive immune deficiency syndromes. (Both have *LOW* circulating immunoglobulins but Wiskott-Aldrich has low T cells too)

- Hereditary angioedema – C1 esterase deficiency
- C3 deficiency – pyogenic bacteria
- C1, C4 or C2 deficiency – opsonization not efficient
- C5–8 deficiency – neisseria Infections
- Paroxysmal nocturnal hemoglobinuria (PNH): Defect in molecule anchoring decay accelerating factor (DAF), which normally degrades C3andC5 convertase on hematopoetic cell membranes therefore in the absence of DAF, complement mediated intravascular lysis of RBC occur (hemoglobinuria; (*clue*: red urine in the morning).
- ↑IgM but deficient IgG and IgA – CD40 ligand deficiency on activated T-cells

- *How to assess different immunodeficiency syndromes in exam*: Look at the organisms in question.

If *recurrent infection with only* Staph. aureus, then you are most probably dealing with *phagocyte dysfunction* (CGD and Chediak-Higashi syndrome) *or C3 deficiency.* If you find the words *neutrophil inclusions* in questions, then go with *Chediak-Higashi*, but if you find the words *negative NBT* (nitro-blue tetrazolium) test in questions, then go with *CGD* (chronic granulomatous disease).

If *no Staph. aureus* infection in the question but infection with *intracellular* (virus, TB, *Candida*) organisms *and/or* sign and symptoms of hypocalcemia (tetany), then go with DiGeorge syndrome. If intracellular (virus, TB) + extracellular (staph, aspergillosis) organisms then go with SCID.

If *low* immunoglobulins, then either Bruton's *or* Wiskott-Aldrich. If low IgM, thrombocytopenia and eczema present, then go with Wiskott-Aldrich.

If staph (extracellular) infection and ask about which complement, then C3 deficiency.

If deficient opsonization (recurrent *encapsulated* organism infection) and ask about which complement, then go with C1, C4, or C2 deficiency. But if they ask which complement is responsible for opsonization, then remember it is C3b.

If disseminated *Neisseria* infection (meningococcal and gonococcal) then go with C5–8 deficiency.

- How does CD8 and CD4 T-cells differentiate in thymus?
- In thymus, cells with LOW affinity for MHC-1 molecule differentiate into CD 8 T-cells (no affinity/high affinity cells are eliminated). Cells with LOW affinity for MHC-2 molecule differentiate into CD 4 T-cells.

- What are first and last events in maturation of B-cells?
- 1st event in pre-B-cells – gene rearrangement of heavy chain
- Last event in mature B-cells – IgM and IgD molecule on the surface of B-cells

- What is normal ratio for T-cells to B-cells?
- *T*-cells to B-cells ratio in the body – *T*hree to one

23. *Primary and Secondary Immune Responses*
- Primary immune response – when antigen presented to our immune system first time – IgM

- Secondary immune response – when same antigen presented to our immune system second time – IgG

24. *Active and Passive Immunities*
    - Natural active immunity – chickenpox
    - Natural passive immunity – mother IgG protects her baby

    - Acquired active immunity – chickenpox vaccine
    - Acquired passive immunity – hepatitis B immunoglobulins

25. How does Superantigen work?

    - *Superantigen* binds to β chain of TCR and MHC-II molecule of APC (antigen presenting cells) stimulating T-cell activation

26. What is responsible for killing of pathogen intramacrophage?

    - γ interferon

27. Which T-cells are involved in T-cell-mediated cytotoxicity and type-4 HS?

    - T-cell mediated cytotoxicity – CD8 cells
    - Type-4 HS – CD4 cells

28. How does destruction occur in TB?

    - TB → macrophage → Th → secrete IL-2 and activate macrophage via γ interferon to become epitheloid cells and multinucleated giant cell → epitheloid cells secrete IL-1 and TNF-α (acute phase response), macrophage releases large numbers of inflammatory mediators that are responsible for tissue damage → fibrosis. So in TB, damage occurs by immune system (DTH), but *NO* endotoxin/exotoxin.

29. What do we check in HIV screening and confirmatory test?

    - We check antibodies in patient, *NOT* antigen.

30. When do we consider western blot test positive?

- The HIV Western blot is considered positive when the patient demonstrates the presence of antibody to *at least two of three* important HIV antigens, which are gp120, gp41, and p24.

31. Important autoantibodies in different diseases:

Autoantibodies	Disease
antiacetylcholine receptor	myasthenia gravis
anti-basement membrane	Goodpasture syndrome
anticentromere	CREST syndrome
antiendomysial and antigliadin	celiac disease
anti-insulin, anti-islet cell	type-1 DM
anti-intrinsic factor, antiparietal cell	pernicious anemia
antimicrosomal	Hashimoto's thyroiditis
antimitochondreal	primary billiary cirrhosis
p-ANCA	*p*olyarteritis nadosa (microscopic polyangitis)
c-ANCA	Wegener's granulomatosis
antiribonucleoprotein	mixed connective tissue disease
anti-TSH receptor	Grave's disease
anti-Scl-70	scleroderma
anti-SS-A, anti-SS-B	Sjogren syndrome
anti-Smith, anti-ds-DNA, ANA (antinuclear antibody)	systemic lupus erythematous (SLE)
antihistone antibody	drug-induced lupus

GENERAL PATHOLOGY

- *Hypoxia*: inadequate oxygenation of tissues
- *Hypoxemia*: ↓in Pao_2 (which is one of the cause of hypoxia)

Physiology: pulmonary art (Sao_2 = 75%) → alveoli (PAo_2 = 100 mmHg, $PAco_2$ = 40 mmHg) → pulmonary vein → LV → systemic circulation (Pao_2 = 95 mmHg, Sao_2 = 97%) → RV → pulmonary art (A = alveoli, a = arteries, P = pressure, S = saturation)

- Causes of hypoxemia: ventilation defect (100% O_2 doesn't ↑Pao_2); perfusion defect (100% O_2 will ↑Pao_2); diffusion defect (interstitial fibrosis)
- *Methemoglobinemia* – Hb with Fe^{+3} (MetHb) – not able to bind with O_2 – *decreased* Sao_2, but *normal* Pao_2 – causes: patient returned from camping who drank mountain water (high amount of nitrites), nitrite- and sulfur-containing drugs (Dapsone, nitroglycerine, sulfa drugs) – *Tx*: methylene blue (activates metHb reductase); vit-C is useful too.
- CO_2 poisoning – automobile exhaust, smoke inhalation – *decreased* Sao_2, but *normal* Pao_2 – inhibits cytochrome oxidase – headache (first symptom), cherry-red discoloration of skin and blood – *Tx*: 100% O_2
- CN poisoning – may result from drug (sodium nitroprusside) – inhibits cytochrome oxidase – *Tx*: amyl nitrite
- Oxygen dissociation curve – shift to the right means it is easy for tissue to extract oxygen from blood (2, 3-BPG [produced during respiratory alkalosis] shift curve to the right)
- Tissues susceptible to hypoxia – watershed areas (area between distribution of anterior and middle cerebral arteries, between superior and inferior mesenteric arteries [splenic flexure],

subendocardial tissue, straight portion of PT in cortex of kidney, thick ascending limb of loop of Henle in the medulla)

- First sign (reversible) of tissue hypoxia – swelling of cell (inactive Na-K ATPase pump)
- Irreversible sign of tissue hypoxia – increase cytosolic Ca^{++} (inactive Ca^{++} ATPase pump) – increase Ca^{++} in mitochondria release cytochrome c, which activates apoptosis
- Ubiquitin – markers for intermediate filament degradation (Mallory bodies in hepatocytes in alcoholic liver disease, Lewy bodies [eosinophilic cytoplasmic inclusions in substantia nigra] in Parkinsonism)
- *Dystrophic calcification*: normal serum calcium/phosphate but deposit of calcium into damaged tissue – atherosclerotic plaques, enzymatic fat necrosis, periventricular calcification in CMV
- *Metastatic calcification*: increased serum calcium and/or phosphate with deposition of calcium in normal tissue – nephrocalcinosis in primary hyperparathyroidism, calcification of basal ganglia in primary hyperparathyroidism (high phosphorous)
- *Atrophy* – decrease *size* of tissue *or* organ – atrophy of muscle in cast for long time (due to lack of stimulation)

- *Hypertrophy* – increase in *size* of tissue or organ – after removing one kidney from body increase in size of other kidney in the body
- *Hyperplasia* – increase in *number* of cells – BPH due to an increase in dihydrotestosteron
- *Metaplasia* – replacement of one cell type by another cell type – goblet cells in stomach
- *Dysplasia* – disordered cell growth – squamous dysplasia of cervix due to HPV infection – increase chance of cancer

- *Types of Cell Necrosis*
- Coagulation necrosis – infarction except brain
- Liquefactive necrosis – infections, brain infarct or infection
- Caseous necrosis – TB and systemic fungi
- Enzymatic fat necrosis – acute pancreatitis
- Fibrinoid necrosis – necrosis of immunologic injury (small vessel vasculitis – type-3 HS)

-   Gummatous – tertiary syphilis

-   *Apoptosis* – programmed cell death – TP53 gene (temporary arrest cell cycle in the G1 phase to repair damage DNA); BAX gene (TP53 activates BAX gene if DNA damage is so much. BAX and cytochrome c promote apoptosis.); BCL2 gene (inhibits apoptosis by preventing leaking of cytochrome c from mitochondria)
-   TP53 and RB suppressor genes – regulate cell cycle (G1 to S phase, RB – sequester specific transcription factor needed for cell cycle progression; TP53 – inhibits Cdk4 to arrest cell cycle in G1 phase)
-   Cyclin D binds to Cdk4 (cyclin-dependent kinase 4) forming a complex that phosphorylates RB protein causing the cell to enter S-phase from G1 phase.
-   Most characteristic features of apoptosis is peripheral aggregation of chromatin (castrated patient's prostate cells show apoptosis)
-   Free radicals cell injury – damage membrane and DNA
-   Reperfusion injury – reperfusion of ischemic tissue produce superoxide free radicals, which irreversibly damage previously injured cells
-   Intracellular iron produce hydroxyl ions which damage parenchymal cells (cirrhosis in hemochromatosis)
-   Fatty liver – clear space pushing the nucleus to the periphery (microscopic)

-   Histamine – vasodilation of arteriole (responsible for redness and heat)
-   Histamine - ↑ permeability of venules (responsible for edema)
-   PGE2 (prostaglandin) – sensitize nerve endings causing pain
-   Neutrophils – primary leukocyte in acute inflammation
-   Monocytes and lymphocytes – primary leukocyte in chronic inflammation
-   Eosinophil – major basic protein
-   Neutrophil – lactoferin, myeloperoxidase, NADPH oxidase
-   Selectins – responsible for "rolling" of neutrophils
-   β_2 integrins – neutrophil adhesion molecule

-   Leukocyte adhesion deficiency – deficiency of selectins or β_2 integrins (CD11a:CD18) – delayed separation of umbilical cord in newborn

- Factors activate ($\downarrow$neutrophils) and inhibit ($\uparrow$neutrophils) adhesion molecule synthesis:
- Activate: C3a, LTB4, endotoxins, IL-1, TNF
- Inhibit: corticosteroids, catecholamine, lithium

- NADPH oxidase produce free radicals of oxygen – superoxide dismutase converts it in to H_2O_2 (called respiratory burst) – myeloperoxidase combine it with Cl and form hypochlorus free radicals, which kills organisms
- Chronic granulomatous disease – absent NADPH oxidase – absent respiratory burst (negative NBT [nitro-blue tetrazolium])
- Myeloperoxidase deficiency – respiratory burst occurs – so able to kill streptococcus species (catalase negative) but *not* staphylococci (catalase positive)
- Job's syndrome – defective chemotaxis (staph infection) and $\uparrow$ IgE (eczema)
- Histiocytes (bone marrow) – monocytes (in blood)
- Monocytes – macrophage (at the site of inflammation)
- Epitheloid cells – activated macrophage is called epitheloid cells
- Giant cells – accumulation of epitheloid cells
- Acute inflammation: purulent (infection); fibrinous (deposition of fibrin rich exudates; e.g., pericarditis); pseudomembranous (damage of mucosal lining produce a shaggy membrane of necrotic tissue) – IgM predominant immunoglobulin
- Chronic Inflammation: destruction of parenchyma (loss of function, repair by fibrosis) – formation of granulation tissue
- Key elements in wound healing – *granulation tissue* (fibronectin [cell adhesion glycoprotein] is required for granulation tissue. Fibroblast [synthesize collagen]; Vascular endothelial growth factor [VEGF] and fibroblast growth factor [FGF] are important for angiogenesis)
- Laminin – key adhesion glycoprotein in basement membrane interacts with type- 4 collagen
- Type-1 collagen has greatest tensile strength. Collagenases (metalloproteinase – require zinc as a cofactor) replace type-3 collagen with type-1 to give strength to the repaired tissue to its original strength.
- Vit-C deficiency – decreased cross-linking of collagen
- Copper deficiency – decrease cross-linking of α-chains in collagen

- Zinc deficiency – defect in removal of type-3 collagen in wound remolding
- Keloids – excessive synthesis of type-3 collagen
- Glucocorticods – interfere with collagen formation and decreased tensile strength – prevent scar formation
- Steroid – increase neutrophils and decrease eosinophils and lymphocytes
- Lung – type-2 pneumocytes repair lung injuries
- Brain – astrocytes and microglial cells repair brain damage
- Schwann cell is a key cell in reinnervation of peripheral nerve transaction
- C-reactive protein – marker of necrosis and disease activity

- ESR – marker of acute and chronic inflammation (increase in fibrinogen, anemia – increase ESR)

- Amyloid – abnormal folding of protein – structure – beta-plated sheet – apple green birefringence in polarized light – amyloid light chain (AL, derived from light chains – e.g., Bence Jones protein); amyloid associated (AA, derived from serum associated amyloid [SAA], an acute phase reactant); β-Amyloid (Aβ, derived from amyloid precursor protein [protein product of chromosome 21] responsible for Alzheimer at early age [around 35] in patient with Down syndrome)

- Decompression sickness (Caisson's disease) – rapid ascent of deep-sea drivers leads to formation of nitrogen gas bubble that occludes vessels lumen and causes thromboembolic events – *Tx*: recompression by forcing nitrogen to solution again by increasing pressure and slow decompression

- Prader-Willi syndrome – microdeletion syndrome with hypogonadism, mental retardation, short stature, and obesity (chromosome 15 deletion is of paternal origin)
- Angelman syndrome – chromosome 15 deletion is of maternal origin (child continuously laughing)
- Cancers caused by radiation – acute leukemia, papillary CA of thyroid

- Dysgeusia, perioral rash, anosmia, poor wound healing – *Zinc deficiency*

- Hemartoma – nonneoplastic overgrowth of tissue – e.g., Peutz-Jeghers polyp
- Choristoma – nonneoplastic normal tissue in a foreign location – e.g., gastric mucosa in Meckel's diverticulum
- Desmoplasia – fibrous tissue formation in the stroma of tumor

- *Important Suppressor Genes*
    - p53 (most cancers; chromosome 17)
    - APC (familial polyposis; chromosome5)
    - BRCA-1 (breast/ovarian cancer, chromosome 17)
    - BRCA-2 (breast cancer, chromosome 13)
    - NF-1 and -2 (neurofibromatosis)
    - Rb (retinoblastoma; chromosome 13)
    - VHL (regulate nuclear transcription, Von Hippel–Lindau syndrome)

- *Oncogene relationships*:
    - ERBB2 (HER) – codes for receptor synthesis – breast cancer
    - RAS – codes for guanosine triphosphate signal transduction (G proteins that transduce signals received from growth factor receptors to the phosphatidyl inositol second messenger system) –30% of all human cancers include cancers of the lung, colon, and pancreas as well as leukemia (20–25% of acute myelogenous leukemia)
    - ABL – produces nonreceptor proteins located on the inner cell membrane surface – t9;22 translocation leads to CML
    - C-myc – is located in the nucleus and produces protein products that activate nuclear transcription – t8;14 translocation leading to Burkitt's lymphoma
    - N-myc – codes for nuclear transcription – Neuroblastoma
    - RET – codes for receptor synthesis – MEN IIa and IIb
    - BCL-2 – anti-apoptosis gene – tl4;18 translocation leads to anti- apoptosis of B lymphocytes causing follicular B cell lymphoma

- HPV (type 16 and 18) – type-16 (E6 gene product inhibits TP53) type-18 (E7 gene product inhibits RB suppressor gene

- *Tumor Markers*
  - AFP (alpha-fetoproteins) – hepatocellular CA (HCC), yolk sac tumor (endodermal sinus tumor of ovaries and testes)
  - Bence Jones protein – multiple myeloma, waldenstrom, macroglobulinemia
  - CA 15-3 – breast CA
  - CA 19-9 – pancreatic CA
  - CA 125 – surface derived ovarian CA
  - CEA – colorectal and pancreatic CA
  - PSA – prostate CA (also increase in BPH)
  - Bombesin – neuroblastoma, small-cell CA, gastric CA, pancreatic CA
  - S-100 – melanoma, neural tumor, astrocytoma
- Down syndrome (trisomy-21) – endocardial cushion defect (atrial and ventricular septal defect)
  - ↑ risk of Hirschprung disease and duodenal atresia
  - ↑ risk for leukemia (acutemegakaryocytic - ‹ 3yrs, ALL - › 3yrs)
  - Alzheimer's disease by age of 35yrs.

- Edward's syndrome (trisomy-18) – VSD, clenched hands with overlapping fingers, "rocker-bottom feet"

- *Patau's syndrome (trisomy – 13)* – VSD, cleft lip and cleft palate
- D E P – 21, 18, 13

- Turner's syndrome – preductal coarctation and bicuspid aortic valve, primary amenorrhea, cystic hygroma

- Most of the spontaneous abortions are due to trisomy 16

- *Marfan syndrome*:
  - Defect in synthesizing *fibrillin*
  - Mitral valve prolapse, aortic dissection.
  - Subluxated lens, arachodactyly.

- *Klinefelter syndrome (47, XXY)*
  - Hypogonadism, infertility, gynacomastia
  - ↑↑FSH and LH, ↓↓Testosterone

- *Kartagenar syndrome:*
  - Immotile cilia syndrome
  - *Recurrent sinusitis*, infertility, and *situs inverses*

- Low protein diet should be given in patient with renal failure and cirrhosis
- Kwashiorkor – inadequate protein intake – edema
- Marasmus – inadequate calorie intake – extreme muscle wasting
- Anorexia nervosa – distorted body image
- Bulimia nervosa – binging and purging (self-induced vomiting)
- Vit-E – decrease synthesis of vit-K dependent coagulation factor

PATHOLOGY

Systemic Pathology

CARDIOLOGY

* Myocardial ischemia / myocardial infarction: *substernal squeezing* chest pain
* Pericarditis: chest pain *relieved by leaning forward*
* Costochondritis: chest pain *reproduced by palpation*
* Dissecting aortic aneurism: *tearing* chest pain *radiating to the back*
* Pneumonia: *pleuritic (increase on inspiration)* chest pain
* Pulmonary embolism: pleuritic chest pain, *dyspnea, tachypnea*
* Esophageal spasm ("nutcracker disease"): *past h/o GERD, gastritis*, pain occurs after eating, *normal EKG*

* Stable angina: chest pain *after* exertion
* Unstable angina: chest pain *at rest* (ST depression) ($D \to E$)
* Myocardial infarction: chest pain *at rest* (ST elevation)
* Prinzmetal angina: chest pain *at rest* (ST elevation – transmural ischemia) (Due to coronary artery spam. Pain may relieve by little exercise like patient gets up and walking and pain is relieved because exercise causes increase in adenosine, which is a potent coronary vasodilator)

* *Complication of MI*: ventricular arrhythmia (MCC of death)

* Rupture (ant. wall, papillary muscles, interventricular septum) – *3–7 days*
* Autoimmune pericarditis (Dressler's syndrome) – *6–8 weeks* post-MI

* EKG changes in acute MI: peak tall T-wave → ST elevation → T-wave inversion → Q-wave
* Inferior wall MI (RC): II, III, aVF
  Anterior wall MI (LAD): $V_2 - V_4$

- Anteroseptal (LAD): $V_1 - V_3$
- Lateral wall MI (LAD/circumflex): I, aVL, $V_4 - V_6$
- Posterior wall MI (posterior descending): $V_1 - V_2$

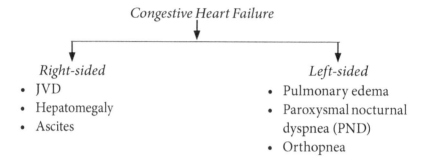

Congestive Heart Failure

Right-sided
- JVD
- Hepatomegaly
- Ascites

Left-sided
- Pulmonary edema
- Paroxysmal nocturnal dyspnea (PND)
- Orthopnea

- *Mitral valve prolapse*: mid to late systolic click
- Presentation → asymptomatic, palpitation, chest pain, syncope, sudden death
- Marfan syndrome

- *Infective endocarditis*: splinter hemorrhages, Roth's spot in eye, Janeway lesions, *valve regurgitation*
- *Strep. viridians* → *most common* overall cause (previously damage valve)
- *Staph. aureus* → *IV drug abuse* (normal/previously damaged valve) *tricuspid valve*
- *Staph epidermidis* → prosthetic devices
- *Strep bovis* → ulcerative colitis / colorectal cancer patient
- Loeffler endocarditis – prominent eosinophil infiltrates

- *Valvular Heart Disease*
- *Stenosis* → Problem in opening of valve; therefore, murmur occurs during opening of the valve
- *Regurgitation* → Problem in closing of valve; therefore, murmur occurs during closing of the valve

- *Austin Flint murmur*: regurgitant stream from incompetent aortic valve hits anterior mitral valve leaflet, producing a diastolic murmur

- *Right-sided murmur increases in intensity with inspiration*

Mitral Stenosis	Aortic Regurgitation	Mitral Regurgitation	Aortic Stenosis
▪ *Diastolic* murmur	▪ *Diastolic* decrescendo	31. *Holosystolic* radiate to the *axilla*	30. *Systolic* ejection radiate to carotid
- Opening snap	- Austin Flint murmur		▪ Chest pain / syncope during exercise in elders
12. *CXR* → double density Right heart border	- *Endocarditis prophylaxis*		• *Endocarditis prophylaxis*

- *Hypertrophic cardiomyopathy*: autosomal dominant (AD), chromosome 14 – disproportionate thickening of interventricular septum – conductance disturbance is responsible for sudden death in athletes

- Valsalva / standing - ↓ preload →↑ obstruction →↑ murmur
- Squatting / hand grip - ↑ preload →↓ obstruction →↓ murmur

- Increase in preload – decrease murmur in mitral valve prolapse and hypertrophic cardiomyopathy.

Acute Pericarditis	Cardiac Temponade	Constrictive Pericarditis
• Chest pain	- Pulsus paradoxus	▢ Kussmaul's Sign
↓	↓	↓
Relieved by leaning forward	↓ SBP more than 10 mmHg on normal inspiration	↑ jugular venous distension with inspiration
▢ *Pericardial friction rub* (Diagnostic)	• Neck vein distension with clear lung	▪ *Pericardial knock*
- *EKG* – diffuse ST segment elevation (In MI – ST elevation is in different leads according to involvement of heart and it is convex)	• Shock (Beck's triad – hypotension, JVP, muffled heart sound)	• *EKG – low voltage*

- *Pericardial Effusion*
- Serosanguineous →TB / neoplasm
- CXR – "water bottle" configuration of cardiac silhouette

- Patent ostium primum (patent foramen ovale) – failure of septum primum to fuse with endocardial cushions
- Atrial septal defect (ASD) – incomplete adhesion between septum primum and septum secondum – wide fixed split S2
- VSD – defect in membranous interventricular septum
- PDA – machinery murmur – associated with congenital rubella – PGE_2 keep it open – it shunts pulmonary artery blood to aorta in fetus

- *Acute Rheumatic Fever*
- Aschoff bodies (pathognomic) (central area of necrosis surrounded by reactive histiocytes [Anitschkow cells])
- Pericarditis, polyarthritis, chorea, erythema marginatum, and subcutaneous nodules (Jones criteria)
- Usually occur 1–3 weeks after a preceding strep. Pyogens pharyngitis

- ■ ↑↑↑ ASO titers
- ■ Treatment of acute infection and monthly penicillin prophylaxis then after.

Location of Murmur	Conditions
upper right sternal border	AS, IHSS
upper left sternal border	PS, PDA
lower left sternal border	VSD
apex	MVP

- • Cardiac myxoma – left atria – mesenchymal tumor – embolic episode, syncopal episode – adult
- • Rhabdomyoma – children – associated with tuberous sclerosis – hemartoma

DERMATOLOGY

- *Urticaria*: Type – 1 HS – I_gE and mast cell mediated – wheals and hives

- *Morbilliform rashes*: rash resembles measles – typical type of drug reaction
    - lymphocyte mediated – maculopapular eruption that blanches with pressure

- *Erythema multiforme*: mycoplasma / herpes simplex – target-like lesions that occur on the palms and soles (iris-like)

- *Stevens-Johnson syndrome*: (erythema multiforme major) – usually involves < 10–15% of the total body surface area—target-like lesions, *mucous membrane involvement* in the oral cavity, conjunctiva, and respiratory tract—hypersensitivity reaction to drugs

- *Toxic epidermal necrolysis*: cutaneous hypersensitivity reaction to drugs – (+) Nikolsky sign – *skin* easily sloughs off – 40–50% mortality rate

- *Staphylococcal scalded skin syndrome*: loss of the *superficial layers* of the epidermis – Toxin mediated – (+) Nikolsky sign

- *Fixed drug reaction*: localized allergic drug reaction that recurs at precisely the same anatomic site on the skin with repeated drug exposure – round, sharply demarcated lesions that leave a hyperpigmented spot at the site after they resolved

- *Erythema nodosum*: multiple painful, red, raised nodules on the anterior surface of the lower extremities – recent streptococcal infection, celiac sprue

- *Toxic shock syndrome*: toxin produced from staphylococcal attached to a foreign body (tampon use in female during menstruation) – fever, hypotension, desquamating rash, vomiting, involvement of mucous membrane – hypocalcemia due to capillary leak leads to ↓ albumin level

- *Impetigo*: *superficial* bacterial infection – up to epidermis – honey-colored crusted lesions (*Strep pyogens*) and *Staph aureus* (bullous impetigo)

- *Erysipeals*: *both dermis and epidermis* involve – shiny red, edematous, tender lesion, fever, chills, bacteremia – *Strep pyogens*

- *Folliculitis, furuncles, carbuncles*: staphylococcus
- Folliculitis → infection of hair follicle
- Furuncles → collection of infected material around hair follicle
- Carbuncles → several furuncles become confluent in to a single lesion
- Hot-tub folliculitis → pseudomonas

- *Necrotizing fasciitis*: very high fever, portal of entry into skin, pain out of proportion to the superficial appearance, presence of bullae, *palpable crepitus* – Group A strep (*Strep pyogens*) – x-ray will show air in the tissue

- *Dermatophyte infection*: microsporum, trichophyton, epidermophyton
- Microsporum - skin, hair, nail
- Trichophyton - hair, nail
- Epidermophyton - skin, nail
- Usually annular lesions expand peripherally and clear centrally

- *Tinea versicolor*: *Malassezia furfur* (*Pityrosporum orbiculare*) – white, scaling lesions that tend to coalesce

- *Pityriasis rosea*: "herald patch" Christmas tree pattern – self-limited – looks like secondary syphilis *except* it spares palm and sole – VDRL / RPR → negative.

- *Pediculosis*: *lice* - *Dx* → direct examination of hair-bearing area

- *Telogen effluvium*: loss of hair in response to excessive physiological stress. (e.g., cancer, malnutrition) – *Tx.*, correct underlying stress

- *Alopecia areata*: autoimmune – *Tx.*, localized steroid injection

- *Solar lentigo*: *freckles* – sun-exposed area in elderly

- *Seborrheic keratosis*: *verrucoid* lesion with *stuck-on appearance* – *no* malignant potential

- *Actinic keratosis*: *precancerous lesion* – sun-exposed area – can progress to squamous cell CA

- *Acanthosis nigricans*: *verrucoid* pigmented skin lesion usually located in *axilla*
- Stomach adenocarcinoma, MEN II b, insulin resistance (DM, obese)

- *Nevocellular nevus (mole)*: nevus cells are modified melanocytes
- Junctional nevus → basal cell layer (childhood)
- Compound nevus → extend into superficial dermis (adolescents)
- Intradermal nevus → compound nevus loses its junctional component (adult)
- Dysplastic nevus (atypical mole) →↑ risk for malignant melanoma – yearly dermatologic examination require

- *Melanoma*: most common *type of* malignancy – sun exposed area - ↑ risk in dysplastic nevus syndrome, xeroderma pigmentosa – asymmetry, borders irregular, color changes, diameter increased – *depth of invasion – best prognostic factor* (< 0.76 mm – do not metastasize, > 1.7 mm – potential for metastasis)

- *Basal cell CA*: most common *skin* cancer – sun exposed area – *upper lip raised papule*, shiny (or) *pearly appearance*

- *Squamous cell CA*: *lower lip* – sun-exposed area, tobacco use, scar tissue in 3rd *degree burn, actinic keratosis – ulcerated lesion*

- *Pemphigus vulgaris* – IgG against desmosomes (intracellular attachment)
- Suprabasal, (+) Nikolsky sign, oral lesions
- Acantholysis of karatinocytes in the vesicle fluid

- *Bullous pemphigoid* – IgG against basement membrane
- Subepidermal vesicle, (—) Nikolsky sign
- No acantholysis of karatinocytes in the vesicle fluid

- *Dermatitis herpetiformis* – IgA-anti-IgA complex deposit at the tips of the dermal papillae
- Subepidermal vesicle with neutrophils, microscopic blisters
- Strong association with celiac disease

- *Psoriasis* – coin-shaped lesions cover with silvery scales – on extensor surface – nail pitting – development of lesion in area of trauma (*Koebner phenomenon*) – bleeding occurs when scale is scraped off (*Auspitz sign*) – neutrophil collection in stratum corneum (*Munro microabscesses*)

- *Atopic dermatitis* – extreme pruritus – flexor surface - ↑ IgE – avoid scratching – Type-1 HS

- *Contact dermatitis* – linear, streaked vesicles (weeping lesion) – type-4 HS

- *Seborrheic dermatitis (dandruff)* – scaly, greasy, flaky skin – pityrosporum ovale

- *Stasis dermatitis* – hyperpigmentation built up from hemosiderin in the tissue – varicose veins for long time

- *Xerosis (asteotic dermatitis)* – dry skin – elderly (due to decrease in lipid)

- *Keratoacanthoma*: rapidly growing, benign crateriform tumor with a central keratin plug – sun-exposed area. Regresses spontaneously with scarring

- *Nummular dermatitis*: coin-shaped lesions (discoid lesions)

- *Pompholyx*: deep-seated vesicles on the palms, fingers, and soles

ENDOCRINOLOGY

- *Hyperprolactinemia*: nonfunctioning pituitary adenoma – microadenoma (women – amenorrhea, galactorrhea) – macroadenoma (men – visual field defect – heteronymous hemianopsia) – dopamine antagonist (phenothiazine, metoclopramide) – dopamine depleting agents (methyldopa, reserpine) – primary hypothyroidism (increases TRH-activated dopamine, which overcomes the normal dopamine inhibition) – diagnosis – prolactin level › 100 ng/ml suggest pituitary adenoma

- *Acromegaly*: ↑↑ GH (gigantism in children) – pituitary adenoma – between 3rd and 5th decade – complaints of inability to wear wedding ring, increase in shoe size – *entrapment neuropathy*, osteoarthritis, hypertension, *impaired glucose tolerance*, CHF (late) – symptoms for an average of 9 years before diagnosis – diagnosis: GH level remains › 5 ng/ml after giving 100gm of glucose orally
- Laron dwarfism – congenital absent of GH receptor - ↑ GH, ↓ IGF-1 and undetectable GH binding protein in blood

- *Hypopituitarism*: loss of function of anterior pituitary – loss of FSH, LH, GH, TSH, and ACTH – *causes*: hypothalamic tumors (craniopharyngioma, meningioma, gliomas), pituitary apoplexy (acute hemorrhage in preexisting pituitary adenoma - emergency) – Sheehan syndrome (postpartum necrosis of pituitary due to loss of blood intrapartum – inability to lactate [1st sign])

- CT head – *no* pituitary + *normal* hormone level – empty sella syndrome

- *Diabetes insipidus*: excessive thirst, polyuria (form dilute urine in the presence of hypernatremia) - central (insufficient ADH) and nephrogenic (unresponsiveness of kidney to ADH) – Diagnosis: (1) increase in urine osmolarity after giving vasopressin – central DI. (2) increase urine osmolarity after dehydration – psychogenic polyuria

- *SIADH*: cancers (small-cell CA of lung), drugs (chlorpropamide, carbamazapine) – continuously form concentrated urine in the presence of hyponatremia

- *Conn's syndrome*: primary hyperaldosteronism – adenoma of zona glomerulosa (adrenal gland) – hypertension (sodium retention), hypokalamia (muscle weakness) – Tx: resection (renal artery stenosis – BUN:Cr >20:1, abdominal bruits. Hypokalamia is *less severe than Conn's* syndrome. For example if hypokalamia in Conn's is in 2-something range, hypokalamia in renal artery stenosis is in 3-something range but less than 3.5; [3.5–5.0 normal range])

- *Hyperthyroidism*: $\downarrow\downarrow$ T3 and T4, $\uparrow\uparrow$ TSH – heat intolerance, weight loss, diarrhea, tremor, arrhythmias; exophthalmos and dermatopathies (only in Grave's disease) – *Grave's disease* - $\uparrow$ RAIU (radioactive iodine uptake), anti- TSH receptor antibodies. *Toxic nodular goiter* (single / multiple) - $\uparrow$ RAIU. *de Quarian Thyroiditis* (subacute granulomatous, giant cell) – $\downarrow$ RAIU – painful (transient hyperthyroidism). *Subacute lymphocytic thyroiditis* - $\downarrow$ RAIU – painless (transient hyperthyroidism). Ectopic thyroid tissue – struma ovarii

- *Hypothyroidism*: $\downarrow\downarrow$ T3 and T4, $\uparrow\uparrow$ TSH (primary) but normal / $\downarrow$ TSH (secondary / tertiary) – cold intolerance, weight gain, amenorrhea, carpal tunnel syndrome, slow, deep tendon reflexes with prolonged relaxation phase, myxedema – *Hashimoto thyroiditis*: antimicrosomal antibody, antithyroglobulin antibody, lymphocytic infiltration – *associated with lymphoma in thyroid gland* – Tx: levothyroxine (T4) in secondary and tertiary first give hydrocortisone then replace thyroid hormone.

- *Reidle thyroiditis*: intense fibrosis of thyroid gland and surrounding structure

- *Papillary CA*: most common thyroid CA – h/o radiation exposure
- *Follicular CA*: elderly – spread hematogenously
- *Medullary CA*: parafollicular cell of thyroid gland - ↑↑↑ Calcitonin – association with MEN type-2b – more malignant then follicular

- *Anaplastic CA*: elderly – highly malignant with rapid and painful enlargement of thyroid gland – poor prognosis

- *Parathyroid hormone*: stimulates osteoclasts and 1-α-hydroxylase (increase production of active form of Vit-D → 1–25-(OH)2-D) – increase Ca+2 level by bone resorption (osteoclast) and by absorption of Ca+2 from gut and kidney (vit-D).

- *Vit-D*: increase absorption of both Ca+2 and Phosphorus (PO4) from intestine and increase absorption of Ca+2 and decrease absorption of PO4 from kidney.

- *Magnesium*: cofactor for adenylate cyclase – cAMP is require for PTH activation – therefore hypomagnesemia can cause hypocalcemia (hypomagnesemia is the most common pathologic cause of hypocalcemia in the hospital)

- *Calcitonin*: inhibit bone resorption
- *Primary hypo- / hyperparathyroidism*: plasma calcium and phosphate levels are changing in opposite direction *EXCEPT* CRF, which causes secondary hyperparathyroidism but in CRF there is hypocalcemia and hyperparathyroidism (moves in opposite direction)

- *Secondary hyperparathyroidism*: increase PTH, decrease Ca+2 level and its excretion, decrease PO4 level and normal/increase its excretion

- *Secondary hypoparathyroidism*: decrease PTH, increase Ca+2 level and its excretion, increase PO4 level and normal/decrease its excretion

- *Hypercalcemia*: primary hyperparathyroidism (one gland hyperplasia), PTH- like substance secretion from CA – osteitis fibrosa cystica, lytic lesions on x-rays – serum Ca+2 level more than 10.2 mg/dl

- *Hypocalcemia*: tetany, muscle cramps/spasm, Chvostek sign (percussion of facial N. leads to contraction of facial muscles), Trousseau's sign (inflation of BP cuff on the arm of patient above SBP for more than 3 mins leads to flexion of metacarpophalangeal joints and extension of interphalangeal joint), QT prolongation on EKG – always check for albumin level (1 gm/dl drop in albumin → calcium level drop by 0.8 mg/dl)

- *Diagnosis of DM*: symptomatic patient (polyuria, ploydipsia, polyphagia) with random blood glucose level › 200 mg/dl *or* fasting blood glucose › 126 mg/dl on two occasion *or* blood glucose › 200 mg/dl at 2 hrs on two occasions

- *HbA1c*: used to follow compliance of the treatment and glucose control in patient with diabetes

- *Insulinoma*: increase in both plasma insulin and C peptide
- *Exogenous insulin administration*: very high insulin level but *low* C peptide

- *Sulfonylureas*: increase in both plasma insulin and C peptide, plasma/urine sulfonylurea (+)

- *Primary hypercortisolism* (*adrenal tumor*) - ↑ cortisol, ↓ ACTH
- *Pituitary Cushing* (*Cushing's disease*) - ↑ cortisol, ↑ ACTH. High dose dexamethasone test - ↓cortisol, ↓ ACTH by 50%

- *Ectopic ACTH secretion* - ↑ cortisol, ↑ ACTH. High-dose dexamethasone test – No suppression of ACTH
- *Signs and symptoms*: buffalo hump, purple striae on abdomen, moon face

- *17 α hydroxylase deficiency*: ↓ cortisol and androgen but ↑ 11 deoxycorticosterone (weak mineralocorticoid, due to which retention of sodium occur and hypertension develop)
- *21 β hydroxylase deficiency*: ↓ cortisol and mineralocorticoid but ↑ androgens
- *11 β hydroxylase deficiency*: ↓ cortisol but ↑ androgens and mineralocorticoid

- Increase ACTH in all of 3 enzymes deficiency (above)
- Male ambiguous genitalia (male pseudohermaphrodite) – 17 α hydroxylase
- Female ambiguous genitalia (female pseudohermaphrodite) – 21 and 11 β hydroxylase
- Female hypogonadism – 17 α hydroxylase
- Precocious puberty in male – 21 and 11 β hydroxylase

- *MEN 1* (Wermer) – pancreas (ZE syndrome), pituitary, hyperparathyroidism (3P)
- *MEN 2a* (Sipple) – hyperparathyroidism, *pheochromocytoma, medullary CA of thyroid*
- *MEN 2b* (3) – *pheochromocytoma, medullary CA of thyroid*, mucosal neuroma (lips/tongue)

- *Presence of Y chromosome* – germinal tissue differentiates into testes
- hCG + LH → leyding cells → testosterone → wallfian duct (epididymis, ductus deference, ejaculatory duct) → 5 α reductase convert testosterone in dihydrotestosteron (DHT), which induces urogenital sinus and genital tubercle to form penis, prostate, and scrotum.
- Sertoli cells → secretes MIF (Müllerian inhibiting factor) which inhibit paramesonephric duct (uterus, uterine tubes, cervix, and upper part of vagina)
- If MIF absent – uterus (paramesonephric duct structure) develops with normal male structure
- If testosterone absent – Wollfian duct regress (male internal structure does *not* develop)

- If 5 α reductase absent – DHT *not* formed. Therefore, male external structures do *not* develop but female external structures develop.
- *Absence of Y chromosome* – germinal tissue differentiates into ovaries. Wollfian (mesonephric duct) regresses and female genitalia develop.
- *Testicular feminization* – androgen receptor insensitivity, *Müllerian duct structure develops in the presence of testes* (no effect of testosterone and DHT)

GESTROENTEROLOGY

- Midline to lateral – sublingual (*m*ucous) – submandibular (mix) – parotid (serous)

- *Dysphagia*
- Dysphagia for solids *not* liquid → *obstruction* – stricture, esophageal CA Plummer-Vinson syndrome
- Dysphagia for solids *and* liquid → *peristalsis problem* – achalasia, systemic sclerosis, CREST, polymyositis

- Achalasia – normal amplitude contraction with high tone of lower sphincter (failure to relax) – absent myenteric ganglion
- Esophageal spasm – high amplitude contraction with normal relaxation of lower esophageal sphincter
- Scleroderma – absence peristalsis wave with very low tone of lower esophageal sphincter

- *Ring and Webs*
- *Schatzki's ring* - more distal and located at the squamocolumnar junction
- *Plummer-Vinson* - more proximal and located in the hypopharynx

- *Esophageal CA*: tobacco + alcohol →SCC →upper 2/3
- GERD and Barrett esophagus →adenocarcinoma →lower 1/3

- *Zenker's diverticulum*: outpocketing of the posterior pharyngeal constrictor muscles at the back of the pharynx
- Bad breath, aspiration pneumonia / lung abscess (anaerobic)

- *Gastroesophageal reflux disease (GERD):*

- Epigastric pain going under sternum, *nonproductive cough at night* (it can cause worsening of asthma at night by irritating bronchus), bad taste in mouth
- Sliding hernia of esophagus – GE junction displaced and reach above
- Paraesophageal hernia – GE junction not displaced

- *Barrett esophagus*: metaplasia (squamous →columnar)

- *Mallory-Weiss tear* →continuous retching followed by largely painless bloody vomiting (mucosal tear)

- *Boerhaave syndrome* →continuous retching followed by severe chest pain, crepitation in the neck, air in mediastinum on CXR (esophageal rupture – usually in distal third, posterolateral segment [where there is *no* serosa] is the most common site)

- *Stomach Histology*
- Parietal cells →HCL and IF
- Chief cells →pepsinogen –$^{H+}$> pepsin
- Mucous cells →mucous, HCO^-_3
- G cells →gastrin
- Vagal stimulation →Ach, gastrin–releasing peptide
- Histamine →enterochromaffin-like cells

- *Zollinger-Ellison syndrome (ZE syndrome)*
- Multiple recurrent ulcers (usually duodenum), steatorrhea
- Associated with MEN – I (parathyroid, pituitary, pancreas)
- *Diagnosis*: elevated gastrin level

- *Gastritis*
- *Type A* →atrophic gastritis (autoimmune), vit-B_{12} deficiency, ↑↑↑ gastrin
- *Type B* →NSAID, *H. pylori*, alcohol
- Increased chance of gastric CA in patient with type-A gastritis

- *Protein-losing enteropathy*: Enlarge rugal folds – hypertrophy of mucous cells (Menetrier disease, ZES, lymphoma)

- *Inflammatory Bowel Disease*
- *Crohn's disease*: oral/perianal involvement, palpable abdominal mass (*granuloma* – characteristic of Crohn), transmural involvement, skip lesions, fistula formation
- *Ulcerative colitis*: rectum involvement, bloody diarrhea, *exclusive mucosal disease*
- CD →vit-B_{12}, vit-K, Ca $^{+2}$, iron deficiency →elevated PT, kidney stones, megaloblastic anemia

- *Lactose intolerance*: lactase deficiency
- Diarrhea associated with gas and bloating after drinking milk
- *Never* has blood/WBC in stool
- *Diagnosis*: stool osmolarity > expected osmolarity

- *Irritable Bowel Syndrome*
- Abdominal pain relieved by bowel movement
- Diarrhea alternating with constipation

- *Carcinoid syndrome*: tumors of the neuroendocrine syndrome
- Tip of vermiform appendix (most common site) but carcinoid tumors of terminal ileum most commonly metastasize (liver)
- Diarrhea, flushing, tachycardia, and hypotension
- *Niacin deficiency* (serotonin and niacin →tryptophan)
- Endocardial fibrosis, tricuspid regurgitation, pulmonic stenosis

- *Diagnosis*: *urinary 5 – HIAA* (5-hydroxyindolacetic acid)

- *Celiac Disease*
- Antigliadin, antiendomysial, anti-transglutaminase antibodies
- Loss of intestinal villi (malabsorption-diarrhea, abd distension, abd pain)
- Celiac disease affect *PROXIMAL* small bowel.
- Function returns if patient is on gluten-free diet
- *Dermatitis herpetiformis →strong association with celiac disease*
- *No* wheat, rye, oat (contains gluten)

- *Whipple's disease: Tropheryma whippeli* bacilli

- PAS–positive macrophage obstruct lymphatic and reabsorption of chylomicrons
- Chronic diarrhea and weight loss

- *Diverticulosis*
- Lack of fibers in the diet
- Right-sided bleed / left-sided obstruct
- Most common cause of lower GI bleed (angiodysplasia – 2nd MCC)

- *Diverticulitis* (left-sided appendicitis)

- *Sigmoid colon*: most common site for diverticulosis, diverticulitis, and polyp
- *Rectosigmoid colon*: most common site for colon CA

- *Volvulus of sigmoid colon* →elderly patient →distended abdomen, similar episodes in past, which resolves itself →parrot's beak appearance (coffee bean sign / omega sign) of large gas shadow on x-ray

- *Mesenteric ischemia* →patient with *history of AF/atherosclerotic disease* present with acute abdomen (pain out of proportion to physical findings like absent rebound tenderness, guarding, rigidity, etc.) and *blood in stool*

- *Mechanical intestinal obstruction* →abdominal pain, constipation, distension, and vomiting (cardinal features of obstruction) →adhesion / indirect inguinal hernia
- Fever, leukocytosis, rebound tenderness in patient with indirect inguinal hernia suggests *strangulation*

- *Meckle's diverticulum* →painless large bloody bowel movement in child (brick red stool) →Technetium scan (^{99m}Tc scan) to identify ectopic gastric mucosa (rule of 2s – 2 ft from ileocecal valve, 2 inches long, 2 years of age, 2% of population; remnant of Vitelline duct [Omphalomesenteric duct])

- *Gastroschisis* → normal cord, *no* protecting membrane (sac) and bowel protruding from this defect

- *Omphalocele* → shiny, thin, membranous sac at the base of the umbilical cord, cord goes to the defect, *not* to the baby →can have multiple defects

- *Meconium ileu* →cystic fibrosis →ground glass appearance on abd x-ray

- *Hirschsprung disease (aganglionic megacolon)* →rectal exam may lead to explosive expulsion of stool and flatus →*x-ray*: distended proximal colon (normal) and "normal looking" distal colon (aganglionic).

- *Intussception* →sausage-shaped mass on the right side of the abdomen, empty-looking right lower quadrant (Dance's sign), *"currant-jelly stool"*

- Classic presentation of acute appendicitis (pain start in midepigastric region and then shifted to RLQ, positive rebound tenderness)

- *Colon cancer*: colonoscopy
- Hyperplastic polyp, juvenile polyp, Peutz-Jeghers →*no* malignant potential
- Tubular polyp (most common neoplastic polyp), villous polyp, familial polyposis, Turcot syndrome, Gardner syndrome →malignant potential

- *Hereditary Nonpolyposis Syndrome (HNPCC, Lynch Syndrome)*
- Mismatch base repair defect
- Colonoscopy every 1–2 years starting at the age of 25 years
- Very high incidence of ovarian and endometrial cancer

- *Familial Adenomatous Polyposis*
- APC gene confers 100% penetrance for the development of adenomas by the age of 35 and colon cancer by the age of 50

- *Cowden Syndrome*
- Hemartomas, rectal bleeding in a child

- *Gardner Syndrome*
- Colon CA + multiple soft-tissue tumors (osteoma, lipoma, fibrosarcoma)

- *Turcot Syndrome*
- Colon CA + *CNS malignancy*

- *Peutz-Jeghers Syndrome*
- Hemartomatous polyp + *hyperpigmented spots* (lips, buccal mucosa, skin)

- *Acute Pancreatitis*
- Midepigastric pain classically radiates straight to the back
- Amylase and lipase (most specific) are extremely elevated

- *Pancreatic head cancer*: palpable gallbladder without significant tenderness

- *Billirubin*: senescent RBC → heme → unconjugated bilirubin (lipid soluble – can accumulate in tissue so large amt in blood can cause problem) → bind with albumin and goes to liver → conjugated in liver (water soluble – easy for our body to excrete) → secreted in bile → 80% excreted in feces and 20% extrahepatic circulation (90% liver and 10% renal [in urine])
- *Jaundice*: ↑ unconjugated (*more hemolysis, liver unable to pick up* [Gilbert syndrome – jaundice with fasting], *liver unable to conjugate* [Crigler-Najjar syndrome – deficient enzyme]) ↑ conjugated (*liver unable to excrete in bile* [Dubin-Johnson syndrome – black liver, OCP], ↓ *extrahepatic bile flow* [gall stone, CA of head of pancreas]) ↑ Both (*liver dysfunction* [hepatitis])
- Pruritus in billiary disease is due to bile salt, which deposits in skin
- For jaundice, we test billirubin in urine with strip test, *not* urobillinogen (UBG). UBG is normally present in urine. UBG is absent in obstructive jaundice, but billirubin (conjugated – water soluble) is present in urine in obstructive jaundice

- *Primary Billiary Cirrhosis*
- Antimitochondrial antibody
- Granulomatous destruction of bile ducts in portal triad
- Middle-aged women, very less elevation of bilirubin, strong association with other autoimmune diseases →Sjogren syndrome, RA, scleroderma
- *Diagnosis*: transaminase are often normal
  ↑↑ alkaline phosphatase and γ-glutamyl transpeptidase
- ↑ risk for hepatocellular carcinoma (HCC)

- *Primary Sclerosing Cholangitis*
- Obliterative fibrosis of intrahepatic and extrahepatic bile ducts
- *Strong association with ulcerative colitis*
- Sx – same as primary billiary cirrhosis (pruritus, etc.)
- Antimitochondrial antibody →*negative*
- ↑ risk for cholangiocarcinoma (CA of bile duct)

- *Hemochromatosis*
- Most common inherited genetic disease
- *Overabsorption of iron* (ferritin [major storage protein] store iron in macrophage in bone marrow and hepatocytes, circulate in small amt in serum [↓ in iron deficiency anemia]; hemosiderin degradation product of ferritin in cell, [doesn't circulate] golden-brown granules in tissue and blue with Prussian blue)
- Intracellular iron produces hydroxyl ions, which damage parenchymal cells
- Cirrhosis, restrictive cardiomyopathy, arthralgia, skin hyperpigmentation, diabetes, hypogonadism
- ↑ infection with *Vibrio vulnificus, Yersinia,* and *L. monocytogens*

- *Wilson Disease*
- Autosomal recessive disease *present with choreoathetoid movements*
- ↓ copper transport into bile and ↓ ceruloplasmin synthesis leads to ↓ excretion of copper from body and ↑ free Cu^{+2} in the body, which is deposited in various tissue and produces damage
- Basal ganglia dysfunction, *Kayser-Fleischer ring (Slit-lamp examination)*, Fanconi syndrome

- *Ruptured hepatic adenoma* →young woman on *birth control pills* present with abdominal pain, low hemoglobin, hypovolemic shock

- *Amebic liver abscess* →h/o travel to Mexico →jaundice, weight loss, right upper quadrant pain, diarrhea

- *Liver problem* →↑↑↑ transaminase *billiary problem* →↑↑↑ alkaline phosphatase *alcoholic liver problem* →↑↑↑ GGT (γ–glutamyl transferase)

- Pericentral vein zone (zone 3) in liver contains the P450 oxidase enzyme system and is most sensitive to ischemic injury
- Periportal zone (zone 1) in liver is most sensitive to toxic injury
- "Ito cells" – site of vit-A storage, located in space of Disse

- Choledochal cyst – congenital benign dilatation of *bile ducts*
- Caroli's syndrome – congenital cystic dilatation of the *intrahepatic biliary tree* – associated with polycystic kidney disease – cholangitis and cholangio CA

- *Gall Stone (Cholelithiasis)*
- Cholesterol (80%) (radiolucent) - ↑cholesterol in bile and ↓bile salt and lecithin
- Pigment stone (20%) (radio-opaque) – calcium bilirubinate (sickle-cell anemia)
- *Billiary colic* →colicky right upper quadrant pain, radiate to the right shoulder, often aggravated after ingestion of fatty food / anticholinergic drug →USG (presence of gall stones, *no* thickening of GB wall)
- *Acute Cholecystitis* →female, forty, fertile, fatty →colicky right upper quadrant pain, radiate to the right shoulder, often aggravated after ingestion of fatty food →USG (presence of gall stones, thickening of GB wall, pericholecystic fluid)

- *Gallbladder Adenocarcinoma*
- Risk factors – cholelithiasis, Caroli's disease, porcelain gallbladder (calcification of GB wall)

- Infant on milk formula – necrotizing enterocolitis – transmural necrosis

- *Diarrhea*:
- Traveler's diarrhea – *E. coli*

- Undercooked hamburger meat – *E. coli O157:H7* (associated with HUS)
- Giardia lamblia – camping, contaminated water source
- HIV Positive, CD4 < 50 cells, acid-fast oocyst – cryptosporidium
- Ingestion of unrefrigerated meat – *Cl. difficile*
- Fried rice – *Bacillus cerius*
- Contaminated shellfish – *V. parahaemolyticus*
- Severe liver disease patient – *V. vulnificus*

- *Reye Syndrome*
- Encephalopathy and microvesicular steatosis in liver
- Recent *viral URI*, varicella, *Aspirin use*
- Ammonia, transaminases are markedly elevated
- Liver biopsy →noninflammatory fatty infiltration, mitochondrial injury

HEMATOLOGY

- *Anemia*: low Hb (<13 in M and <12 in F) / low hematocrit (<40 in M and <37 in F)

Microcytic (MCV < 80)	Normocytic	Macrocytic (MCV > 96)
• Iron deficiency	• Hemolytic anemia	• B12 deficiency
* Thalasemia	* ACD	• Folate deficiency
- Sideroblastic		- Alcohol related
- Lead poisoning		▪ Liver disease
• Anemia of chronic diseases (ACD)		(3) Chemotherapy/drugs

- *MCHC*: mean corpuscular Hb concentration (avg. Hb concentration in RBC)
  ↓ MCHC → central area of pallor – microcytic
  ↑ MCHC → No central area of pallor – spherocytosis
  N MCHC → megaloblastic anemia

- Hb A - α, β   Hb F - α, γ   Hb A_2 - α, δ
  a) Daily requirement of iron – 1 mg/day in M, 2–3 mg/day in F

- *Iron Deficiency Anemia*
  b) *Low* serum ferritin, serum iron, *high* TIBC
  c) Blood loss (menstruation), dietary deficiency

- *ACD (Anemia of Chronic Diseases)*
  d) *Normal/elevated* serum ferritin
  e) *Both* serum iron and TIBC →*low*
  f) *Pathophysiology*: Inflammatory cytokines increase production of hepcidin from liver. Hepcidin, in turn, stops ferroportin

from releasing iron stores—inflammatory cytokines increase the production of white blood cells. Bone marrow produces both red blood cells and white blood cells from the same precursor stem cells. Therefore, the upregulation of white blood cells causes fewer stem cells to differentiate into red blood cells. So decreased iron release and decreased RBC production is responsible for anemia. (Ferroportin: a transmembrane protein that transports iron from the inside of a cell to the outside of it—located on the surface of enterocytes in the duodenum, hepatocyte and macrophage.)

- *Sideroblastic Anemia*
    g) Normal serum ferritin
    h) *Very high* transferrin saturation

- *High* serum iron and *low* TIBC
- Prussian blue stain of RBC in the marrow will show ringed sideroblast
- Vit-B$_6$ deficiency: ↓ protoporphyrin and ↓δ ALA
- Iron deficiency: ↑ protoporphyrin and N δ ALA
- Lead poisoning: ↑ protoporphyrin and ↑δ ALA

- *Thalassemia*
- Underproduction of alpha/beta globin chain
- Mild-moderate anemia with *very low MCV*
- Target cells, normal serum iron and RDW

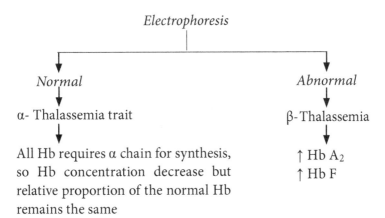

Electrophoresis

Normal

Abnormal

α- Thalassemia trait

β-Thalassemia

All Hb requires α chain for synthesis, so Hb concentration decrease but relative proportion of the normal Hb remains the same

↑ Hb A$_2$
↑ Hb F

- "Crew haircut" on skull x-ray is distinctive radiological change seen most often in patient with sickle-cell anemia and thalassemia major.

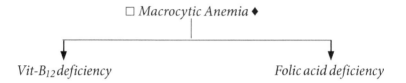

□ *Macrocytic Anemia* ◆

Vit-B$_{12}$ deficiency   *Folic acid deficiency*

25. Peripheral Blood smear: Hypersegmented Neutrophils seen in *Both*

26. *How to differentiate*: Low B$_{12}$ level

         Low RBC folic acid level

         ↑ *Methylmalonic acid*
level is seen in only B$_{12}$

- Schilling test is occasionally used to determine etiology of B$_{12}$ def
- *Schilling test*: oral administration of radioactive Vit – B$_{12}$
- Reabsorption →pure vegan
- B$_{12}$ +IF →reabsorption →pernicious anemia
- B$_{12}$ +antibiotics →reabsorption →bacterial overgrowth
- B$_{12}$ +pancreatic extract →reabsorption →chronic pancreatitis
- *Important*: Vit-B$_{12}$ and folic acid are required for DNA synthesis in all cells, so their deficiency affects all bone marrow cells, not just RBC.

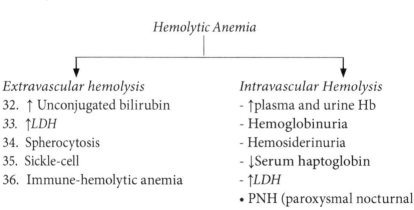

Hemolytic Anemia

Extravascular hemolysis	*Intravascular Hemolysis*
32. ↑ Unconjugated bilirubin	- ↑plasma and urine Hb
33. ↑LDH	- Hemoglobinuria
34. Spherocytosis	- Hemosiderinuria
35. Sickle-cell	- ↓Serum haptoglobin
36. Immune-hemolytic anemia	- ↑LDH
	• PNH (paroxysmal nocturnal hemoglobinuria)
	• G6PD

- *Sickle-cell anemia*: autosomal-recessive
- Substitution of valine for glutamic acid at sixth position on β-globin chain

- *Hereditary spherocytosis*: autosomal dominant
- RBC membrane protein defect (spectrin, ankyrin)
- Osmotic fragility test and ↑ *MCHC*

- *Autoimmune Hemolytic Anemia*
- *Coomb's test*
- Warm – antibody (I_gG), cold – antibody (I_gM)
- Drug-induced →penicillin, quinidine, α-methyldopa

- *Paroxysmal Nocturnal Hemoglobinuria (PNH)*
- *Loss of anchor for DAF* (decay accelerating factor)
- More complements bind to RBC and intravascular hemolysis occurs
- *Presentation: hemoglobinuria in first morning urine*

- *G6PD deficiency*: ↓synthesis of NADPH and GSH (glutathione)
- X-linked recessive
- Hemolysis in the presence of *oxidant stress*
- Oxidant stress →infection, fava beans, drugs (sulfa, dapsone, primaquine, quinidine, nitrofurantoin, INH)
- Diagnosis →Heinz bodies, bite cells, G6PD level

- *Pyruvate kinase deficiency*: ↓synthesis of ATP
- Autosomal recessive
- PK gives 2 ATPs – its deficiency produce membrane damage – RBC with thorny projection (echinocytes)

◆ Leukemia ◆

ALL	AML	CML	CLL
• Children (< 14 years)	• 15–39 years	• 40–60 years	• > 60 years
• Thrombocytopenia	• Thrombocytopenia	• Thrombocytopenia thrombocytosis in 40%	• Thrombocytopenia
• Pre-B cells - CALLA, CD10 and TdT positive	• t (15; 17) in M3	• Philadelphia chromosome, t (9; 22)	• CD19 Antigen
• T cells - CD10 and TdT negative	• DIC in M3	• Basophillia	• Predominantly B lymphocytes.
• t (12; 21) – good prognosis	• Auer rods in M2 and M3		• "Smudge cells"
CALLA (common ALL antigen)	• CNS in M4 and M5 M3- premyelocytic M4- myelomonocytic M5- monocytic • Vit-A – useful in premyelocytic (M3)		

*   *Adult T-cell lymphoma*: HTLV-1 (human T-cell leukemia virus – 1)
-      Activation of TAX gene – inhibits TP53 suppressor gene
-      ↑ CD4 T-cells
-      Skin infiltration and lytic bone lesion (lymphoblast release osteoclast activating factor, hypercalcemia)
-      Negative TdT

*   *Hairy cell leukemia*: only leukemia *without* lymphadenopathy
-      B-cell leukemia
-      *Positive TRAP stain* (tartrate-resistant acid phosphate)

*   *Infectious mononucleosis*: EBV – CD21 receptor on B-cells – heterophile antibody (IgM to sheep's RBC) – danger of rupture of spleen

*   *Myeloid stem cells*: RBC, granulocytes, mast cells, and platelets – polycythemia vera affect myeloid stem cells so increase everything in polycythemia vera – myelofibosis (teardrop cells, extramedullary hematopoesis)

*   *Aplastic anemia*: pancytopenia (Everything is decreased, including RBCs, platelets, and WBCs.)

◆ *Plasma Cell Disorder* ◆

Multiple Myeloma	Monoclonal Gammopathy of Uncertain Significance
• *Bone pain*, infection, anemia, renal failure	• *No* systemic manifestation like multiple myeloma
• *Electrophoresis* – IgG monoclonal spike	• IgG monoclonal spike on electrophoresis
• *X-ray* – punched out lytic lesion (osteoclast activating factor)	• *No* lytic bone lesion on x-ray
• Hypercalcemia	• Normal lab test (creatinine, calcium)

• *Bence-Jones protein* (acidification of urine is required to test BJ protein)	
• Bone marrow biopsy - >10% plasma cells	• Bone marrow - < 5% Plasma cells

* *Waldenstrom's macroglobulinemia (lymphoplasmatic lymphoma)*: M spike with IgM, BJ protein – *no* lytic lesions like multiple myeloma

• BJ proteins – kappa or lambda light chains

♦ *Lymphomas* ♦

Hodgkin's Lymphoma	Non-Hodgkin's Lymphoma
• Reed-Sternberg cells	• Reed-Sternberg cells *absent*
• Lymphadenopathy is more common (cervical, supraclavicular, axillary)	• Extralymphatic involvement is more common (spleen, liver, stomach)
• B-cells lineage involve	• Both B and T cell lineages involve
• Lymphocyte predominant (best prognosis)	• HIV, EBV → *Burkitt lymphoma*, t (8;14)
• Mixed celluarity	• *H. pylori* → gastric lymphoma (mucosa associated lymphoid tissues in stomach)
• Nodular sclerosing (Female) → lacunar cells	• CNS involvement is more common in HIV- positive patient
• Lymphocyte depletion (worst prognosis)	• *Follicular lymphoma* – t (14;18), over expression of BCL2 anti-apoptosis gene

• *RS cells* – CD15, CD 30 positive - B-lymphocyte with somatic hypermutation	• *Sjogren syndrome* – salivary gland and GI lymphoma • *Hashimoto's thyroidits* – thyroid malignant lymphoma

- Mycosis fungoides – cutaneous (begins in skin) T-cell lymphoma (*not* a fungal infection)

◆ *Bleeding Disorders* ◆

- Tissue thromboplastin → factor 7 → extrinsic pathway (PT) → warfarin
- Subendothelial collagen, HMWK → factor 12 → intrinsic pathway (PTT) → heparin
- Common final pathway → factor 10, 5, 2, 1 (2-prothrombin)
- Heparin →⊕ AT III → neutralize 9, 10, 11, 12, prothrombin and thrombin
- Thrombin → convert fibrinogen into fibrin monomers (fibrin monomers then aggregate, which are soluble)
- Thrombin →activate fibrin stabilizing factor (13; once fibrin monomers aggregate, factor-13 stabilizes them by making them insoluble)
- Plasmin →cleaves insoluble fibrin monomers and fibrinogen into fibrin degradation products (FDP)
- D-dimers →fragments of cross-linked insoluble fibrin monomers
- Protein C and S (vit-K dependent) →inactivate 5 and 8 →enhance fibrinolysis
- tPA – synthesized by endothelial cell, TxA_2 –synthesized by platelets
- $_vWF$ – synthesized by endothelial cell and platelets - Func.[n] →platelet adhesion and prevent degradation of factor VIII:C
- Platelet storage →$_vWF$ and fibrinogen (1)
- Platelet receptors →glycoprotein (gp) 1b – $_vWF$; GP2b:3a – fibrinogen
- Platelet factors →PF_3 →prothrombin complex (V, Xa, PF_3, Ca^{+2}). PF_4 →heparin neutralizing factor

- *Hemostasis in small vessel injury*: injury →tissue thromboplastin (activates extrinsic pathway) and exposed collagen (activates intrinsic pathway) → endothelial cells synthesize vWF so injury makes it expose to platelets, and platelets start attaching to them, and ADP from platelets help aggregating them (temporary plug) →platelets have fibrinogen at gp2b:3a →activated thrombin (by intrinsic and extrinsic pathway) converts fibrinogen to fibrin monomers that aggregate and make soluble plug →thrombin also activates factor-13, which converts the soluble plug into an insoluble plug →bleeding stops →tPA activates plasmin, which dissolves fibrin monomers and blood flow is reestablished to the tissue

- *Idiopathic Thrombocytopenic Purpura*
- Sign of bleeding from superficial areas of body
- Absent spleenomegaly, prolonged bleeding time
- Idiopathic antibody (IgG) production to the platelets' receptors (gp2b:3a)
- *Diagnosis*: antiplatelet antibody
  Bone marrow →megakaryocytosis – indicate problem with platelate destruction, *not* with production

- *Thrombotic thrombocytopenic purpura (TTP)* – deficiency in vWF cleaving metalloprotease in endothelial cells leads to ↑↑vWF → more platelets attach to vWF, which leads to thrombosis and thrombocytopenia (due to platelet consumption in thrombosis) – microangiopathic anemia, renal, and CNS involvement – schistocytes (fragmented RBCs), helmet-shaped cells

- *Hemolytic uremic syndrome (HUS)* – microangiopathic anemia, thrombocytopenia, and renal involvement (*no* CNS involvement)

- Schistocytes – TTP, DIC, aortic stenosis

- *Von Willebran disease (VWD)*: autosomal – dominant
- Sign of bleeding from superficial areas of body
- *Low* level of $_v$WF, factor VIII: C
- *Ristocetin platelate aggregation test*: abnormal
- *Elevated* PTT, normal PT

- ■ *Hemophilia*: autosomal – recessive
- Hemophilia A – factor 8 deficiency, hemophilia B – factor 9 deficiency
- Sign of deep bleeding →hemarthrosis, hematoma, GI bleeding
- May become apparent at the time of circumcision
- *Diagnosis*: *elevated* PTT, normal PT
- *Mixing study*: 50% patient's blood + 50% normal blood →PTT corrected →hemophilic →if PTT is *not* corrected →antibody inhibition of the factor
- *Treatment*: *desmopressin*, specific factor replacement

- ■ *Vit–K deficiency*: ↓production of factor 2, 7, 9, 10
- Both PT and PTT are *elevated*
- *Diagnosis*: correction of PT and PTT after giving vit-K
- *Treatment*: *fresh frozen plasma* in severe bleeding

- ■ *Liver disease*: ↓production of all factors *except* $_v$WF and factor 8
- *Both* PT and PTT are elevated
- *Diagnosis*: H/O liver disease and *no* correction of PT and PTT after giving vit-K

- ■ *DIC (Disseminated Intravascular Coagulation)*
- Platelates, ↑↑PT and PTT, ↑*D- dimmers* and FDP$_S$, low fibrinogen level *schiztocytes* on peripheral blood smear
- *Treatment*: fresh frozen plasma, platelet transfusion

MUSCULOSKELETAL

Joint aspiration

Cell count   Gram stain   Microscopic Polarization

Cell count	Gram stain		Microscopic Polarization
• *< 2,000 – OA,* traumatic	(+) organism	(-) organism	Needle-shaped / (-) birefringent – monosodium urate (gout)
• *Up to 50,000 –* inflammatory (RA, gout, pseudogout) • *>75,000* (without crystal) – Septic	Staph aureus	N. gonorrhea	Rhomboid / (+) birefringent – calcium pyrophosphate (pseudogout)

- *Rheumatoid Arthritis (RA)*
  - Polyarticular symmetric
  - Inflammatory synovitis
  - Bone erosions
  - *MCP and PIP* involvement
  - Swan-neck deformity
  - Boutonniere deformity
  - Radial deviation of the wrist with ulnar

- *Osteoarthritis (OA)*
  - Monoarticular asymmetric
  - Noninflammatory
  - Nonerossive
  - *PIP and DIP* involvement
  - Osteophytes and unequal joint space
  - Bouchard's node (PIP)
  - Heberden's node (DIP) deviation of the digits

- ■ *Ankylosing spondylitis: positive HLA B-27,* M>W, 2nd - 3rd decade
  - Chronic lower back pain, *morning stiffness >1 hrs improvement with exercise*
  - Anterior uveitis, aortic insufficiency, 3rd degree heart block
  - *X-ray* →sacroilitis and eventual fusing of the sacroiliac joint, bamboo spine

- ■ *Reactive arthritis*: infectious diarrhea (*C. jejunii*) + arthritis
- - Urethritis (chlamydia)/conjunctivitis + arthritis →Reiter syndrome

- ■ *Psoriatic arthritis*: DIP joint + pitting of nail + skin lesions

- ■ *Enteropathic Arthritis (Ulcerative colitis / Crohn's disease)*
- - Inflammatory bowel disease + arthritis + pyoderma gangrenosum + erythema nodosum

- ■ *Gout*: deposit of uric acid crystals in joints – most common site first toe (podagra) – precipitating factors are alcohol, steroid withdrawal, diuretics, pyrazinamide, ethambutol, following anticancer treatment

- ■ *Pseudogout*: deposit of calcium pyrophosphate in joints – most common site knee joints – preexisting joint damage is a precipitating factor – *causes*: hyperparathyroidism, hemochromatosis, hypophosphatemia, hypomagnesemia

- ■ *Septic arthritis*: *gonococcal*—migratory polyarthropathy, tenosynovitis (inflammation of tendon sheath); *staphylococci*— preexisting joint damage (e.g., RA patient)

- ■ *SLE*: antinuclear Ab, anti-Smith, and anti-ds-DNA Ab (most specific)
- - nonerosive arthritis, malar rash, photosensitivity, renal, CVS (Libman-Sack endocarditis – sterile vegetation on MV), CNS involvement (psychosis)
- - Antiphospholipids antibody – anticoagulant, recurrent abortion
- - Anticardiolipin antibody – give false VDRL and RPR test

- ■ *Scleroderma*: excessive collagen deposition – Raynaud's phenomenon (blue discoloration of fingers on exposure to cold), skin thickening, dysphagia – anti–scl-70 Ab

- ■ *CREST Syndrome*: anticentromere antibody

      ☐   Calcinosis, *R*aynaud's phenomena, *E*sophagus (dysphagia), *S*cleroductly (claw- like finger), *T*elangiectasia (dilated blood vessels)

- ■ *Sjogren syndrome*: anti-Ro (SS-A) and anti-La (SS-B) antibodies, dry eye (constant sensation of foreign body in eye), dental caries, parotid enlargement (lymphatic infiltration of glands – lip biopsy - most specific) – also gives positive RA factor

- Juvenile rheumatoid arthritis: salmon pink evascent rash

- *Osteochondroma* →most common benign tumor →metaphysis

- *Osteoma* →facial bones →associated with Gardner's polyposis syndrome

- *Giant cell tumor* →epiphysis →females

- *Osteogenic sarcoma* →metaphysis of distal femur, proximal tibia "sunburst" appearance on x-ray →male (10–25 years) →familial retinoblastoma

- *Ewing's sarcoma* →diaphysis and metaphysis of proximal femur, ribs, pelvic bones →"onion skin" appearance on x-ray

- Erb's palsy – *upper trunk* (C_5, C_6) → axillary N. and musculocutaneous N. → muscles of shoulder and arm → *arm*: medially rotated and adducted → *forearm*: extended and pronated ("waiter's tip")

- Klumpke's palsy – *lower trunk* (C_8, T_{11}) → loss of muscles of hand

NEPHROLOGY

- Prerenal azotemia - ↑ BUN but creatinine near normal (N, 0.6–1.2)
- Postrenal azotemia - ↑ BUN and ↑ creatinine
- Renal azotemia – BUN/Cr ≤ 15 (because more ↑↑ in creatinine)
- Cortical necrosis of both kidneys sparing medulla – DIC
- Sickle-cell anemia affects medulla most severly and can cause papillary necrosis.
- Renal papillary necrosis (SADD) – *s*ickle-cell anemia, *a*cute pyelonephritis, *d*rugs (Aspirin + acetaminophen), *d*iabetes

* *Nephritic Type Glomerular Disease* (Moderate proteinuria and RBC cast)

- IgA glomerulonephritis (Buerger's disease, Buerger's disease – thromboangiitis obliterans – male – smoking cigarettes, both are different disease) – episodic bouts of hematuria *1–3 days* following URTI, slow progression to CRF (40–50%), mesangeal IgA deposit with granular immunoflurocence
- Post-streptococcal – hematuria *1–3 weeks* following group A *Strep pyogens* infection
    - Skin infection - ↑ anti-DNAase B titer
    - Pharynx infection - ↑ ASO titer
    - Diffuse proliferative (usually resolve, CRF is uncommon)
- Diffuse proliferative (SLE) – sub*endo*thelial immune complex (IC) (anti-ds DNA Ab) deposit with granular IF, "wire looping" of capillaries (CRF most common cause of death in SLE)
- Rapidly progressive – crescent formation, associated with Goodpasture syndrome (linear IF, lower resp tract involvement, hemoptysis followed by ARF), polyarteritis nodosa (p-ANCA; GIT involvement – mesenteric artery, bowel ischemia, bloody

diarrhea), Wegner's granulomatosis (c- ANCA; upper and lower resp tract involvement, perforation of nasal septum)

* *Nephrotic Type Glomerular Disease* (Proteinuria› 3.5 g/24 hrs and fatty cast)

- Minimal change disease – children – EM show fusion of podocytes (selective proteinuria – Albumin *not* globulin), negative IF
- Focal Segmental – HIV, Heroin IV abuse, NSAID, Hodgkin's lymphoma – negative IF, non-selective proteinuria
- Diffuse Membranous – Adults – captopril, HBV, malaria, syphilis – subepithelial deposit with granular IF – "spike and dome" pattern
- Type-1 MPGN – HCV, HBV, cryoglobulinemia – subepithelial deposit – EM show "tram track" (progress to CRF)
- Type-2 MPGN – C3 nephritic factor (C3NeF), Ab binds to C3 convertase and prevent its degradation and sustain activation of C3 leads to very low C3 level. "dense deposit disease" (progress to CRF)

- Only in SLE, there is subendothelial deposit. In all others, there is subepithelial deposit.
- Only in Goodpasture syndrome, there is linear deposit. In all others, there is granular deposit.
- Polyarteritis nodosa – p-ANCA – HbsAg (+) in 30% of cases
- Lichen planus – association with hep. C
- Glomerular basement membrane (GBM) – type-IV collagen – heparan sulfate (negative charge to GBM) – positive charge LMW proteins are permeable – albumin has strong negative charge so it is not permeable (loss of negative charge → loss of albumin in urine)
- Glomerular nodule – DM / amyloid (chronic disease) both show red on H&E stain but with Congo red stain – amyloid – "apple-green" birefringence nodule. DM nodule is composed of type-4 collagen and protein

- Ethylene glycol poisoning – metabolic acidosis ($\uparrow$ anion gap) + oxalate crystalluria
- Cystinuria – staghorn calculi, positive nitropruside cyanide test
- Staghorn calculi – *Proteus* infection

* **Acid-Base Disturbances**

- (Na + K) – (HCO3 + Cl) = 8–14 (normal anion gap)
- Only chronic acidosis/alkalosis is compensated *not* acute
- Chronic resp. acidosis – compensated by metabolic alkalosis (HCO3 – 22–28) PCo2 - › 45 mmHg, HCO3 - ≤ 30 mEq/L – acute resp. acidosis
  HCO3 - › 30 mEq/L – chronic resp. acidosis
- Chronic resp. alkalosis – compensated by metabolic acidosis PCo2 - ‹ 33 mmHg, HCO3 - ≥ 18 mEq/L – acute resp. alkalosis
  HCO3 - ‹ 18 mEq/L (but›12 mEq/L) – chronic resp. alkalosis

* *Renal Tubular Acidosis (Normal Anion Gap Acidosis)*

- Type-1 – secondary to autoimmune diseases, lithium, analgesics, sickle-cell disease
  Inability to secrete H+ in urine, urine pH - › 5.4 Patient usually gets renal stone
  Acid load test – after giving ammonium chloride, urine pH still remain elevated (normally it should be decreased)

- Type-2 – renal threshold for absorbing HCO3 is lowered from normal of 24 mEq/L to 15 mEq/L
  Initially pH › 5.5 and then it goes back to ‹5.5 Patient usually gets bone lesion (osteomalacia, rickets)

  Both type-1 and type-2 get hypokalamia.

- Type-4 is the only renal tubular acidosis that produce hyperkalamia due to destruction of JG apparatus - ↓ rennin - ↓ aldosterone
  Causes – hyaline arteriosclerosis in afferent arteriole in DM, Legionnaire's disease

- Intake of salt = output of salt (95% renal and 5% sweat)
- Hyponatremia – Na ‹135 in the absence of hyperglycemia
- SIADH – oral hypoglycemic and carbamazapine
- *Diagnosis* – urine osm › serum osm (urine osm › 40 is typical)
- *Treatment* – Fluid restriction, loop diuretics and normal saline, hypertonic saline, lithium/demeclocycline in SIADH. Rapid

correction of hyponatremia results in central pontine myelinosis—destruction of brain stem present with paraparesis, dysarthria, or dysphagia.

- Hypernatremia – loss of hypotonic fluids (sweating, burns, fever), central DI and nephrogenic DI

- Hypokalamia – U wave on ECG, alkalosis, ↑ aldosterone

- Hyperkalemia – peaked T wave on ECG, acidosis, ↓ aldosterone

- Hypercalcemia – loop diuretics/hypercalciuria – thiazide diuretics

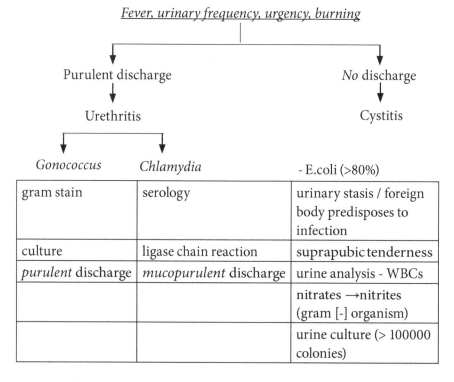

Fever, urinary frequency, urgency, burning

Purulent discharge   *No* discharge

Urethritis   Cystitis

Gonococcus   *Chlamydia*   - E.coli (>80%)

gram stain	serology	urinary stasis / foreign body predisposes to infection
culture	ligase chain reaction	suprapubic tenderness
purulent discharge	*mucopurulent* discharge	urine analysis - WBCs
		nitrates →nitrites (gram [-] organism)
		urine culture (> 100000 colonies)

- *   *Pheochromocytoma*
- A neuroendocrine tumor of the medulla of the adrenal glands
- Signs and symptoms of sympathetic hyperactivity (increase HR, HTN, etc)
- *Diagnosis*: urinary vanillylmandelic acid (VMA)

- CT scan/MRI – to localize tumor
- *Treatment* – alpha-blockade followed by surgical removal

* *Important Urinary Cast*
- Waxy, broad cast – signs of end stage renal disease
- WBC cast – acute pyelonephritis, acute tubulointerstitial nephritis (drug)
- Renal tubular cell cast (muddy brown granular cast) - ATN

* *Juvenile Polycystic Kidney Disease*
- Autosomal recessive
- Bilateral enlarged kidney at birth
- Maternal oligohydramnios

* *Adult Polycystic Kidney Disease*
- Autosomal dominant
- Bilateral enlarged kidney around 20–25 years of age
- Cyst also present in liver (40%)
- Intracranial berry aneurysm (10–30%, present with subarachnoid hemorrhage), HTN, sigmoid diverticulosis, MVP

* *Renal Cell CA (Clear Cell CA, Hypernephroma, Grawitz Tumor)*
- Derived from proximal tubule (PT)
- Risk factors – smoking, Von Hipple-Lindau syndrome, adult polycystic kidney disease (APKD)
- Hematuria, flank mass, and CVA tenderness
- Metastasize to lung (cannonball appearance on x-ray), left-sided varicocele

* *Wilms Tumor*
- Derived from mesonephric mesoderm (unilateral flank mass)
- Histology: abortive glomeruli and tubules, primitive blastemal cells, rhabdomyoblasts
- Hypertension in child, autosomal dominant (chromosome-11)
- WAGR Syndrome (Wilms tumor, aniridia, genital abnormalities, retardation)

* *Neuroblastoma*
- N-myc gene amplification
- Small blue cell tumors (Ewing sarcoma, lymphoma, neuroblastoma, small cell CA of lung)
- Composed of malignant neuroblast, presence of Homer-Wright rosettes
- *Neurosecretory granules on electron microscopy*
- Hypertension in child
- ↑↑↑ *Urinary VMA* (vanillylmandelic acid), HVA, metanephrines

• Potter's syndrome – absent of both kidney – oligohydroamnios – failure of ureteric buds to develop

• Pathogenesis of DM: nonenzymatic glycosylation (glucose + AA) → ↑vessel permeability to protein and ↑athrogenesis; osmotic damage → aldolase reductase (glucose → sorbitol) → sorbitol draws water into tissues causing damage (e.g., retinopathy); diabetic microangiopathy → ↑synthesis of type-IV collagen in basement membrane and mesangium

• *Alport Syndrome*
- X-linked dominant disorder
- *Asymptomatic hematuria, sensorineural hearing loss*
- *Renal biopsy*: glomerular sclerosis, thickened basement membrane tubular atrophy fibrosis and foam cells.

• *Hemolytic Uremic Syndrome (HUS):*
- *E. Coli (O157: H7)* →produces *verotoxin* →endothelial cell injury
- Endothelial injury of the kidney results in localized clotting →RBCs and intra- renal platelate damage causes microangiopathic anemia and thrombocytopenia
- Approximately one week after *E. Coli (O157: H7)* infection, patient develop oliguria, signs and symptoms of anemia
- ↓Hb level m drop in platelate count, hematuria, proteinuria, helmet cells on peripheral smear
- *D/D*: TTP, which involves CNS whereas HUS involves kidney.

- *Henoch-Schonlein Purpura*
- IgA – mediated vasculitis of small vessels
- Nonthrombocytopenic purpura in children
- Usually follows an URI
- Tetrad of *abd. pain, rash, renal involvement, and thrombocytopenia.*
- *Palpable purpuric rash on buttocks*

NEUROLOGY

- *CSF*: Lat ventricle → foramen of Monro → 3rd ventricle → aqueduct of Sylvius → 4th ventricle (obstruction to CSF flow will give hydrocephalus)
- Arnold-Chiari malformation – herniation of cerebellum – hydrocephalus
- Arnold-Chiari malformation type 2 – syringomyelia, myelomeningocele
- Syringomyelia is associated with Arnold-Chiari malformation in most cases.

- *Meningitis*: infection of covering of brain – fever, headache, stiff neck, and focal neurologic deficiency
- *Causes*
  - Newborn (< 1 month) →group B streptococci, *E. coli*, *L. monocytogenes*
  - 1 month – 18 years old →*N. meningitides*
  - >18 years old →*Strep pneumoniae*
  - *Staph aureus* →recent neurosurgery
  - *L. monocytogenes* →immunocompromised (neonates and elderly patients)
  - *Cryptococcus* →HIV positive, *CD$_4$$^+$ < 100 cells*
  - RMSF →*rash* on wrist, ankle →*spreads toward body*
  - Neisseria →*petechial rash*
  - Cause of viral meningitis in pediatric population in the United States – arbovirus and enterovirus
  - *CN – 8 deficits* is more common longterm neurological deficit

- *CSF findings of bacterial meningitis* – low glucose (<40 mg/dl), increase WBC count (Neutrophils)

- *CSF findings of viral meningitis* – increase WBC (lymphocytes), normal glucose
- *CSF findings of cryptococcal meningitis* – low WBC count (<50 cells/L) (lymphocytes), low glucose

- *Encephalitis*: infection of parenchyma of brain – fever, headache, stiff neck, and altered mental status
- *Causes*
    - HSV (temporal lobe, most common)

* *Brain Abscess*
- Headache, fever, focal neurologic deficit
- HIV positive →toxoplasmosis / lymphoma (90% of cases)
* Transverse myelitis – rapidly progressing lower extremity weakness following URI, accompanied by sensory loss and urinary retention – Dx: MRI
* Epidural abscess – patient with h/o IV drug abuse

- *Subfalcine herniation*: cingulate gyrus herniates under falx cerebri (compress anterior cerebral artery)

- *Uncal herniation*: medial portion of temporal lobe herniates through tentorium cerebellli (compresses midbrain and posterior cerebral artery)
- *Tonsillar herniation*: cerebellar tonsils herniates through foramen magnum (produces cardiorespiratory arrest)

- **Guillain-Barré Syndrome**
    - Autoimmune destruction of myelin
    - *Begins in lower extremities and move upward*
    - Patient usually c/o pain / tingling dysesthesia
    - Associated with *C. jejunii*

- **Myasthenia Gravis**
    - Antibodies produce against Ach receptors
    - *C/o diplopia, ptosis*, difficulty swallowing
    - *Symptoms are improved with rest*

- *Eaton-Lambert myasthenic syndrome* →increasing muscle strength on repetitive contraction. Association with malignancy, especially small-cell CA
- Botulism →dilated pupils and EMG shows an incremental increase in muscular fiber contraction (opposite to myasthenia gravis)

■ *Huntington Disease*
- Autosomal dominant
- Affect caudate nucleus
- CAG trinucleotide repeat expansion
- Chorea and behavioral disturbance
- Onset in 4th or 5th decade

■ *Parkinson's Disease*
- Degeneration of substantia nigra (↓dopamine)
- Imbalance between dopamine (↓↓) and cholinergic (↑↑) transmitters
- Bradykinesia, cogwheel rigidity, resting tremor (pill rolling), postural instability
- Shy-Drager syndrome – Parkinsonism + orthostatic hypotension

■ *Multiple Sclerosis*
- Focal areas of demyelination
- Optic neuritis, scanning speech, intention tremor, nystagmus
- Bilateral internuclear ophthalmoplegia (demyelination of MLF, pathognomic)
- *Blurry vision and double vision* →common initial manifestations of the disease →*resolve spontaneously*
- CSF show oligoclonal bands (70 –90%)

■ Marcus Gunn phenomenon – dilatation of right pupil with dilatation of left pupil occurs (paradoxical dilatation) in patient with right optic neuritis/right retinal detachment

• *Alzheimer's disease*: defect in degradation of β-amyloid protein by secretase leads to accumulation of amyloid protein in neuron and damage neurons – mutation in Tau protein (maintain microtubule in neuron) leads to formation of neurofibrillary tangles – microscopic (senile plaques [amyloid protein] and neurofibrillary tangles) – problem in memory (affect hippocampus [old brain] short term memory loss) and visuospatial abilities (early); hallucination and personality change (late)

- *Pick disease: frontotemporal dementia* →pick body (intracytoplasmic spherules composed of paired helical filaments) →present with personality change
- *Lewy body dementia*: Lewy body (intracytoplasmic spherules that stain brightly eosinophilic) →fluctuating cognitive impairment that can be confused with delirium
- *Creutzfeldt-Jakob disease (CJD)*: Shorter and more aggressive course, present with dementia and myoclonus
- *Vascular dementia*: h/o multiple strokes – multi-infarct dementia
- *Binswanger's disease*: involves subcortical white matter, slow course
- *Normal pressure hydrocephalus*: dementia, gait abnormality, and urinary incontinence

- *Krabbe's disease*: presence of globoid cells (multinucleated histiocytic cells) in degenerating white matter in brain – galactocerebrosidase deficiency

■ *Subacute combined degeneration*: vit – B$_{12}$ deficiency
- deficit of vibration and proprioception with pyramidal signs like plantar extension and hyperreflexia

■ *Ant. Spinal Artery Infarct*
- Acute onset of flaccid paralysis that evolves into a spastic paresis over days to weeks
- Loss of pain and temp. sensation with sparing of vibration and position sense.

- Tabes *dorsalis: dorsal* column of spinal cord – tertiary syphilis

- *Tuberous Sclerosis*
- Infantile spasm (*Tx*: ACTH and prednisone)
- Rhabdomyoma of heart (echocardiography)
- Ash-leaf spots (hyperpigmented lesions), shagreen patches ("orange-peel" lesions), sebaceous adenomas
- Angiofibroma on the face
- Angiolipomas in the kidney

- Astrocyte proliferations in subependyma (look like "candlestick drippings" in the ventricles)

- *Neurofibromatosis (NF)*
- Café au lait spots (tan/light brown flat lesion), axillary freckling, Lisch nodules, optic nerve gliomas, *acoustic neuroma (CN-8, feature of NF-2,* all other NF-1)
- Association with pheochromocytoma, Wilms tumor

- *Duchenne Muscular Dystrophy*
- Pseudohypertrophy of the calves
- *Gower sign* (child places hands on the knees for help in standing)
- *Deficiency* of dystrophin

- *Becker Muscular Dystrophy*
- *Defective* dystrophin
- Less serious than Duchenne muscular dystrophy

- *Warding-Hoffman Disease*
- Infantile spinal muscular atrophy
- Atrophy of anterior horn cells in the spinal cord and of motor nuclei in the brainstem
- Severe hypotonia and absent tendon reflexes
- Legs tend to lie in a frog-leg position

- *Charcot-Marie-Tooth Disease*
- Hereditary motor-sensory neuropathy
- Peroneal muscular atrophy
- Peroneal and tibial nerve most commonly affected
- Wasting of the lower legs, giving them stork-like appearance.
- Sural nerve biopsy →"onion bulb" formation (interstitial hypertrophic neuropathy)

- *Friedreich Ataxia*
- Expanded GAA triplet repeats
- Ataxia (before 10 years of age), disarthric speech, nystagmus, absent tendon reflexes (lower extremities affected more than upper)

- *Ataxia Telangiectasia*

- Mutation in DNA repair enzyme, thymic hypoplasia
- Cerebellar ataxia, telangiectasia of skin and eye

- *CNS tumors*: Adult (*above* tentorium cerebelli), children (*below* tentorium cerebelli). Most common (adult – glioblastoma multiforme, meningioma; children – astrocytoma, medulloblastoma).

  * Oligodendroglioma – "fried egg cell," round nuclei and clear cell – cerebral hemisphere
  * Choroid plexus papilloma – papillary growth in ventricle
  * Ependymoma – pseudorosettes and structure resembling ependymal canal
  * Glioblastoma multiforme – hemorrhagic tumor (multiple area of necrosis and cystic degeneration)
  * Pilocytic astrocytoma – bipolar cells – cerebellum of young children
  * Medulloblastoma – most common in children – only CNS tumor with both neural and glial components – affect granular cell layer of cerebellum
  * Meningioma – associated with neurofibromatosis – parasagital location
  * *Craniopharyngioma* →remnant of Rathke's pouch (*resembles amblioblastoma*) →calcified lesion above the sella on x-ray →bitemporal hemianopsia

- ■ *CNS bleeds*:
  * Epidural: skull fracture – rupture middle meningeal artery
  * Subdural: tear of bridging veins – fluctuating levels of consciousness
  * Atherosclerotic stroke: usually pale infarct (since no reperfusion)
  * Embolic stroke: hemorrhagic infarct extends to surface of the brain
  * Intracerebral bleed: *hypertension* most common cause – rupture of lenticulostriate Charcot-Bouchard aneurysms – hematoma (not an infarct) – globus pallidus/putamen area most common sites

- Subarachnoid bleed: ruptured congenital berry aneurysm (junction of communicating branch with anterior cerebral artery) – severe occipital headache – common in patient with polycystic kidney disease

PULMONOLOGY

Obstructive Pulmonary Disease	Restrictive Pulmonary Disease
• ↑airway resistance	• ↑in lung recoil
• ↓expiratory flow rate	• ↓in all lung volume
• ↑TLC, ↓FEV$_1$ / FVC	• ↑or N FEV$_1$/ FVC

- A – a gradient = 150 – 1.25 × PCO$_2$ – PaO$_2$
- Normal →5 –15 mmHg

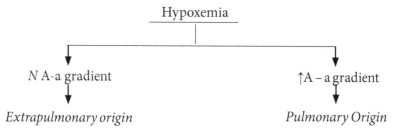

Hypoxemia

N A-a gradient → Extrapulmonary origin

↑A – a gradient → Pulmonary Origin

- PAO$_2$ =% O$_2$ (713) – arterial PCO$_2$ / 0.8

- PAO$_2$ = 0.21 (713) – 40 / 0.8 = 100 mmHg
- PaO$_2$ = 95 mmHg
- A-a gradient = 5 mmHg

- Atelectasis – most common cause of fever in 1st 24-hrs post operatively

- Bacterial pneumonia →consolidation →dull to percussion, ↑vocal framitus
- Pneumothorax →hyperresonant to percussion, ↓breath sound
- Pleural effusion →dull to percussion, ↓breath sound, ↓vocal framitus

- Atelectasis →dull to percussion, absent breath sound, loss of framitus pneumothorax →opposite side
- Deviation of trachea atelectasis (upper lobe) →same side
- Atelectasis (lower lobe) →elevation of diaphragm (same side)

- Trachea → right and left main bronchus → terminal bronchioles → respiratory bronchioles → alveolar duct (AD) → alveoli

- *Asthma*: reversible airway obstruction

- *COPD (Emphysema and Chronic Bronchitis)*
- Nonreversible airway obstruction

- *Emphysema*: cigarette smoking and alpha$_1$-anti-trypsin deficiency (AAT) - ↑compliance (more dilated alveoli) and ↓elasticity (failure to keep airway lumen open – essential for expiration so air trapped during expiration) – centriacinar (distended respiratory bronchioles – air trapped in AD and alveoli), panacinar (distended whole respiratory unit [resp bronchioles, AD, and alveoli] – air trapped in whole unit)
- *Chronic Bronchitis*: productive cough for at least 3 months for 2 consecutive years – smoking cigarette and cystic fibrosis - ↑mucus in bronchi obstruct terminal bronchioles and narrowing of lumen due to chronic inflammation and fibrosis

- ■ *Lung abscess*: alcoholic, *extremely bad odor (like decomposing dead animal)*

- ■ *Pneumonia*
- Following flu →*Staph aureus* (abscess)
- HIV positive (CD4+ < 200 cells) →PCP
- California, desert of Arizona →coccidiomycosis
- Young (*school children*) →*Mycoplasma*
- Alcoholics →*Klebsiella*
- Smoker, COPD →*H. influenzae*
- Elderly pt., CXR – lobar consolidation →*Strep pneumoniae*
- Neutropenia, steroid use, cavitatory lesion →*Aspergillus*

- Exposure to animal at the time of giving birth →*Coxiella Burnetti* (Q-fever)
- Birds →*Chlamydia psittaci*
- Elderly, smoker, Air–conditioning →*Legionella*

• TB: alveolar macrophage → $CD4^+$ T-cells → macrophage release IL-12 (stimulates T_H1 cells) and IL-1 (fever; activate T_H1 cells) → T_H1 release IL-2 (self stimulation of T_H1) and - interferon (activate macrophage to kill tubercular bacilli) → inflammatory mediators release from macrophage are responsible for tissue damage (*no* endotoxin or exotoxin) → lipid from tubercular bacilli leads to caseous necrosis

• *Bronchiactasis*
- Permanent dilation of bronchi and bronchioles.
- Chronic infection (gram [-] organisms, destruction of cartilage and elastic tissues)
- Persistent cough with purulent copious sputum production, wheezes, crackles

• *Idiopathic Pulmonary Fibrosis*
- Involve only lung *except* clubbing
- Unknown etiology, occurs in 5th decade
- CXR – reticular/reticulonodular disease
- Chest CT – ground glass appearance
- PFT- restrictive pattern

• *Sarcoidosis*
- 20–40 year-old women
- Presence of nonspecific noncaseating granuloma in the lung and other organs
- CXR – *bilateral hilar adenopathy*
- Hypercalcemia (↑ 1-α-hydroxylase by macrophage leads to ↑ Vit–D)
- ↑ ACE (60% of patients)
- Ophthalmoscopic examination (uveitis and conjunctivitis - >25% of the cases)

- *Pneumoconiosis*:
- CXR – small irregular opacities, interstitial densities, ground glass appearance, honeycombing
- Asbestosis → H/O exposure, usually involve lower lung fields
- CXR – diffuse /local pleural thickening, pleural plaques, *calcification at the level of diaphragm*
- Lung biopsy – barbell-shaped asbestos fiber (Best diagnostic test)
- ↑↑↑ Risk of bronchogenic CA
- ↑ Risk of pleural/peritoneal mesothelioma

- *Coal Miner's / Coal Worker's Pneumoconiosis (CWP)*
- Usually involves upper half of lung
- Increase levels of IgA, IgG, C3, anti-nuclear Ab, RF
- *Caplan syndrome* – rheumatoid nodule in the periphery of the lung in a patient with RA and CWP

- *Silicosis* → hyaline nodule, usually involves upper lobe
- Strong association with TB, Pt should go yearly PD and if PPD >10mm then INH for 9 months

- *Pulmonary Thromboembolism*
- Sudden onset of dyspnea along with tachycardia
- ECG → right axis deviation
- H/O long term immobility

- *Adult Respiratory Distress Syndrome (ARDS)*
- ↑Permeability of the alveolar – capillary membrane and pul. edema
- Alveolar macrophage → cytokines → neutrophil → damage capillary membrane
- CXR – diffuse interstitial infiltrates; whiteout of both lung fields
- Swan-Ganz catheter – *normal* cardiac output and capillary wedge pressure ↑ pulmonary artery pressure

- *Sleep apnea*: daytime somnolence
- *Obstructive sleep apnea* → floppy airway, obese patient
- *Central sleep apnea* → inadequate ventilatory drive

- *Bronchogenic Carcinoma*
- Squamous cell CA → centrally located → hypercalcemia – PTH-like substance
- Small cell CA → centrally located → SIADH, Eaton-Lambert, venocaval obstruction syndrome
- Large Cell CA → peripherally located
- Adenocarcinoma → peripherally located → pleural effusion with high hyaluronidase level in effusion fluid. Bronchoalveolar CA is subtype.

- *Pancoast tumor* – Hornor's syndrome, phrenic N involvement (chest movement asymmetry, a dangerous sign in patient with Miscellaneous
- *Edema*: transudate (↑ hydrostatic pressure and ↓ oncotic pressure) exudates (↑ vascular permeability)

- *Shock*: low perfusion pressure to tissues – hypovolemic (low circulatory volume); cardiogenic (heart is not pumping well) and septic (vasodilation leads to blood flow too quickly and give less time for tissue to extract oxygen)
- *Cardiogenic shock* – low CO and *High* PCWP
- *ARDS* – *normal* PCWP (pulmonary capillary wedge pressure)
- *Septic shock* – high CO, low PCWP and *normal mixed venous O2*
- *Hypovolemic shock* – *low* CO, *low* PCWP, *low* mixed venous O2

- High PCWP and low CVP (central vein pressure) – *LV dysfunction*
- High PCWP and high CVP – *cardiac temponade*
- Respiratory distress and high CVP – *tension pneumothorax*

- Abdominal aortic aneurism – atherosclerosis – (rupture - left flank pain, hypotension, pulsatile mass) – below renal artery origin is most common site

- Syphilitic aneurism – aortic arch aneurism, tertiary syphilis, vasculitis of vasa- vasorum, aortic valve regurgitation, brassy cough due to stretching of left. recurrent laryngeal N by aneurism

- Aortic dissection – cystic medial degeneration (elastic tissue fragmentation) – Marfan syndrome and EDS (Ehler-Danlos syndrome) – usually occurs within 10cm of the aortic valve – cardiac tamponade most common cause of death – aortic regurgitation, widening of aortic valve root on echo – loss of upper extremity pulse due to compression of subclavian artery

- Ehler-Danlos syndrome: defect in type-I and type-III collagen – poor wound healing, aortic dissection, hypermobile joints

- Atherosclerosis – fibrous cap (pathognomic lesion)
- Lines of Zahn – laminated thrombi with alternate pale and red area (heart and aorta)

- Arteriosclerosis – hardening of arterioles
- Hyaline arteriosclerosis – protein deposition in arterial wall – DM (basement membrane leak proteins into vessel wall due to nonenzymatic glycosylation of basement membrane protein); HTN (increase pressure push protein into vessel wall)
- Hyperplastic arteriosclerosis – smooth muscle cell hyperplasia – "onion skin" appearance

- Churg-Strauss syndrome – vasculitis + *eosinophilia*

- Capillary hemangiomas in newborn regress with age

- Sturge-Weber syndrome – Nevus flammeus (birth mark) on face in distribution of ophthalmic branch of CN 5 – ipsilateral malformation of pia mater vessel overlying occipital and parietal lobes

- Kawasaki syndrome – child with cervical lymphadenopathy, fever, *desquamating rash on palm, sole, and mouth* – coronary artery aneurysm/thrombosis

- Takayasu's arteritis (pulseless disease) – young Asian girl – granulomatous vasculitis of aortic arch

- Temporal arteritis (giant cell arteritis) – focal granulomatous inflammation – vasculitis of superficial temporal artery and ophthalmic artery

- Kaposi's sarcoma – HHV-8 – malignant tumor of endothelial cells – raised, red-purple flat lesions to plaque and nodules

- Bacillary angiomatosis – benign capillary proliferation involving skin and viscera in AIDS – simulate Kaposi's sarcoma – *Bartonella henselae* (causative agent)

- Von Hippel–Lindau disease – autosomal dominant – cerebellar hemangioblastomas, pheochromocytoma, renal adenocarcinoma (high incidence)

- *Rhabdomyosarcoma*
- Tumor of striated muscles
- Head, neck, and genitourinary tract.
- Grapelike mass protruding through vagina (Sarcoma botryoides)

MISCELLANEOUS

- *Edema*: transudate (↑ hydrostatic pressure and ↓ oncotic pressure) exudates (↑ vascular permeability)

- *Shock*: low perfusion pressure to tissues – hypovolemic (low circulatory volume); cardiogenic (heart is not pumping well) and septic (vasodilation leads to blood flow too quickly and give less time for tissue to extract oxygen)
- *Cardiogenic shock* – low CO and *High* PCWP
- *ARDS* – *normal* PCWP (pulmonary capillary wedge pressure)
- *Septic shock* – high CO, low PCWP and *normal mixed venous O2*
- *Hypovolemic shock* – *low* CO, *low* PCWP, *low* mixed venous O2

- High PCWP and low CVP (central vein pressure) – *LV dysfunction*
- High PCWP and high CVP – *cardiac temponade*
- Respiratory distress and high CVP – *tension pneumothorax*

- Abdominal aortic aneurism – atherosclerosis – (rupture - left flank pain, hypotension, pulsatile mass) – below renal artery origin is most common site

- Syphilitic aneurism – aortic arch aneurism, tertiary syphilis, vasculitis of vasa- vasorum, aortic valve regurgitation, brassy cough due to stretching of left. recurrent laryngeal N by aneurism

- Aortic dissection – cystic medial degeneration (elastic tissue fragmentation) – Marfan syndrome and EDS (Ehler-Danlos syndrome) – usually occurs within 10cm of the aortic valve – cardiac tamponade most common cause of death – aortic regurgitation, widening of aortic valve root on echo – loss of upper extremity pulse due to compression of subclavian artery

- Ehler-Danlos syndrome: defect in type-I and type-III collagen – poor wound healing, aortic dissection, hypermobile joints

- Atherosclerosis – fibrous cap (pathognomic lesion)
- Lines of Zahn – laminated thrombi with alternate pale and red area (heart and aorta)

- Arteriosclerosis – hardening of arterioles
- Hyaline arteriosclerosis – protein deposition in arterial wall – DM (basement membrane leak proteins into vessel wall due to nonenzymatic glycosylation of basement membrane protein); HTN (increase pressure push protein into vessel wall)
- Hyperplastic arteriosclerosis – smooth muscle cell hyperplasia – "onion skin" appearance

- Churg-Strauss syndrome – vasculitis + *eosinophilia*

- Capillary hemangiomas in newborn regress with age

- Sturge-Weber syndrome – Nevus flammeus (birth mark) on face in distribution of ophthalmic branch of CN 5 – ipsilateral malformation of pia mater vessel overlying occipital and parietal lobes

- Kawasaki syndrome – child with cervical lymphadenopathy, fever, *desquamating rash on palm, sole, and mouth* – coronary artery aneurysm/thrombosis

- Takayasu's arteritis (pulseless disease) – young Asian girl – granulomatous vasculitis of aortic arch

- Temporal arteritis (giant cell arteritis) – focal granulomatous inflammation – vasculitis of superficial temporal artery and ophthalmic artery

- Kaposi's sarcoma – HHV-8 – malignant tumor of endothelial cells – raised, red-purple flat lesions to plaque and nodules

- Bacillary angiomatosis – benign capillary proliferation involving skin and viscera in AIDS – simulate Kaposi's sarcoma – *Bartonella henselae* (causative agent)

- Von Hippel–Lindau disease – autosomal dominant – cerebellar hemangioblastomas, pheochromocytoma, renal adenocarcinoma (high incidence)

- *Rhabdomyosarcoma*
- Tumor of striated muscles
- Head, neck, and genitourinary tract.
- Grapelike mass protruding through vagina (Sarcoma botryoides)

PHARMACOLOGY

* General Pharmacology
1. Which form of the drug contributes to concentration gradient?
   - Only free drug forms contribute to the concentration gradient.

2. Which form of the drug can cross cell membranes?
   - Only nonionized (uncharged) form of a drug crosses biomembranes.

3. How P^H and P^{Ka} will affect drugs?
   - P^H and P^{Ka} will help us determine if drugs are in nonionized form or ionized form. If $P^H - P^{Ka}$ value is negative, weak acids are in nonionized form and can absorb better. For example, if $P^H - P^{Ka}$ value is -2, 99% of weak acids are in nonionized form means they can cross cell membrane easily. If value is 0, 50% of drugs are in nonionized form, and 50% of drugs are in ionized form.
   - If $P^H - P^{Ka}$ value is positive, weak bases are in nonionized form and can absorb better.

4. In which medium weak acid will cross cell membranes?
   - In acidic medium (means weak acid is absorbed better in stomach).

5. In which medium will a weak base cross cell membranes?
   - In basic medium, a weak base will cross cell membranes.

6. Which drug form is reabsorbed from the kidney?
   - Only a nonionized form is reabsorbed. (Both ionized and nonionized form filtered through glomerulus.)

7. How will acidification and alkalization of urine affect elimination of drug?

- Acidification of urine causes increased ionization of weak bases, which means increased elimination of weak bases.
- Alkalization of urine causes increased ionization of weak acids, which means increased elimination of weak acids.

8. What are the things we use to acidify and alkalize urine?

- NH_4Cl, vit- C, cranberry juice to acidify urine
- $NaHCO_3$, acetazolamide to alkalize urine

9. Which route has 100% bioavailability (f)?

- IV route

10. What is the relationship between distribution of drug (V_d) and plasma concentration of drug?

- Increase V_d – decrease plasma concentration of drugs
- Increase plasma protein binding – decrease V_d

11. What should I remember for drug with high V_d?

- Drugs with high V_d value raise the possibility of displacement by other agents and therefore change in pharmacologic activities.

12. What is loading dose? How will it affected by bioavailability?

- Variables are used to calculate the loading dose: Cp = desired peak concentration of drug
  Vd = volume of distribution of drug
  F = bioavailability
- The required loading dose may then be calculated as
  $LD = Cp \times Vd / F$.
- Bioavailability (f) affects LD in the following way:
- If f = 0.5 then LD should double ($\times 2$)
- If f = 0.25 then LD should quadruple ($\times 4$)

13. What is the renal clearance of drug?

- $K = Cu \times Q / C_P$ (Cu = concentration in urine, Q = urine flow, Cp = plasma concentration)

14. What is infusion rate?
- Drug $_{\text{Infusion rate}}$ = steady state concentration (C_{ss}) × clearance

15. What is maintenance rate?
- Drug $_{\text{maintenance rate}}$ = steady state concentration (C_{ss}) × clearance × dosing interval

16. What is elimination constant?
- Ke (elimination constant) = 0.7/ $T_{1/2}$ = clearance / Vd

17. What is elimination half-life?
- $T_{1/2}$ = 0.7 / Ke

18. What is steady state and on what does it depend?
- Steady state: rate in = rate out. It depends on $T_{1/2}$

19. At which half-life do we attain clinically significant steady state?
- 4–5 times $T_{1/2}$

20. What is zero-order elimination? Give two important examples
- There are circumstances where a sufficient quantity of drug is ingested, which saturates the metabolic enzymes in the liver, and so is eliminated from the body at an approximately constant rate (amount)
- *Examples*: large amounts of ethanol, salicylates (Aspirin), at toxic dose

21. What is first-order elimination? How it differs from zero-order?
- Constant proportion (percentage) of the drug is eliminated per unit time
- *Difference*: The amount of drug eliminated per unit time is same in zero-order, which means if 50 mg is eliminated in one hour, then 50 mg will be eliminated after each hour. If 200 mg in the body, zero-order will follow like this: 200 – 150 – 100 – 50 – 0. Percentage of the drug eliminated per unit time is same in first-order means if 50% of drug is eliminated in one hour, then 50% will be eliminated after each hour. If 200 mg in the body, first-order will follow like this: 200 – 100 – 50 – 25 – 12.5

22. What happen to elimination when you increase drug dose in first-order elimination?
   - Increased drug dose in first-order will increase elimination. (That's not what happens in zero-order.)

23. What is potency? What is efficacy?
   - *Efficacy*: Ability of a drug to induce a biological response in its molecular target. (It does not matter how much is required.)
   - *Potency*: An amount of drug is required to achieve maximal response.
   - *Example*: If 100 mg of drug X produces a maximal effect and 10 mg of drug Y produces the same maximal effect, then both drug X and Y have same efficacy, but drug Y is more potent then drug X.

24. What is full agonist? What is partial agonist?
   - *Full agonist*: binds and activates receptors and shows full efficacy at that receptor
   - *Partial agonist*: binds and activates receptor but shows partial efficacy at that receptor compare to full agonist
   - *Inverse agonist*: binds and activates receptor but shows the reverse action of that receptor

25. What happens if a partial agonist is given to the patient who already received a full agonist?
   - Response will decrease b/c the partial agonist displaces the full agonist from the receptor. Here it will work as antagonist.

26. What is antagonist? Competitive, noncompetitive?
   - *Antagonist*: Binds to the receptor but doesn't provoke any response, but blocks or decreases the agonist-mediated response.
   - *Competitive*: Reversibly binds to receptors at the same binding site as the endogenous agonist binds, but without activating the receptor. (Increased level of agonist may replace competitive antagonist and reverse its action.)
   - *Example*: Atropine for ACh receptors
   - *Noncompetitive*: Binds to a distinctly separate binding site from the agonist on the receptor and exerts its action to that

receptor. (Increased level of agonist doesn't have any effect on noncompetitive antagonist.)

- *Example*: Phenoxybenzamine at alpha-receptors
- (Learn how to identify effects of the agonist, the antagonist, and the partial agonist on graph.)

27. What are the difference between physiological antagonist and pharmacological antagonist?

- *Physiological antagonist* works on different receptors. (*Example*: ACh causes decrease in heart rate through M2 receptor whereas epinephrine causes increase in heart rate through beta-receptors. ACh and epinephrine are antagonists to each other's action and both work at different receptors.)
- *Pharmacological antagonist* works on same receptors as endogenous agonist works. (*Example*: Atropine binds to same receptor where ACh binds but exerts an opposite effect than Ach.)

28. What is therapeutic index (TI)? Importance of it? Give 2 examples of drugs with low TI.

- It is the ratio given by the toxic dose divided by the therapeutic dose.
- Importance: drugs with narrow TI should be monitored more frequently, as slight fluctuations in their level can produce toxic effects.
- *Examples*: lithium, warfarin, theophylline

29. How intracellular receptors differ from membrane-bound receptors?

- Intracellular receptors act via modifying gene expression, so it takes time for them to exert their effect.
- *Example*: steroids, hormones

30. Give examples of receptors that use cGMP.

- H_1, M_3, NO (nitrous oxide) (cGMP is present in vascular smooth muscles. It relaxes smooth muscles and produce vasodilation)

31. Give examples of receptors that work through transmembrane enzymes. How?
  - Insulin, EGF, PDGF, ANF; they stimulate the tyrosine kinase domain in cytoplasm to exert their action.

32. How cytokines work?
  - Erythropoietin, somatotropin, interferon; they stimulate the tyrosine kinase domain in cytoplasm to exert their action.

* ANS (Autonomic Nervous System)
  - What are the ANS receptors and neurotransmitters? Where are they located?
  - Nicotinic, muscarinic, alpha, and beta receptors
  - *Neurotransmitters*: ACh (act on nicotinic and muscarinic receptors), epinephrine, and norepinephrine (act on alpha and beta receptors)
  - N_N – Cell bodies in ganglia of both PANS and SANS and in the adrenal medulla
  - N_M - Skeletal muscles
  - M_{1-3} – Located on the organ and tissues innervated by PANS and on thermoregulatory sweat glands which are innervated by *SANS*
  - Alpha and Beta – Located on the organ and tissues innervated by SANS
  - *Easy way to remember important muscarinic location*: only heart has M_2, all other places have M_3, GI glands have M_1;
  - Now remember, M_2 is operated through Gi so it has inhibitory effect on the organ. So whenever ACh stimulate M_2, it causes decrease in heart rate and decrease in conduction velocity (AV block); M_{1-3} operated through Gq so they have stimulating effect whenever they are stimulated through ACh (*location of M3* – eye: miosis [constriction of pupils] through contraction of *sphincter muscles* of pupil and accommodation for near vision through contraction of *ciliary muscles*; bladder: voiding of urine through contraction of detrusor muscles; sphincters: contraction of all sphincters in the body except LES (lower esophageal sphincter), which relax; blood vessels: dilation of blood vessels through nitrous oxide and EDRF; GIT: increase motility of stomach, increase secretions of GI glands

- *Easy way to remember important alpha receptors' location:* α_2 present at only three locations: 3P (platelets, pancreas, and prejunctional nerve terminal) All other places have α_1.
- Now remember, α_2 works through Gi, so whenever they stimulate, they have inhibitory effects. So they decrease norepinephrine secretion at prejunctional nerve terminals, decrease release of pancreas, and causes aggregation of platelets
- α_1 receptors work opposite to Ach, so they produce mydriasis (dilatation of pupils), vasoconstrictions, and urinary retention; other important location vas deference in male
- *Easy way to remember important beta receptors location:* β_1 presents on heart and kidney; all other places have β_2.
- Now remember both beta receptors work through Gs so they have stimulatory effect on the organ whenever they are stimulated; β_1 increases every thing means it increases heart rate, conduction velocity, force of contraction, and release of renin.
- Stimulation of β_2 receptors causes vasodilation, relaxation of uterus, bronchial dilation; other important locations are skeletal muscles (increase contractility – tremors), liver (increase glyconeogenesis), and pancreas (increase insulin secretion)

Cholinergic	*Anti-Ch*	α_1 Receptor	α_2 Receptor	β_1 Receptor	β_2 Receptor
miosis (all cholinergic action occur through M3 except in heart where it is M2)	mydriasis

atropine enter in CNS will produce confusion, hallucination | mydriasis | ↓insulin secretion | increase everything (HR, force of contraction, conduction velocity renin secretion) | ↑insulin secretion |
AV block (M2)	urinary retention	urinary retention	↓ NE		dilation of bronchi
vasodilation		constriction of vessels			*vasodilation*
voiding of urine	dry mouth				relaxation of uterus

- Agonists of above receptors produce the same effect as the above receptors.
- Indirect agonists produce the same effect as agonists but have a different mechanism.
- Antagonists of above receptors produce opposite effects than above receptors

- What is an important thing about thermoregulatory gland, and which ANS receptors are present there?
- Thermoregulatory glands contain muscarinic receptors, but they are innervated by SANS.

- Which neurotransmitter is present at preganglionic fibers of both PANS and SANS?
- ACh (acetylcholine)

- What are the neurotransmitters for postganglionic fibers of PANS and SANS?
- Postganglionic PANS – ACh
- Postganglionic SANS – NE, E, DA

- Which is dominant in the tissue with dual innervation (PANS and SANS)? What is an exception to this rule?
- For effector tissues with dual innervation, PANS is dominant.
- Exception: Blood vessels – only SANS →produce vasoconstriction

- Synthesis and degradation of ACh
- Choline + acetyl Co-A → choline acetyltransferases → ACh
- Choline acetyltransferases is found in neurons
- ACh → acetylcholinesterase → choline + acetate
- Choline is taken up for reuse
- Acetylcholinesterase is found in synaptic cleft

- Which drug inhibits choline uptake?
- Hemicholinum (decrease ACh formation)

- Which drug inhibits Ach release?

- *Botulinum* toxin

- Give the name of drugs which directly stimulates Ach receptors
- Pilocarpine, bethanechol, methacholine

- Give the names of indirectly acting cholinomimetics drugs
- Neostigmine, physostigmine, edrophonium, pyridostigmine, donepezil (by *reversibly* inhibiting acetylcholinesterase, they increase effect of ACh)
- Echothiophate, organophosphate insecticides (by *irreversibly* inhibiting acetylcholinesterase, they increase effect of ACh)

- Give the names of muscarinic receptor antagonists
- Atropine, ipratropium, scopolamine (hyoscine)

- Give the names of nicotinic receptor antagonists (ganglion blockers)
- Mecamylamine, hexamethonium

- Give the names of neuromuscular blockers
- Succinylcholine, atracurium, tubocurarine, vecuronium

- Difference between succinylcholine and other neuromuscular blockers
- Succinylcholine is a depolarizing neuromuscular blocker
- Others are nondepolarizing neuromuscular blockers

- Why do we use pilocarpine in acute angle closure glaucoma?
- It causes constriction of pupils by which it pulls ciliary process and increases aqueous drainage so it decreases IOP fast.

- Use of drugs that directly stimulate Ach receptors
- *Pilocarpine*: acute glaucoma, sweat test for diagnosis of cystic fibrosis
- *Bethanechol*: urinary retention, postop ileus
- *Methacholine*: diagnosis bronchial hyperactivity in COPD

- Use of drugs that indirectly stimulate Ach receptors (AchE inhibitors)

- *Physostigmine*: glaucoma, anticholinergic overdose (atropine)

- *Neostigmine, pyridostigmine*: myasthenia gravis
- *Edrophonium*: to differentiate myasthenia from cholinergic crisis
- *Donepezil, tacrine* (enter in CNS): Alzheimer's disease

- Use of anticholinergic drugs
- *Atropine* (enter in CNS): anti-AchE inhibitors overdose, bradycardia, heart block, pupillary dilation with cycloplegia
- *Ipratropium*: COPD
- *Scopolamine*: motion sickness

- Use of neuromuscular blockers
- Endotracheal intubation

- Important side effects of succinylcholine
- Malignant hyperthermia (Tx., dantrolene – inhibits release of Ca^{++} from sarcoplasmic reticulum – relax all muscles), hyperkalemia

- Important side effects of atracurium
- It releases histamine (vasodilation, rash, bronchial constriction)

- Treatment of overdose of nondepolarizing neuromuscular blockers
- Physostigmine, neostigmine

- Difference between physostigmine and neostigmine, pyridostigmine
- Physostigmine can enter in CNS that's why it is used in anticholinergic overdose

- Treatment of AchE inhibitors poisoning
- Atropine and pralidoxime (2-PAM, as early as possible; 2-PAM will reactivate acetylcholinesterase)

- How anticholinergic drugs are helpful in Parkinsonism? Which symptom is not improved by anticholinergic drugs?

- In Parkinsonism, there is imbalance between ACh and DA (dopamine). There is increase in ACh so giving anticholinergics will reduce tremors and rigidity symptoms of Parkinsonism. It has *no* effect on bradykinesia.

- What is the difference between atropine and phenylephrine when it comes to use for eye dilatation?
- Atropine - mydriasis and cycloplegia (spasm of accommodation)
- Phenylephrine (α_1 – agonist) →mydriasis *without* cycloplegia

- How ANS works to control BP
- ($\downarrow\alpha_1$) $\downarrow$TPR →$\uparrow$*BP* →*reflex bradycardia*
- ($\downarrow\beta_1$) $\downarrow$TPR →$\downarrow$*BP* →*reflex Tachycardia*

- Difference between norepinephrine and epinephrine
- Norepinephrine (NE) – $\alpha_1 \alpha_2 \beta_1$ (*no* β_2 action)
- Epinephrine (E) – $\alpha_1 \alpha_2 \beta_1 \beta_2$ (acts on all adrenergic receptors, low dose of E – beta action is predominant, high dose of E – alpha action is predominant)

- What is epinephrine reversal?
- High dose epinephrine ($\uparrow$BP through α action)

  $\downarrow$

  Then if α blocker given

  $\downarrow$

  Fall in BP occur ($\downarrow$BP, because α activity is blocked but β activity remains)

- Use of epinephrine
- Anaphylaxis, cardiac arrest, laryngospasm, status asthmatics

- Give names of alpha and beta receptors' agonists
- α_1 agonist: methoxamine, phenylephrine
- α_2 agonist: clonidine (mixed α_1 and α_2 actions), methyldopa
- β_2 agonist: salmeterol, salbutamol, terbutaline, metaproterenol, dobutamine ($\beta_1 > \beta_2$), dopamine

- Give names of alpha and beta receptors' antagonists
- *α_1 antagonist:* prazosin, terazosin, doxazosin

- α_2 *antagonist:* yohimbine, benzylpiperazine
- *α nselective α antagonist:* phenoxybenzamine (noncompetitive), phentolamine (competitive)
- *Nonselective α antagonist:* propranolol, timolol, pindolol (ISA), sotalol
- *Selective β_1 antagonist:* acebutolol (ISA), metoprolol, atenolol, esmolol

- Use of alpha agonists:
- *Methoxamine:* paroxysmal supraventricular tachycardia
- *Phenylephrine:* nasal decongestant
- *Clonidine:* antihypertensive, opioid detoxification, also use in conjunction with methylphenidate in ADHD
- *Methyldopa* (alpha methylnorepinephrine is an active form of methyldopa which *act centrally*): gestational hypertension

- Use of alpha antagonists:
- *Phenoxybenzamine:* As an anti-HTN in pheochromocytoma
- *Doxazosin:* BPH (benign prostatic hypertrophy), anti-HTN
- *Yohimbine:* postural hypotension, impotence

- Use of beta agonists:
- Salmeterol, salbutamol: bronchial asthma
- Terbutaline, ritodrine: premature labour

- Use of beta antagonists:
- HTN, CHF, MI, angina, arrhythmia, migraine prophylaxis, glaucoma, essential tremor, portal HTN, social anxiety

- Important side effect of clonidine
- Rebound HTN on abrupt withdrawal

- Important side effect of alpha-blocker
- First dose syncope

- Important contraindications of beta-blockers
- Bronchial asthma, COPD, PVD

- Important side effects of nonselective beta-blockers

- Sexual dysfunction, delayed hypoglycemia, alter plasma lipids, fatigue, heart block, depression

- *Dopamine receptor locations*:
- D_1 *(peripheral)*: renal, mesenteric, coronary vessels
- D_2: central nervous system

- Difference between dopamine and dobutamine
- Dopamine has effects on renal vasculature, which is an advantage over dobutamine

- What is an important thing to remember about indirect-acting adrenoceptor agonists?
- Indirect agonist act only on effector tissues innervated by SANS. Denervated tissues are nonresponsive. (E.g. if the heart is transplanted, then SANS fibers are not present there, so in that part, indirect-acting adrenoceptor agonists give *no* response.)

- What is tachyphylaxis?
- Tachyphylaxis means a rapid loss of pharmacologic activity; chronic use of decongestant produces tachyphylaxis b/c NE store may become depleted.

- What is the main difference between phenoxybenzamine and phentolamine?
- Phenoxybenzamine (noncompetitive), phentolamine (competitive)

- Name of nonselective beta-blockers with ISA (intrinsic sympathomimetic action)
- Pindolol

- Name of selective beta-1 antagonist with ISA
- Acebutolol

- Usefulness of beta-blockers with ISA
- Less bradycardia and minimal change in plasma lipids

- Drugs with both alpha-1 and beta-blocking activity
- Labetalol, carvedilol

* CVS (Cardiovascular System)
- Mechanism of different classes of antiarrhythmic drugs
- *Class 1*: block Na^+ channels (increase action potential duration by decreasing Vmax)
- *Class 2*: beta-blockers (AV block so useful in supraventricular tachycardia)
- *Class 3*: block K^+ channels (prolong repolarization and refractory period so useful in re-entrant tachycardia)
- *Class 4*: block Ca^{++} channels (decrease conduction through AV node and shorten phase-2 [plateau] – decrease contractility)

- Name of drugs according to different classes (class 1 to 4)
- Class 1a: quinidine, procainamide
- Class 1b: lidocaine, phenytoin
- Class 1c: flecainide, propafenone
- Class 2: propranolol, esmolol, sotalol
- Calss 3: amiodarone, sotalol
- Class 4: verapamil, diltiazem

- What are important characteristics of quinidine?
- Also blocks K^+ channel, M_2 receptors, and alpha-1 receptors
- Use of quinidine
- Atrial fibrillation (AF, quinidine itself increases risk of arrhythmia therefore prior digitalization is required), also used in malaria

- Important AE (adverse effects) of quinidine
- Immune thrombocytopenia, immune hemolysis, cinchonism (quinidine intoxication: tinnitus [characteristic], occular dysfunction), torsade de pointes (*increase QT interval*)

- Important use of procainamide
- WPW syndrome (Wolff-Parkinson-White)

- What is the characteristic of lidocaine?
- Not useful orally due to rapid first-pass metabolism

- Use and AE of lidocaine
- *Use*: post-MI ventricular arrhythmia, arrhythmia due to digoxin
- *AE*: seizures in overdose

- Antiarrhythmic use of phenytoin
- Arrhythmia due to digoxin overdose

- What are important things I should remember about amiodarone?
- Mimic all 4 classes, long half-lives
- *AE*: interstitial lung disease (pulmonary fibrosis), thyroid dysfunction (hypothyroidism / hyperthyroidism), increase LDL, torsade de pointes

- What is an important thing I should remember about sotalol?
- Mimic both class 2 and 3

- What is the main difference between verapamil and nifedepine
- Verapamil is more cardioselective.

- Different Classes of Calcium Channel Blockers (CCB)
- Dihydropyridine: nifedepine, amlodepine, felodepine – less cardioselective – more effect on vasculature, so useful in HTN – SE: vasodilation and hypotension causes reflex tachycardia
- Phenylalkylamine: verapamil – more cardioselective – reverse cardiospasm, so use in treating angina
- Benzothiazepine: diltiazem – intermediate – both cardioselective and vasodilator – use in controlling HR in atrial arrhythmias – less reflex tachycardia due to both effects
- Effect of cardioselective CCB on heart: reduces heart rate (cardiodepressant!) mainly through AV block, that's why it's used in atrial arrhythmias

- Where shouldn't we use calcium channel blockers (CCB)?
- WPW syndrome (digoxin is C/I too), CHF

- Mechanism and Use of Adenosine

- *Mechanism*: Inhibits adenyl cyclase by which it reduces cAMP, and so it causes cell hyperpolarization by increasing outward K+ flux. It is a potent coronary vasodilator.
- *Use*: DOC for paroxysmal supraventricular tachycardia (PSVT)

- Drugs causing torsade. Treatment of torsade.
- Drugs that block K^+ ion channel produce torsade, like quinidine, procainamide, amiodarone, sotalol
- *Tx.*, magnesium

- Safe antihypertensive drug in pregnancy and renal dysfunction
- Methyldopa

- Antihypertensive (HTN) drug that is contraindicated in pregnancy
- Angiotensin-converting enzyme inhibitors (ACEI)

- Mechanism of water retention when we use anti-HTN drugs
- Water retention (↓BP →increase in ADH release and renin-angiotensin system activity →Na and water retention)

- Between alpha- and beta-blockers, which affects plasma lipid level?
- Beta-blockers (Alpha-blockers have no effect on plasma lipids.)

- Name and mechanism of vasodilators
- *Hydralazine, nitroprusside*: increase cGMP via release of nitrous oxide
- *Minoxidil*: K^+ channel agonist; chemical structure similar to nitrous oxide so may be nitrous oxide agonist

- Drugs for HTN emergency
- Nitroprusside, labetalol

- Side effect of hydralazine
- Drug-induced lupus erythematous

- Side effects of nitroprusside
- Rebound HTN, cyanide poisoning

- Side effect of minoxidil for which this drug is used clinically
- Hypertrichosis (used clinically in hair loss)

- Side effect of diazoxide for which this drug is used clinically
- Insulinoma (decrease insulin release)

- Which CCB is used in subarachnoid hemorrhage?
- Nimodipine (produce constriction of cerebral vasculature)

- Name of ACEI and AT-1 receptor blockers
- ACEI: captopril, enalapril, lisinopril
- AT-1 antagonist: losartan

- Which are the most important side effects of ACE inhibitors?
- Dry cough (increase bradykinin), hyperkalemia

- Contraindication of ACEI
- Anaphylaxis (angioedema)
- Renal artery stenosis

- What is the difference between ACEI and AT-1 receptor blocker?
- Dry cough is not seen with AT-1 receptor blockers.

- What are the side effects of loop and thiazide diuretics in regards to pH and potassium?

- Both loop and thiazide diuretics produce alkalosis and hypokalemia.

- What are the side effects of carbonic anhydrase (CA) diuretics in regards to pH and potassium?
- CA inhibitor diuretics produce acidosis and hypokalemia.

- What are the side effects of K+-sparing diuretics in regards to pH and potassium?
- K^+-sparing diuretics produce acidosis and hyperkalemia.

- What is the mechanism of action of mannitol? Important uses?

- *M/A*: Filtered but *not* reabsorbed. It draws more water with it in urine.
- *Use*: To decrease intracranial pressure, to decrease occular pressure in acute glaucoma, to prevent renal failure in hemolysis and rhabdomyolysis.

- In which condition mannitol is C/I?
- Pulmonary edema

- What is the site of action of CA inhibitors? Important uses and AE?
- *M/A*: block formation of H_2CO_3; indirectly block Na/H transporter in PCT
- *Use*: glaucoma, benign intracranial hypertension (pseudotumor cerebri), high altitude sickness
- *AE*: renal stone, numbness, and tingling in fingers and toes

- What is the mechanism and site of action of loop diuretics? Important AE?
- *M/A*: inhibits Na^+- K^+-2Cl$^-$ symporter in thick ascending loop of Henle
- *AE*: ototoxicity (ethacrynate), hypomagnesemia, hypocalcemia (increased Ca loss in urine)

- What is the mechanism and site of action of thiazide diuretics?
  - *M/A*: inhibits Na^+- K^+-2Cl$^-$ symporter in DCT
  - *AE*: hyperglycemia, hyperlipidemia, hypercalcemia (decrease Ca in urine)

- What is the relationship between GFR and thiazide diuretic?
- $\downarrow$GFR α $\downarrow$ activity

- How will I identify loop and thiazide diuretics from urine analysis?
- Loop causes hypocalcemia by loosing more Ca^{++} in urine, whereas thiazide causes hypercalcemia by $\uparrow$ Ca^{++} Absorption and is the *only* diuretic that absorb Ca^{++}. Therefore thiazide is given to patients with h/o Ca^{++} stone.

- What is the mechanism and site of action of K+-sparing diuretics? Important AE of Spironolactone

- *Spironolactone*: competitive antagonist of aldosterone; prevent potassium and hydrogen secretion
- *Amiloride, Triamterene*: directly block epithelial Na channel in DCT
- *A/E*: gynacomastia, hirsutism, sexual dysfunction (spironolactone), renal stones

- What is the main difference between mechanism of action of reserpine and guanethidine?
- *Reserpine*: blocks the vesicular monoamine transporter (VMT, decreases NE in sympathetic neurons by decreasing its uptake, which leads to ↓CO and ↓PVR)
- *Guanethidine*: blocks the release of norepinephrine in response to arrival of an action potential, so decreases NE in synaptic cleft, which leads to ↓ CO and ↓PVR)

- Important side effects of reserpine
- Severe depression, hypotension, hyperprolactinemia

- Important side effects of guanethidine
- Hypotension, sexual dysfunction

- What is the MA of ACEI in CHF?
- ↓preload and ↓afterload

- What is the mechanism of action (MA) of digitalis?
- Inhibits Na / K ATPase

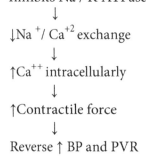

↓

↓Na^+/ Ca^{+2} exchange

↓

↑Ca^{++} intracellularly

↓

↑Contractile force

↓

Reverse ↑ BP and PVR

- Is digitalis prolongs survival of patient with CHF?
- No. (ACEI prolongs survival of patient with CHF.)

- Uses of digitalis (vagomimetic effect)
- In reentrant cardiac arrhythmias and to slow ventricular rate in atrial fibrillation

- Symptoms of digitalis toxicity; treatment of the same
- Nausea, vomiting, anorexia, diarrhea, abdominal pain, hallucinations, heart block, bradycardia, tachycardia
- *Tx.*, lidocaine, phenytoin, digitalis fab antibodies, cardioversion

- What increases digitalis toxicity?
- Hypokalemia (K^+ and digitalis both competes for Na-K ATPase), Hypomagnesemia (Most diuretics cause hypokalemia and hypomagnesemia, so electrolytes should be monitored frequently for those who are on diuretics and digitalis)

- In which condition should CCB and digitalis be avoided?
- WPW syndrome

- Which drug has shown to reduce mortality in patient with CHF when use in conjunction with ACEI?
- Spironolactone

- What is the MA of nitrates? What is the MA of sildenafil (Viagra)?
- Nitrates: venous and arterial vasodilation through NO
- Sildenafil: inhibits cGMP specific phosphodiesterase 5 (PDE-5) – increase in cGMP, which causes vasodilation

- What happen if we use Viagra and nitrates together?
- Excessive fall in BP occurs.

- Use of sildenafil besides erectile dysfunction
- Pulmonary HTN

- What is the half-life of nitrates?
- Around 5 hours

- Are beta-blockers helpful in Prinzmetal's angina?
- No. (Prinzmetal's angina is caused by spasm of coronary vessels and beta-blockers don't relieve spasm.)

- What is the MA of CCB in angina?
- Decreased contractility, decreased preload and afterload (vasodilation), decreased vasospasm

- Which drugs are useful in hyper-TGs?
- Niacin, atrovastatin, gemfibrozil

- Which is the only statin to lower TG?
- Atrovastatin

- What are the MA and side effects of bile acid sequesters?
- M/A: They serve as ion-exchange resins, so they bind with bile acids and prevent its reabsorption to enter in enterohepatic circulation
- AE: Decrease absorption of fat-soluble vitamins (A, D, E, K)

- What are the main AE of HMG co-A reductase inhibitors?
- Myositis, myopathies, and rhabdomyolysis (increased risk with fibrates)

- What are the important effects of nicotinic acid? Important AE?
- It blocks breakdown of fats in adipose tissue by which it decreases level of VLDL (a precursor of LDL).
- AE: facial flushing and itching, dyspepsia, hyperglycemia

- What are the MA and important AE of gemfibrozil?
- MA: increases activity of peroxisome proliferators-activated receptor alpha, which is involved in metabolism of carbohydrates and fat; also increases lipoprotein lipase synthesis – decreases VLDL, LDL, and TGs
- AE: gallstones, hypokalemia, rhabdomyolysis with statins

* CNS (Central Nervous System)
  - MA of barbiturates and benzodiazepines

- *MA*: Both bind to GABA$_A$ receptors at different sites and potentiate its effect. GABA$_A$ receptor is potential CNS inhibitor. Barbiturates produce their pharmacological effects by increasing the length of time the chloride ion channel remains open at the GABA$_A$ receptor, whereas benzodiazepines increase the opening frequency of the chloride ion channel at the GABA$_A$ receptor.

- Which benzodiazepines are metabolized outside the liver (meaning they don't require phase-1 metabolism)? What's the advantage of them?
- Lorazepam, oxazepam
- *Advantage*: can be used safely in liver dysfunction and elderly people

- Nonbenzodiazepine drugs that activate benzodiazepine receptors
- Zolpidem

- Drug use in barbiturates withdrawal
- Diazepam

- DOC for status epileptics
- Lorazepam

- Important C/I of barbiturates
- Porphyria

- M/A of buspirone and indication
- 5 HT1A presynaptic receptor, partial agonist
- *No* action on GABA
- *Indication*: Generalized anxiety disorder (GAD)

158. DOC for social and performance anxiety
- Propranolol

- DOC for alcohol overdose. M/A of it
- Fomepizole

- *MA*: long acting inhibitors of alcoholic dehydrogenase (ADH)

- Reason for giving ethanol in methanol poisoning
- Ethanol inhibits formation of formaldehyde that form formic acid (toxic to eyes)

- M/A of disulfiram. Use of it. Drug causing disulfiram-like reaction when used with alcohol.
- Normally alcohol is converted into acetaldehyde by alcohol dehydrogenase, which is then converted into acetic acid by acetaldehyde dehydrogenase. Disulfiram inhibits acetaldehyde dehydrogenase by which it increases the level of acetaldehyde, which produces unpleasant symptoms after drinking alcohol.
- *Use*: alcohol detoxification
- *Drugs causing disulfiram-like effects with alcohol*: metronidazole, cephalosporins, oral antidiabetic agents

- M/A of different antiepileptic drugs
- *MA*: The major molecular targets of anticonvulsant drugs are (1) voltage- gated sodium channels (carbamazapine, phenytoin, Valproic acid); (2) components of the GABA system, including $GABA_A$ receptors (benzodiazepines, barbiturates); and (3) voltage-gated calcium channel (ethosuximide, valproic acid)

32. Safe antiepileptic drug during pregnancy
- Phenobarbital

33. DOC for absence (petit mal) seizure
- Ethosuximide

31. Usually a DOC for all other seizure
- Valproic acid

32. Important drug interaction of all anticonvulsants
- Decrease efficacy of oral contraceptives
- Important AE of all anticonvulsants

- *Phenytoin*: horizontal nystagmus, gingival overgrowth, megaloblastic anemia (folic acid depletion), fetal hydantoin syndrome (teratogenic)
- *Carbamazapine*: SIADH, teratogenic (supply folic acid)
- *Valproic acid*: thrombocytopenia

- *Ethosuximide*: GI distress

- DOC for trigeminal neuralgia
- Carbamazapine, gabapentin

- M/A of newer anticonvulsants
- Block AMPA receptor – lamotrigine, topiramate
- Block NMDA receptor – felbamate

- M/A of general anesthetics
- *MA*: Inhibits excitatory function of some CNS receptors (glutamate, 5-HT receptors), some stimulate inhibitory receptors (GABA$_A$)

- Importance of blood-gas ratio for inhaled anesthetics
- High blood-gas ratio – quick redistribution in adipose tissue
- Quick redistribution in fat – require high dose to maintain blood level
- High dose – late recovery
- *Importance*: high blood-gas ratio – late recovery, low blood-gas ratio – fast recovery

- Important AE of halothane and Tx of that adverse reaction. M/A of drug that is used to Tx adverse reaction of halothane.
- Malignant hyperthermia in *genetically susceptible* individuals (Tx., dantrolene – inhibits release of Ca^{++} from sarcoplasmic reticulum – relax all muscles)

- Which inhaled anesthetic produce dose related depression of myocardial contractility?
- Enflurane (another side effect – lower threshold for seizure so it should not be used in patient with h/o epilepsy)

- Name and uses of IV anesthetics
- *Thiopental*: ultra short acting barbiturate used as IV in general anesthesia; Rapid recovery b/c redistribution from CNS to peripheral tissues (exhibits zero-order kinetics)
- *Propofol*: rapid onset and recovery, *produce amnesia*, useful for minor out-patient procedure like colonoscopy, *AE*: dystonia

- What is a neuroleptic anesthesia?
- Droperidol and fentanyl combination is used to achieve pain control for minor procedures, which is called neuroleptic anesthesia. Sometimes N_2O (laughing gas) is also added in this combination.

- Which drug produce dissociative anesthesia?
- Ketamine (blocks NMDA receptors, also binds opioid μ [mu] and σ [sigma] receptors)

- M/A of local anesthetics. Two groups of local anesthetics.
- *MA*: reversibly decrease the rate of depolarization and repolarization by inhibiting Na influx through sodium channels in neuronal cells
- Amino amide: lidocaine, bupivacaine
- Amino esters: procaine, cocaine

178. How pH affects action of local anesthetics
- Acidosis such as caused by inflammation at the wound reduces the action of local anesthetics

179. What is the main AE of amino ester group of local anesthetics?
- Amino ester group of anesthetics metabolized to PABA through pseudocholinesterase. Allergic reaction to PABA is the most important side effect.

180. C/I of Morphine
- Raised intracranial pressure so head trauma
- Asthma (bronchial constriction)
- Renal failure (accumulate metabolite morphine-6-glucuronide)
- Billiary colic (contract billiary apparatus)

- ◼ Important characteristic of morphine
- ◼ Predominantly act on µ receptors (agonist)
- ◼ Miosis (constriction of pupils), constipation

- ◼ Name of partial opioid agonist
- • Nalbuphine, pentazocin

- ◼ Which drug is an exception to all opioids? How?
- • Meperidine (It causes muscarinic receptor block, so it is useful in billiary colic. It causes mydriasis, whereas all others produce miosis.)

13. DOC for opioid overdose

- • Naloxone

* Antimicrobial Drugs
    - Best initial antibiotics for different microorganisms
    - *Staph aureus*: dicloxacillin, oxacillin (penicillins) / cefadroxil, cefalaxin (1ˢᵗ generation cephalosporins)
    - • If patient is allergic to above groups – macrolide, newer fluoroquinolone
    - • If patient has MRSA – vancomycin / linezolid
    - • *Streptococcus*: penicillin (if sensitive) / ceftriaxone / levofloxacin
    - • *Strep pneumonia*: penicillin G / ceftriaxone / levofloxacin
    - • *Strep viridans*: penicillin G / ceftriaxone
    - • *Strep pyogens*: ampicillin / ampicillin + sulbactam
    - • *Strep meningitis*: ceftriaxone

    - • *Listeria monocytogens*: ampicillin
    - • *Legionella pneumonia*: erythromycin
    - • *Rickettsia in children*: chloramphenicol, erythromycin
    - • *Rickettsia in adults*: doxycycline
    - • *Lyme disease in children < 9 years of age*: amoxicillin
    - • *Lyme disease in children >9 years of age and adults*: doxycycline
    - • *Lyme disease in pregnant women*: amoxicillin
    - • *Disseminated Lyme disease (Bell's palsy, cardiac involvement, CNS involvement)*: ceftriaxone

- *Syphilis*: penicillin G
- *Gonococcus*: ceftriaxone
- *Chlamydia, mycoplasma*: macrolides / doxycycline
- *C.Jejunii*: erythromycin
- *H Influenzae*: 2nd or 3rd generation cephalosporin
- *E coli*: ciprofloxacin / ampicillin
- *Pseudomonas*: piperacillin, ticarcillin (antipseudomonal penicillin)
- *Klebsiella*: 2nd or 3rd generation cephalosporin
- *Cryptococcus*: amphotericin B (severe), fluconazole (prophylaxis)
- *Candida*: fluconazole
- *Dermatophytes*: terfinabine (oral) / meconazole (local)
- *PCP*: trimethoprim + sulfamethoxazole
- *Actinomycetes*: penicillin
- *Nocardia*: sulfonamides
- *Anaerobes*: metronidazole / clindamycin
- Penicillin and aminoglycosides have synergistic effects, so a combination of both (penicillin + aminoglycosides) is used in enterobacteraceae and *Pseudomonas* infections

- M/A of penicillins
- Inhibit formation of peptidoglycans cross-link in cell wall synthesis, which weakens the cell wall, and death occurs due to osmotic pressure

- Mechanism of resistance to penicillins
- Enzymatic hydrolysis of beta lactam ring by beta lactamase (penicillinase) enzyme
- Due to possession of altered penicillin-binding proteins (this mode is seen in MRSA and penicillin resistant in streptococci)

- Difference between benzathine penicillin and benzylpenicillin (penicillin G)
- *Benzathine penicillin*: slowly absorbed into the circulation, IM use, prolonged antibiotic action over 2–4 weeks after a single IM dose, useful in prophylaxis of rheumatic fever
- *Benzylpenicillin (penicillin G)*: IV use, achieves high concentration quickly, increased antibacterial activity

- Important AE of penicillins. What is Jarisch-Herxheimer reaction?

- *AE*: allergic reactions, interstitial nephritis (methicillin)
- *Jarisch-Herxheimer reaction*: occurs most often in secondary syphilis and with penicillin therapy, characterized by fever, fatigue, and transient worsening of any mucocutaneous symptoms, and usually subsides within 24 hours, *Tx.*, acetaminophen

- Name of beta lactamase–resistant penicillin
- Dicloxacillin, oxacillin, methicillin

- Name of cephalosporins according to different generation
- *First generation*: cefadroxil, cefalexin, cefazolin
- *Second generation*: cefaclor, cefuroxime
- *Third generation*: cefdinir, cefotaxime, ceftriaxone, ceftizoxime
- *Fourth generation*: cefepime

- Coverage of all generation of cephalosporin
- *First*: penicillinase-producing staph, *E. coli*, *Klebsiella*, *Proteus*
- *Second*: increased activity against gram-negative organism
- *Third*: hospital-acquired infections, antipseudomonal activity (cefoparazone, ceftazidime), less gram-positive activity
- *Fourth*: same gram-positive as first generation, greater resistance to penicillinase, antipseudomonal

- M/A of cephalosporin / mechanism of resistance
- Same as penicillin

194. Important AE of cephalosporin
- Allergic reaction, hypoprothrombinemia, disulfiram-like reaction

- Which drug group should we use for patients allergic to penicillins and cephalosporins?
- For gram (+) infection, give macrolides.
- For gram (-) infection, give imipenem (carbapenem).

- ☐ Reason for using cilastatin with imipenem. AE of imipenem.
- Imipenem is hydrolysed by a dehydropeptidase enzyme in the kidney. This enzyme is inhibited by cilastatin by which it increases the activity of imipenem.
- *AE*: seizure

- ☐ M/A of vancomycin. Mechanism of resistance to vancomycin.
- *MA*: It prevents incorporation of N-acetylmuramic acid (NAM)- and N- acetylglucosamine (NAG)-peptide subunits into the peptidoglycans (early stage of wall synthesis) It is *not* active against gram negative organisms.
- *Mechanism of resistance*: alteration to the terminal amino acid residue of NAM and NAG

- ☐ Can vancomycin penetrate CNS?
- No

- ☐ Important use and AE of vancomycin
- *Use*: MRSA, pseudomembranous colitis
- *AE*: Red man syndrome (nonspecific mast cell degradation – Tx., antihistamines), ototoxicity, nephrotoxicity

- ☐ Do cephalosporin and penicillins have cross-allergenicity?
- Yes

- ☐ What is an important feature of aztreonam?
- No cross-allergenicity with penicillin and cephalosporins

- ☐ M/A of macrolides / mechanism of resistance of macrolides
- *MA*: Inhibition of protein synthesis by binding to 50S subunit of ribosome. It prevents peptidyl translocation of t-RNA (same for clindamycin).
- *Mechanism of resistance*: (1) post-transcriptional methylation of 23S ribosomal RNA, (2) production of drug-inactivating enzymes, (3) active ATP-dependent efflux proteins that transport the drug outside of the cell

◻ Should the erythromycin dose be reduced in patient with renal dysfunction?
• No

◻ Does macrolide have any effect on a P450 metabolism system?
• Yes

◻ Important AE of macrolide
• QT prolongation (torsade de pointes)

◻ Name of important antimicrobial agents that should be avoided in pregnancy
• Aminoglycosides
• Fluoroquinolones (ciprofloxacin)
• Tetracyclines
• Erythromycin and clarithromycin (azithromycin is safe in pregnancy)

◻ M/A of tetracycline / mechanism of resistance
• *MA*: inhibits protein synthesis by binding 30S ribosomes by which it inhibits binding of aminoacyl t-RNA to mRNA-ribosome complex
• *Mechanism of resistance*: (1) enzymatic inactivation, (2) active efflux of drug, and (3) ribosomal protection

◻ Important organism coverage of tetracycline
• Brucella, vibrio, Lyme disease, rickettsia, chlamydia, tularemia, plague, anthrax

◻ Important use of demeclocycline
• SIADH

◻ Effect of antacid on absorption of tetracycline
• Tetracycline binds to aluminum, magnesium, iron, and calcium, which reduce its absorption

◻ Which tetracycline can be used safely in renal dysfunction?
• Doxycycline

☐ Important AE of tetracyclines
• Teeth discoloration, steatosis, phototoxicity, pseudotumor cerebri, ototoxicity (minocycline)

☐ Important AE of clindamycin
• Pseudomembranous colitis (Tx., metronidazole [DOC], vancomycin)

☐ Important use of clindamycin
• Acne, malaria, MRSA, bacterial vaginosis in early stage of pregnancy

☐ M/A and resistance of aminoglycosides
• *MA*: Inhibits protein synthesis by binding 30S ribosome. It prevents translocation of the peptidyl-tRNA from the A-site to the P-site.
• *Resistance*: enzymatic inactivation

☐ Why are anaerobes resistant to aminoglycosides?
• It requires more energy for uptake, and anaerobes don't have much energy. (No oxygen!)

☐ Use of neomycin. Is it useful systemically?
• Neomycin is used orally in hepatic encephalopathy to ↓NH3 production by intestinal bacteria, otherwise it has no systemic use. It is used locally.

☐ Name important nephrotoxic antimicrobial drugs
• Aminoglycosides
• Amphotericin B
• Foscarnet

☐ Use of aminoglycosides
• TB, plague, infective endocarditis

☐ M/A and resistance of chloramphenicol
• *MA*: It inhibits peptidyl transferase and binds to 23S rRNA of 50S subunit and prevents peptide bond formation.

- *Resistance*: reduced membrane permeability, mutation of the 50S ribosomal subunit, and elaboration of chloramphenicol acetyltransferase

☐ AE of chloramphenicol. Is dose reduction required in LIVER dysfunction?
- Aplastic anemia, bone marrow suppression (reversible once drug is stopped), gray baby syndrome in newborns (hypotension, cyanosis)

☐ Drugs use for vancomycin resistant organisms
- Linezolid, daptomycin

☐ M/A of sulfa drugs
- *MA*: Inhibits folic acid synthesis by competitively inhibiting dihydropteroate synthesis (prevent formation of PABA to dihyropteroate)

☐ Uses and important AE of sulfa drugs
- *Use*: PCP (*Pneumocystis jirovecii* pneumonia), UTI, inflammatory bowel disease (sulfasalazine), *Nocardia* infection, trachoma (sulfacetamide), burn patient (silver sulfadiazine), toxoplasmosis (sulfadiazine + pyrimethamine), Whipple's disease (sulfamethoxazole + trimethoprim)
- *E*: allergies, known to increase level of warfarin (sulfamethoxazole/trimethoprim), Steven Johnson syndrome, agranulocytosis, kernicterus in the newborn if used during last 6 weeks of pregnancy

☐ Which other drugs have sulfa component?
- Thiazide diuretics, celecoxib, and glipizide/glyburide

☐ M/A of trimethoprim and pyrimethamine
- Both inhibit folic acid synthesis by inhibiting dihydrofolate reductase

☐ M/A of fluoroquinolones

- Inhibits DNA gyrase, topoisomerase II, and topoisomerase IV. These enzymes are necessary to separate replicated DNA. By inhibiting them, it prevents cell division.

☐ Important side effect in adults
- Achilles tendon rupture (tendonitis), delirium in elderly patients

☐ Effect of antacid on absorption
- Aluminum, iron, calcium binds with it and prevents its absorption

☐ M/A of amphotericin B and nystatin
- It binds with ergosterol (important substance in fungal cell wall) and forms pores in the fungal cell wall that leads to leakage of K^+ and fungal death.

☐ How can we prevent AE of amphotericin?
- Important AE of amphotericin B are fever, chills, hypotension, nausea, vomiting. It occur *due to release of histamine and increase prostaglandin synthesis,* so it can be prevented by acetaminophen, Aspirin, diphenhydramine, and/or hydrocortisone

☐ M/A of azoles
- Inhibits synthesis of ergosterol

☐ AE of ketoconazole
- Inhibit synthesis of testosterone (useful in prostate cancer, also useful in androgenic alopecia), glucocorticoids (useful in Cushing's disease), gynacomastia

☐ Important use of fluconazole
- *DOC* for candidiasis, *prophylaxis* of cryptococcal meningitis; first-line drug for coccidioidomycosis and histoplasmosis

☐ Which is the only azole that can penetrate in CNS?
- Fluconazole

▢ Drug use for topical fungal infection
• Miconazole and clotrimazole

▢ What is the M/A of flucytosin?
• *MA*: It is a fluorinated pyrimidine analog. (1) It intrafungally converted into the cytostatic fluorouracil and *interacts as 5-fluorouridinetriphosphate with RNA synthesis.* (2) It *inhibits fungal DNA synthesis* by conversion into 5-flourodeoxyuridinemonophosphate.

▢ AE of flucytosin
• Bone marrow suppression, GI toxicity

▢ What are M/A and AE of gresiofulvin?
• *MA*: It inhibits mitosis by binding to tubulin and interfering with microtubule function.
• *AE*: disulfiram-like reaction with ethanol, phototoxicity

▢ What is the M/A of terbinafine?
• It inhibits synthesis of ergosterol by inhibiting squalene epoxide enzyme.

▢ M/A and uses of metronidazole
• *MA*: It inhibits nucleic acid synthesis. (It is converted in anaerobic organisms by the redox enzyme pyruvate-ferredoxin oxidoreductase. The nitro group of metronidazole is chemically reduced by ferredoxin [or a ferredoxin-linked metabolic process] and the products are responsible for disrupting the DNA helical structure, thus inhibiting nucleic acid synthesis.)
• *Use*: amoebic dysenosis, bacterial vaginosis, *Trichomonas* vaginitis (give metronidazole to *both* partners), diarrhea due to *Giardia*, *H. pylori* regimen, anaerobic infections

▢ Important AE of antitubercular drugs
• *Rifampin*: thrombocytopenia, orange-colored body fluids, hepatitis
• *INH*: neuropathy (prevented by vit-B6 [pyridoxine]), hemolysis in G6PD patients, drug-induced lupus, hepatitis
• *Ethambutol*: optic neuritis

- *Pyrazinamide*: hepatitis, arthralgia

- ☐ M/A antitubercular drugs
- *Rifampin*: inhibits RNA transcription by inhibiting DNA-dependent RNA polymerase
- *INH*: Activated by catalase-peroxidase enzyme KatG to form isonicotinic acyl anion or radical, which binds with NADH radical and inhibit mycolic acid synthesis. (Mutations of the catalase gene is the reason of resistance.)
- *Pyrazinamide*: Pyrazinamidase enzyme in M. tuberculosis converts it into pyrazinoic acid, which inhibits fatty acid synthesis. (Mutations of the pyrazinamidase gene is the reason of resistance.)
- *Ethambutol*: Inhibits formation of cell wall.

- ☐ M/A and use of acyclovir
- *MA*: It is selectively *converted into acyclo-guanosine monophosphate* (acyclo-GMP) *by viral thymidine kinase*. Subsequently, the monophosphate form is further phosphorylated *into the active triphosphate form*, acyclo-guanosine triphosphate (acyclo-GTP), *by cellular kinase of host cell*. Acyclo-GTP is a very potent inhibitor of viral DNA polymerase. It has approximately 100 times greater affinity for viral than host cellular polymerase. As a substrate, acyclo-GMP is incorporated into viral DNA, resulting in *chain termination*.
- *Use*: HSV and VZV infections

245. Does acyclovir have any effect on postherpetic neuralgia?
- *No*. It reduces the severity and duration of herpes zoster, but does *not* reliably prevent postherpetic neuralgia.

- ☐ Drugs use in shingles
- Famciclovir and valacyclovir

- ☐ M/A of ganciclovir

- *MA*: It competitively inhibits the incorporation of dGTP by viral DNA polymerase, resulting in the termination of elongation of viral DNA
- *Use*: CMV infections (cytomegalovirus)

☐ What are the characteristics of foscarnet?
- *MA*: selectively inhibits the pyrophosphate binding site on viral DNA polymerase at concentration that do not affect human DNA polymerases
- *Use*: acyclovir and ganciclovir resistant viruses

☐ Important AE of foscarnet when it is used with pentamidine
- Hypocalcemia

250. Difference between NRTI and non-NRTI
- NRTI must be activated by cell kinase to act

- Important AE of zidovudine
- Hematotoxicity (anemia, bone marrow suppression)

- Drugs that increase zidovudine toxicity
- Aspirin, trimethoprim, cimitidine

253. Use of lamivudin
- Hepatitis B

■ M/A and important AE of protease inhibitors
- *MA*: inhibits viral replication by inhibiting HIV-1 protease
- *AE*: nephrolithiasis, hyperlipidemia, bizarre alterations in body shape

■ Only teratogenic anti-HIV drug name
- Efavirenz

■ M/A of amantadine. Other use of amantadine. Is amantadine useful against influenza B? AE of amantadine?

- *MA*: Amantadine interferes with a viral protein, M2 (an ion channel), which is required for the viral particle to become "uncoated" once it is taken inside the cell by endocytosis
- *Other use*: Parkinsonism
- No. It is not useful against influenza B.
- *AE*: livedo reticularis (reaction that results in skin mottling and purpurish mesh network of blood vessels, also seen with atropine)

- ■ Difference between amantadine and zenamivir, oseltamivir
- Oseltamivir and zenamivir are active against both influenza A and B viruses
- Both are neuraminidase inhibitor

- ■ M/A and use of ribavirin. Is it used in hep C?
- *MA*: inhibit RNA-dependent replication in RNA viruses
- *Use*: RSV (respiratory syncytial virus)
- Yes. It is used in conjunction with α-interferon

- ■ Important Antiprotozoal Drugs
- Mebendazole, albendazole: by selectively and *irreversibly blocking uptake of glucose*, and it is a *spindle poison*, which induces chromosomes; *use*: pinworm, whipworm, tapeworm hookworm, roundworm
- Pyrantel pamoate: acts as a *depolarizing neuromuscular blocking agent*, thereby causing sudden contraction, followed by paralysis of the helminths; *use*: hookworm, roundworm
- Anti-leishmaniasis: meglumine antimoniate and sodium stibogluconate
- Praziquantel: praziquantel increases the permeability of the membranes of parasite cells for calcium ions and thereby induces contraction of the parasites resulting in paralysis in the contracted state; *use*: liver fluke, Schistosomiasis
- Antimalarial drugs: quinine, chloroquine, pyrimethamine, mefloquine, proguanil, sulphdoxine, primaquine, atovaquone; *prophylaxis*: mefloquine and chloroquine

- * Anticoagulants, Thrombolytics, and Antiplatelets:
    - ■ M/A and important AE of heparin

- *MA*: binds to antithrombin III which inactivate thrombin and factor Xa
- *AE*: thrombocytopenia, osteoporosis

- ■ Drug use in heparin-induced thrombocytopenia
- Bivalirudin (direct inhibitor of thrombin)
- Fondaparinux (Xa inhibitor, it has no affinity to PF-4)

- • Can heparin be used in pregnancy?
- • Yes

- • How do we monitor patient on heparin / warfarin
- • Heparin – aPTT
- • Warfarin – PT

- • Antagonist of heparin and warfarin
- Heparin: protamine sulfate
- Warfarin: vit-K, fresh frozen plasma

- • M/A of warfarin
- *MA*: it inhibits vit-K epoxide reductase by which it reduces synthesis of vit-K dependent factors (2, 7, 9, and 10)

- • Most important AE to keep in mind when we give warfarin
- Warfarin necrosis (skin necrosis occurs due to deficiency of protein C), Teratogenic (contraindicated in pregnancy)

- • M/A of thrombolytics. Difference between streptokinase and alteplase.
- *MA*: Activate plasminogen which clears the cross-linked fibrin mesh.

- *Difference*: Streptokinase is *not* clot-specific, can cause allergic reaction, activity may decrease if recently used or recent strep infection

- • Antagonist of thrombolytics
- Aminocaproic acid, tranexamic acid

- Difference between Aspirin, clopidogrel, and abciximab
- *Aspirin*: irreversible inactivation of the cyclooxygenase (COX); low- dose Aspirin use irreversibly blocks the formation of thromboxane A_2 in platelets, producing an inhibitory effect on platelet aggregation
- *Clopidogrel*: an irreversible blockade of the ADP receptor on platelet cell membranes
- *Abciximab*: block glycoprotein IIb/IIIa receptor on the platelet

* Endocrine Pharmacology
- M/A of propyl thiouracil (PTU) and methimazole?
- *MA*: PTU inhibits the enzyme thyroperoxidase, which normally acts in thyroid hormone synthesis. Also acts by inhibiting the enzyme 5'- deiodinase, which converts T_4 to the active form T_3.

- Which one is safe in pregnancy out of above two drugs?
- PTU (extensively plasma protein bound)

- AE of PTU
- Agranulocytosis

- Use of propranolol in hyperthyroidism
- Propranolol treats symptoms of hyperthyroidism like palpitations, trembling, and anxiety, which are mediated by beta adrenergic receptors

- M/A and important AE of ^{131}I
- *MA*: The radioactive iodine is picked up by the active cells in the thyroid and destroys them. Since iodine is only picked up by thyroid cells.
- *AE*: Hypothyroidism

- Name and use of GH agonist
- *Somatotropin*: short stature

- Name and use of somato*statin*

- *Octreotide*: more potent inhibitor of GH, glucagon, and insulin; *use*: acromegaly, carcinoid syndrome, VIPomas, esophageal varices

- Name and use of ACTH agonist
- *Cosyntropin*: used in ACTH stimulation test to evaluate and diagnose cortisol disorder, infantile spam

- Name and use of GNRH agonist
- *Leuprolide, nafarelin*: prostate cancer, endometriosis, fibroids, precocious puberty, breast cancer

- Name and use of prolactin-inhibiting hormones (dopamine agonist)
- *Bromocriptine*: hyperprolactinemia

- Use of oxytocin
- Labor induction, lactation

- Use of vasopressin
- *Desmopressin (analog)*: binds V2 receptors in renal CD, which increase water reabsorption, also stimulate release of factor VIII through V1a receptor; *use*: bedwetting, central DI, vWD, hemophilia

- M/A and use of cyproheptadine
- *MA*: 5–HT$_2$ antagonist, H1 blocking action too
- *Use*: carcinoid, GI tumors, postgastractomy, anorexia nervosa

- Use of megestrol acetate
- Use in cachexic patient to improve appetite

- Name of drugs that block steroid receptors
- Spironolactone, mifepristone

- Name of drugs that inhibit steroid synthesis
- Metyrapone, ketoconazole

- Important AE of estrogen, progesterone, and androgens

- *Estrogen*: endometrial hyperplasia, ↑*gall bladder diseases*, *cholestasis*, ↑blood coagulation (↓antithrombin III)
- *Progesterone*: ↓HDL and ↑LDL, glucose intolerance
- *Androgen*: premature closer of epiphysis, cholestatic jaundice
-
- Name and M/A of antiandrogens
- Flutamide - androgen receptor blocker
- Finasteride - 5 α reductase inhibitor; *use*: BPH, male-type baldness
- Ketoconazole - synthesis inhibitor
-
- M/A and use of anastrozole, danazol, clomiphen citrate, tamoxifen, and raloxifen. Difference between tamoxifen and raloxifen.
- *Anastrozole*: inhibits aromatase enzyme which convert androgens to estrogen; *use*: breast CA
- *Tamoxifen*: competitively binds to estrogen receptors and inhibits estrogen effects (*antagonist* in *breast tissue* and *partial agonist* in *endometrium*); *use*: breast CA, anovulatory infertility, gynacomastia
- *Raloxifene*: estrogen agonist at bone and antagonist on breast and uterus; *use*: to prevent osteoporosis in postmenopausal women (*can be used in patient with h/o breast CA in family*)
- *Difference between tamoxifen and raloxifene*: raloxifene has antiestrogenic effect on uterus
- *Danazol*: inhibits ovarian steroidgenesis resulting in decreased secretion of estradiol; also has weak androgenic activity; *use*: endometriosis, fibrocystic breast disease (C/I in pregnancy)
- *Clomiphen citrate*: inhibiting the action of estrogen on the gonadotrope cells in the anterior pituitary gland, which leads to increased FSH leading to increased ovulation; *use*: infertility ("pregnancy drug")

289. Insulin forms that can be used as IV

- Regular insulin

- M/A of sulfonylureas

- *MA*: block k$^+$ channel →depolarization of beta cells →insulin release
- Important AE of chlorpropamide (1st generation sulfonylurea)
- SIADH, disulfiram-like reaction with ethanol
- *C/I of sulfonylureas*: sulphonylureas should be avoided where possible in severe hepatic and renal impairment and in porphyria, breastfeeding, and pregnancy

- M/A and important AE of metformin
- *MA*: suppression of hepatic gluconeogenesis ("euglycemic"), so it decreases postprandial blood glucose
- *AE*: lactic acidosis in patient with *renal dysfunction*

- M/A of acarbose
- It *inhibits alpha-glucosidase enzymes* in the brush border of the small intestines, so it decreases carbohydrate digestion, which leads to a decreased blood glucose level

- M/A of thiazolidinediones
- Bind to nuclear peroxisome proliferators activating receptors (PPAR) involved in transcription of insulin–responsive gene →sensitization of tissues to insulin; ↓hepatic gluconeogenesis and TGs; increase HDL

- M/A of repaglinide
- Block k$^+$ channel →depolarization of beta cells →insulin release

---

Incretin: a group of gastrointestinal hormones includes glucagon-like peptide-1 (GLP-1) and gastric inhibitory peptide (GIP). It causes an increase in the amount of insulin released from the pancreas, *even before blood glucose levels become elevated.* GIP inhibits gastric emptying, so it also decreases absorption of food into blood.

Dipeptidyl peptidase-4 (DPP4): It inactivates incretin.

- M/A of exenatide (Byetta)
- It is an incretin mimetic, so it enhances glucose-dependent insulin secretion by the pancreatic beta-cell, suppresses inappropriately elevated glucagon secretion, and slows gastric emptying.
- The only disadvantage is it must be administered by SC injection!

- M/A of sitagliptin (Januvia)
- It inhibits DPP-4, so it enhances incretin activities.
- Its advantage over exenatide is it can be used orally.

- M/A of bisphosphonates
- They inhibit osteoclast action and the resorption of bone, so it is useful in osteoporosis.

- Important AE of alendronate. Why do we ask patients to take alendronate with a full glass of water?
- Esophageal ulcers (esophagitis)

* Anticancer Drugs
- Do anticancer drugs kill a fixed percentage of tumor cells or fixed number of tumor cells?
- Anticancer drugs kill a fixed percentage of tumor cells.

- Drugs known as spindle poisons
- Vincristine, vinblastine (Both act on M-phase of cell cycle.)

- AE of methotraxate, cyclophosphamide, and doxorubicin. How can we prevent it?
- *Methotraxate*: nephrotoxicity (hydrate well to prevent it), folate deficiency (give *folinic acid* to prevent it)
- *Cyclophosphamide*: hemorrhagic cystitis (give mesna, a sulfhydryl donor that binds acrolein, to prevent it)
- *Doxorubicin*: dilated cardiomyopathy (give dexrazoxane to prevent it)

- M/A of azathioprine, 6-MP and 5-FU
- Azathioprine →6MP (purine antimetabolite) →bioactivated by HPGR transferase (6MP is used in ALL)
- 5–FU (pyrimidine antimetabolite) bioactivated to inhibits thymidylate synthase (used in basal cell CA and keratosis)

- M/A of cyclosporine
- *MA*: It binds to cyclophilin of immunocompetent lymphocytes, especially T-lymphocytes. This complex inhibits calcineurin, which under normal circumstances is responsible for activating the transcription of IL-2. It also inhibits lymphokine production and interleukin release and therefore leads to a reduced function of effector T-cells.
- *Use*: to prevent rejection in organ transplant

- M/A and AE of bleomycin
- *MA*: It induces DNA strand breaks. DNA cleavage by bleomycin depends on oxygen and metal ions.
- *AE*: pulmonary fibrosis

* Drugs for Gout
  - Give names of drugs that used in acute gouty attack (NSAID)
  - Indomethacin, Colchicine

  - M/A and important AE of Colchicine
  - *MA*: It inhibits microtubule polymerization by binding to tubulin so it inhibits mitosis ("mitotic poison") and also inhibits neutrophil motility and activity, leading to a net anti-inflammatory effect
  - *AE*: diarrhea, agranulocytosis

  - Difference between allopurinol and probenecid
  - Allopurinol inhibits uric acid synthesis by inhibiting xanthine oxidase whereas probenecid increases uric acid elimination in urine.

309. Relationship between probenecid and GFR
- It is ineffective if GFR< 50 ml/min

- Does allopurinol have any effect on 6-MP metabolism?
- It inhibits 6MP metabolism.

* Drugs for Rheumatoid Arthritis (RA)
  - Name of drugs that are used in treatment of RA
  - Methotraxate, sulfasalazine, hydroxychloroquine, steroids, leflunomide, anti-TNF (infliximab, etanercept), NSAIDs (best initial drug)

  - When will you start DMARD (disease modifying antirheumatic drug)?
  - Within 3 months for any patient with established RA and ongoing inflammation

  - Best initial DMARD
  - Methotraxate

  - Important points to remember before starting Tx with anti-TNF
  - Screening for tuberculosis

* Drugs for Asthma
  - Name of drugs that used in treatment of asthma
  - Beta agonists, cromolyn, corticosteroids, antileukotrienes

  - M/A of theophylline
  - It inhibits phosphodiesterase (PDE) →↑ cAMP →*antagonize adenosine* (adenosine is bronchoconstrictor)

  - M/A of cromolyn. Is cromolyn useful in an acute attack of asthma?
  - Prevents degranulation of pulmonary mast cells and ↓release of mediators (histamine) that attract inflammatory cells.
  - No. It is not useful for acute attack. It is used to prevent asthma attacks.

  - Difference between zafirlukast and ziluton.
  - *Zafirlukast*: leukotriene receptor antagonist. Used to prevent asthma attack.

- *Ziluton*: Inhibits lipoxygenase

* Miscellaneous
  - Name and use of different PGs
  - *PGE1*: alprostadil; treatment of erectile dysfunction, is a vasodilator
  - *PGE2*: dinoprostone; as a vaginal suppository, to prepare the cervix for labour; also used as an abortificient
  - *PGE2$_\alpha$*: carboprost; used in postpartum bleeding (Atonic PPH)

* Difference between Aspirin (ASA) and other NSAIDs
  - Aspirin irreversibly inhibits COX

* Reason for using low Aspirin
  - At low dose, it irreversibly blocks only the formation of thromboxane A$_2$ in platelets

* How Aspirin is eliminated from the body at high toxic dose
  - Zero-order kinetics

* Symptoms specific for salicylism
  - Tinnitus

* Treatment of Aspirin overdose
  - Alkalization of urine facilitate its renal elimination

* Give the name of a selective COX-2 inhibitor and advantage of it over other NSAIDs
  - Celecoxib
  - Advantage: it has less GI side effects

* Difference between acetaminophen and other NSAIDs
  - Acetaminophen has *no* Peripheral COX inhibition
  - Inhibits COX in CNS – lacks anti-inflammatory effects, but equivalent analgesic and antipyretic activity to ASA

* Tx of acetaminophen overdose
  - N–acetylcystine (give as soon as possible)

* Name of antiemetic drugs according to different groups
  * 5-HT$_3$ antagonist – *ondansetron*
  * DA antagonist – prochlorperazine, metoclopramide
  * H$_1$ antagonist – meclizine, promethazine
  * M antagonist – scopolamine (motion sickness)

* Use of Cisapride. Why is it withdrawn from market?
  * Prokinetic drugs, used in GERD
  * Due to arrhythmias, it was withdrawn from the market

* M/A of sucralfate. Important things to remember about it.
  * *MA*: coats stomach surface and prevents it from acid exposure
  * Never use with antacid / PPI (Antacid and PPI inhibits action of sucralfate.)

Printed in the USA
CPSIA information can be obtained
at www.ICGtesting.com
LVHW090041131123
763722LV00029B/21